Clinical Cases
Pathology

Second Edition

EUGENE C. TOY, MD
The John S. Dunn Senior Academic Chief and Program Director
Obstetrics and Gynecology Residency Program
The Methodist Hospital, Houston
Clerkship Director and Clinical Associate Professor
Department of Obstetrics and Gynecology
University of Texas Medical School at Houston
Houston, Texas

MARGARET O. UTHMAN, MD
Professor and Vice Chairman for Education
Assistant Dean for Educational Programs
University of Texas Medical School at Houston
Houston, Texas

ED UTHMAN, MD
Adjunct Professor, Department of Pathology
University of Texas Medical School at Houston
Pathologist, Brown and Associates Medical Laboratories
Houston, Texas

EARL J. BROWN, MD
Associate Professor
Department of Pathology
East Tennessee State University–James H. Quillen College of Medicine
Johnson City, Tennessee

Mc Graw Hill Education

McGraw Hill Education (India) Private Limited
NEW DELHI

McGraw Hill Education Offices
New Delhi New York St Louis San Francisco Auckland Bogotá Caracas
Kuala Lumpur Lisbon London Madrid Mexico City Milan Montreal
San Juan Santiago Singapore Sydney Tokyo Toronto

McGraw Hill Education (India) Private Limited

Clinical Cases: Pathology, Second Edition

Notice

Medicine is an ever-changing science. As new research and clinical experience broaden our knowledge, changes in treatment and drug therapy are required. The authors and the publisher of this work have checked with sources believed to be reliable in their efforts to provide information that is complete and generally in accord with the standards accepted at the time of publication. However, in view of the possibility of human error or changes in medical sciences, neither the authors nor the publisher nor any other party who has been involved in the preparation or publication of this work warrants that the information contained herein is in every respect accurate or complete, and they disclaim all responsibility for any errors or omissions or for the results obtained from use of the information contained in this work. Readers are encouraged to confirm the information contained herein with other sources. For example and in particular, readers are advised to check the product information sheet included in the package of each drug they plan to administer to be certain that the information contained in this work is accurate and that changes have not been made in the recommended dose or in the contraindications for administration. This recommendation is of particular importance in connection with new or infrequently used drugs.

McGraw Hill Education (India) Edition 2013

RZZYCDRORYDRR

Reprinted in India by arrangement with The McGraw Hill Companies, Inc., New York

Sales territories: India, Pakistan, Nepal, Bangladesh, Sri Lanka and Bhutan

Library of Congress Cataloging-in-Publication Data

Clinical Case: Pathology / Eugene C. Toy …[et al.].—2nd ed.
p. ; cm
Obstetrics and gynecology
Includes index.
ISBN 978-0-07-148666-8 (pbk. : alk. paper)
ISBN 0-07-148666-6 (pbk. : alk. paper)
I Pathology—Case studies. I. Toy, Eugene C. II. Title: Pathology.
[DNLM: 1. Pathology, Clinical—Case Reports. 2. Pathology, Clinical—Problems and Exercises. QZ 18.2 C337 2008]
RB112.C345 2008
616.07—dc22 2008003377

ISBN-13: 978-93-5134-341-7
ISBN-10: 93-5134-341-3

Published by McGraw Hill Education (India) Private Limited, P-24, Green Park Extension, New Delhi 110 016, and printed at Rajkamal Electric Press, Kundli-131028, Haryana

DEDICATION

To my dear wife, Terri, my first and only true love.
She encourages me each day and is my enduring inspiration.

—ECT

To Dr. Aubrey Hough, my chairman during residency training,
and to Dr. Harvey Rosenberg
who gave me my first (and only) faculty position.

—MOU

For those who taught me the basics of pathology:
Sidney A. Coleman, MD, Robert Joseph Peace, MD, and Fred Shipkey, MD.

—EU

To Darlene, who has showed me how to once again dream of good things.

—EJB

❖ CONTENTS

CONTRIBUTORS

John E. Bertini, Jr, MD, FACS
Academic Chief
Department of Urology
St. Joseph Medical Center
Houston, Texas
Testicular Cancer

Tri A. Dinh, MD
Assistant Professor of Obstetrics and Gynecology
Division of Gynecologic Oncology
Weill Medical College of Cornell University
Attending Physician
The Methodist Hospital, Houston
Houston, Texas
Paget Disease

Alaina J. Johnson
Medical Student
Class of 2008
University of Texas Medical School at Houston
Houston, Texas
Principal Manuscript Reviewer
Alzheimer Disease
Hepatitis
Pneumococcal Pneumonia
Nephrotic Syndrome
Temporal Arteritis

Alan L. Kaplan, MD
Professor
Department of Obstetrics and Gynecology
Weill Medical College of Cornell University
Chairman, Department of Obstetrics and Gynecology
The Methodist Hospital, Houston
Houston, Texas
Ovarian Teratoma

Raymond H. Kaufman, MD
Professor
Department of Obstetrics and Gynecology
Weill Medical College of Cornell University
Professor Emeritus
Department of Obstetrics and Gynecology
Baylor College of Medicine
Houston, Texas
Cervical Cancer

Aaron Han, MD, PhD
Consultant Pathologist and Chief
Department of Pathology and Laboratory Medicine
American Hospital Dubai
Dubai, United Arab Emirates
Colon Adenomas
Ventricular Septal Defect

Laura Han, MD
Pediatrician, Private Practice
Dubai, United Arab Emirates
Ventricular Septal Defect

Eric Haufrect, MD
Clinical Professor
Department of Obstetrics and Gynecology
Weill Medical College of Cornell University
Vice Chairman
Department of Obstetrics and Gynecology
The Methodist Hospital, Houston
Houston, Texas
Fibrocystic Changes

George T. Kuhn, MD, FACOG
Chairman
Department of Obstetrics and Gynecology
St. Joseph Medical Center
Houston, Texas
Pulmonary Embolus

Sonia Robazetti Hodgson, MD, CCRC
Research Coordinator
Department of Obstetrics and Gynecology
The Methodist Hospital, Houston
Houston, Texas
Cervical Cancer

Samuel W. Law II, MD
Clinical Associate Professor
Department of Obstetrics and Gynecology
Weill Medical College of Cornell University
Medical Director of Labor and Delivery
Department of Obstetrics and Gynecology
The Methodist Hospital, Houston
Houston, Texas
Syphilis

Claudel Jean-Pierre, MD
Assistant Professor
Department of Obstetrics and Gynecology
Weill Medical College of Cornell University
Faculty
Division of Maternal Fetal Medicine
Department of Obstetrics and Gynecology
The Methodist Hospital, Houston
Houston, Texas
Neural Tube Defects

John T. Patlan, MD
Assistant Professor of Medicine
Department of General Internal Medicine
University of Texas–MD Anderson Cancer Center
Houston, Texas
Hepatitis

Waverly F. Peakes, MD
Residency Coordinator
Obstetrics and Gynecology Residency Program
The Methodist Hospital, Houston
Houston, Texas
Prolactin Adenoma

Keith O. Reeves, MD
Clinical Professor of Obstetrics and Gynecology
Weill Medical College of Cornell University
Attending Physician
The Methodist Hospital, Houston
Houston, Texas
Appendicitis

Priti P. Schachel, MD
Assistant Professor
Department of Obstetrics and Gynecology
Weill Medical College of Cornell University
The Methodist Hospital, Houston
Houston, Texas
Ovarian Teratomas

Anna Sienko, MD, FRCP(C)
Associate Professor
Department of Pathology
Weill Medical College of Cornell University
Staff Pathologist
The Methodist Hospital, Houston
Houston, Texas
Syphilis

Jeané Simmons Holmes, MD, FACOG
Assistant Clinical Professor
Obstetrics and Gynecology Residency Program
The Methodist Hospital, Houston
Houston, Texas
Human Immunodeficiency Virus
Stroke

ACKNOWLEDGMENTS

The inspiration for this basic science series originated at an educational retreat led by Dr. Maximilian Buja, who at that time was Dean of the Medical School. It has been a joy to work with Dr. Margaret Uthman and her husband, Dr. Ed Uthman, and Dr. Earl J. Brown who are accomplished mentors, scientists, and teachers. Likewise, I would like to thank the hard work of the other contributors. I especially thank Alaina Johnson, a fourth year medical student, for her time and expertise in helping to edit this book, adding high yield tables and reviewing the manuscript for readability. I appreciate McGraw-Hill for believing in the concept of teaching by clinical cases, and I owe a great debt to Catherine Johnson, who has been a fantastically encouraging and enthusiastic editor. Alaina wishes to acknowledge God, for giving her the grace and strength to pursue a career in medicine, and her parents, Allan and Kelly, for their constant encouragement, sacrifice, and dedication to helping her achieve her goals. At the Methodist Hospital, I appreciate Drs. Mark Boom, Karin Pollock-Larsen, H. Dirk Sostman, and Judy Paukert, and Mr. John Lyle and Mr. Reggie Abraham. At St. Joseph Medical Center, I would like to recognize our outstanding administrators: Phil Robinson, Pat Mathews, Laura Fortin, Dori Upton, Cecile Reynolds, and Drs. John Bertini and Thomas V. Taylor. I appreciate Marla Buffington's advice and assistance. Without the help from my colleagues in the Southwest Community Clinic, Bernie King, Cornell McKenzie, Carlissa Bowler, Kathy Hinze, Laura P Fernandez, and Sr. Roseanne Popp, MD, this book could not have been written. Most important, I am humbled by the love, affection, and encouragement from my lovely wife, Terri, and our four children, Andy, Michael, Allison, and Christina.

Eugene C. Toy

INTRODUCTION

Often, the medical student will cringe at the "drudgery" of the basic science courses and see little connection between a field such as pathology and clinical problems. Clinicians, however, often wish they knew more about the basic sciences, because it is through the science that we can begin to understand the complexities of the human body and thus have rational methods of diagnosis and treatment.

Mastering the knowledge in a discipline such as pathology is a formidable task. It is even more difficult to retain this information and to recall it when the clinical setting is encountered. To accomplish this synthesis, pathology is optimally taught in the context of medical situations, and this is reinforced later during the clinical rotations. The gulf between the basic sciences and the patient arena is wide. Perhaps one way to bridge this gulf is with carefully constructed clinical cases that ask basic science-oriented questions. In an attempt to achieve this goal, we have designed a collection of patient cases to teach pathology-related points. More important, the explanations for these cases emphasize the underlying mechanisms and relate the clinical setting to the basic science data. We explore the principles rather than emphasize rote memorization.

This book is organized for versatility: to allow the student "in a rush" to go quickly through the scenarios and check the corresponding answers and to provide more detailed information for the student who wants throught-provoking explanations. The answers are arranged from simple to complex: a summary of the pertinent points, the bare answers, a clinical correlation, an approach to the pathology topic, a comprehension test at the end for reinforcement or emphasis, and a list of references for further reading. The clinical cases are arranged by system to better reflect the organization within the basic science. Finally, to encourage thinking about mechanisms and relationships, we intentionally did not primarily use a multiple-choice format at the beginning of each case. Nevertheless, several multiple-choice questions are included at the end of each scenario to reinforce concepts or introduce related topics.

HOW TO GET THE MOST OUT OF THIS BOOK

Each case is designed to introduce a clinically related issue and includes open-ended questions usually asking a basic science question, but at times, to break up the monotony, there will be a clinical question. The answers are organized into four different parts:

PART I

1. **Summary**
2. A **straightforward answer** is given for each open-ended question.
3. **Clinical Correlation**—A discussion of the relevant points relating the basic science to the clinical manifestations, and perhaps introducing the student to issues such as diagnosis and treatment

PART II

An **approach to the basic science concept** consisting of three parts:

1. **Objectives**—A listing of the two to four main principles that are critical for understanding the underlying pathology to answer the question and relate to the clinical situation
2. **Definitions of basic terminology**
3. **Discussion of topic**

PART III

Comprehension Questions—Each case includes several multiple-choice questions that reinforce the material or introduce new and related concepts. Questions about the material not found in the text are explained in the answers.

PART IV

Pathology Pearls—A listing of several important points, many clinically relevant, reiterated as a summation of the text and to allow for easy review, such as before an examination.

We would like to recognize a great physician, educator, administrator, colleague, and leader, Dr. Maximilian Buja, who served as Dean of the University of Texas Health Science Center–Houston Medical School from 1995 to 2003 before being appointed Executive Vice President for Academic Affairs. Dr. Buja, a pathologist, continues to contribute greatly to the pathology course at the medical school by lecturing on the basic principles of cell injury and inflammation as well as on cardiovascular pathology. He led an educational retreat in 2002 which inspired the concept for this series, joining the clinical case to the basic sciences. Dr. Buja has taught thousands of medical students and serves as a role model and mentor for many pathology residents and scientists.

SECTION I

Applying the Basic Sciences to Clinical Medicine

PART 1. APPROACH TO LEARNING PATHOLOGY

Pathology is best learned by a systematic approach, first by learning the **language** of the discipline and then by understanding the **function** of the various processes. Increasingly, the understanding of cell and organ function plays an important role in the understanding of disease processes and the treatment of disease. Initially, some of the "language" must be memorized in the same way that the alphabet must be learned by rote; however, the appreciation of the way the "pathology words" are constructed requires an understanding of mechanisms, in essence, an awareness of "how things are put together and work together."

PART 2. APPROACH TO DISEASE

Physicians usually approach clinical situations by taking a history (asking questions), performing a physical examination, obtaining selected laboratory and imaging tests, and then formulating a diagnosis. The conglomeration of the history, physical examination, and laboratory tests is called the **clinical database.** After a diagnosis has been reached, a treatment plan is usually initiated, and the patient is followed for a clinical response. Rational understanding of disease and plans for treatment are best acquired by learning about the normal human processes on a basic science level, and likewise, being aware of how disease alters the normal physiologic processes is understood on a basic science level. In short, clinical problem solving involves three basic steps: (1) making a diagnosis, (2) initiating a therapy, and (3) monitoring the patient's response.

PART 3. APPROACH TO READING

There are **seven key questions** that help to stimulate the application of basic science information to the clinical setting.

1. **Given histologic findings in an organ, what are the most likely clinical manifestations?**
2. **Given clinical symptoms, if a tissue biopsy is taken, what histologic findings are most likely to be seen?**
3. **Given clinical findings, if the microscopic photograph is shown, what is the most likely diagnosis?**
4. **Given a histologic description, what would be the most likely complication to the organ in question?**
5. **Given a gross description of a pathologic lesion, what is the most likely diagnosis?**
6. **Given autopsy findings, what is the most likely diagnosis?**
7. **Given histologic findings, what is the most likely explanation?**

1. **Given histologic findings in an organ, what are the most likely clinical manifestations?**

   This is a fundamental principle in the understanding of the discipline of pathology. The student first must understand the **normal** histologic structure in an organ in the context of its function. Then the student must be able to relate the **abnormal** histology to clinical findings, both subjective (patient complaints) and objective (physical examination findings). The organ or system is highly organized both on the gross and on the microscopic level. There also must be awareness of the mechanism that causes disruption of the normal cellular architecture.
2. **Given clinical symptoms, if a tissue biopsy is taken, what histologic findings are most likely to be seen?**

   This is the converse of the first question and requires going backward from clinical manifestations to the probable disease process to probable histologic findings. The student must be able to translate the clinical picture to the cellular characteristics. This also requires being aware of what symptoms various cellular alterations will produce in the patient; for instance, some changes will be silent and not cause symptoms, whereas other changes will produce dramatic manifestations.
3. **Given clinical findings, if the microscopic pictograph is shown, what is the most likely diagnosis?**

   This sequence of analysis is very similar to the practice of "real-life" medicine, the role of the pathologist. The clinical history and physical examination are critical to putting the pathologic findings into context. For instance, if endometrial curettings are sent to the pathologist and on microscopy reveal crowded, complex glands, abnormal epithelial nuclei, and loss of nuclear polarity, the pathologist may render a diagnosis of cancer. However, when the information is given that the patient is 6-week pregnant, the diagnosis of an Arias-Stella reaction is made, an expected finding in the endometrium in light of the human chorionic gonadotropin levels of pregnancy. The next logical step is to propose a treatment. Thus, the student should be able to shift back and forth between the basic science and the clinical areas

Pathophysiology ↔ Histologic findings ↔ Diagnoses ↔ Treatment

4. **Given a histologic description, what would be the most likely complication to the organ in question?**

   This analysis requires that the student be able to relate the histologic findings of one organ to a disease process and then extrapolate the probable changes to another organ. The student should become proficient at working back and forth between histologic changes and clinical findings and disease processes. The best way to acquire this skill is to think in terms of mechanisms of disease and not just memorize key words. It is the understanding of the underlying pathophysiology of the disease that allows the physician-scientist to make rational predictions of the natural history of a disease process.

5. **Given a gross description of a pathologic lesion, what is the most likely diagnosis?**

   The student of pathology also must be able to process the visual picture of the organ, biopsy specimen, or cytology, as well as the written description. Because the pathologist often communicates with clinicians by using written reports, the student should be able to take the written description and apply that information to the clinical setting, such as making a diagnosis. For instance, if the description is that of an ovarian cyst with sebaceous material, hair, and teeth, the most likely diagnosis is a benign cystic teratoma.

6. **Given autopsy findings, what is the most likely diagnosis?**

   This question is similar to the analysis performed by working back from gross pathologic description to the diagnosis. In cases of a patient's death, an autopsy often will be helpful in explaining the circumstances surrounding the death, or the etiology. The student of pathology must be able to correlate the postmortem examination with the probable diagnosis and be able to speculate about the interaction between disease and host. For example, the case may involve a 30-year-old female who suddenly collapses and dies, and the autopsy reveals a dilated aortic root and aortic dissection; other findings include long extremities and long fingers. The most likely diagnosis is Marfan syndrome.

7. **Given histologic findings, what is the most likely explanation?**

   The student once again is challenged to relate the histologic findings in the context of scientific explanation and not just memorize the histologic findings of a certain disease. For example, the histologic specimen may reveal a pulmonary lesion with an area of central necrosis surrounded by epithelioid and multinucleated giant cells. The explanation would be that the organism is probably *Mycobacterium tuberculosis,* which evades phagocytosis from macrophages because it has complement C3b antigen on its cell wall. It is incorporated into the macrophage, and the tuberculosis bacterium blocks fusion of the lysosome with the phagosome, allowing the bacterium to multiply within the macrophage. The responding T cells produce cytokines such as interferon type II (IF-2) to activate other T cells and interferon γ (IFN-γ), which activates macrophages, transforming them into epithelioid cells and multinucleated giant cells. Thus, it is delayed or cell-mediated immunity that is required to address the infection. The monocyte response, dictated by the type IV hypersensitivity reaction of cell-mediated immunity, leads to the caseous necrosis (acellular debris in the center), as well as the granulomatous reaction. The cell-mediated immune response also explains the need to wait 48 to 72 hours for a skin response to the purified protein derivative (PPD) test to assess for prior exposure (sensitivity) to tuberculosis.

PATHOLOGY PEARLS

- There are seven key questions to stimulate the application of basic science information to the clinical arena.
- Medicine is both an art and a science.
- The scientific aspect of medicine seeks to gather data in an objective manner, understand physiologic and pathologic processes in light of scientific information, and propose rational explanations.
- A skilled clinician must be able to translate back and forth between the basic sciences and the clinical sciences.

REFERENCES

Kumar V, Abbas AK, Fausto N. Acute and chronic inflammation. In: Robbins and Cotran Pathologic Basis of Disease, 7th ed. Philadelphia, PA: Elsevier Saunders, 2005:48–83.

Mark DB. Decision making in medicine. In: Kasper DL, Fauci AS, Longo DL, et al., eds. Harrison's Principles of Internal Medicine, 16th ed. New York: McGraw-Hill, 2004:6–13.

Mitchell RN. Acute and chronic inflammation. In: Mitchell RN, Kumar V, Abbas AK, et al. Pocket Companion to Robbins and Cotran Pathologic Basis of Disease, 7th ed. Philadelphia, PA: Saunders, 2006, 27–51.

SECTION II

Clinical Cases

CASE 1

A 42-year-old policeman has been seen by his family physician for a 5-year history of "heartburn." He has been intermittently taking ranitidine, a histamine-2 blocking agent, with some relief. An upper endoscopic examination that was performed recently revealed some reddish discoloration and friability of the lower esophageal region. A biopsy of the lower esophagus was performed, and the microscopic examination revealed columnar cells containing goblet cells.

- **What is the most likely diagnosis?**
- **What is a long-term complication of this process?**
- **What is the most likely mechanism of this process?**

ANSWERS TO CASE 1: BARRETT ESOPHAGUS

Summary: A 42-year-old man has a 5-year history of "heartburn" unrelieved by a histamine-2 blocking agent. Upper endoscopy reveals reddish discoloration of the distal esophagus, which on biopsy shows columnar epithelium with goblet cells.

- **Most likely diagnosis:** Barrett esophagus.
- **Long-term complication of this process:** Adenocarcinoma of the esophagus.
- **Most likely mechanism:** Repeated acid reflux to the distal esophagus leading to metaplasia of the normal squamous epithelium into columnar epithelium.

CLINICAL CORRELATION

The normal esophagus is lined by nonkeratinized squamous epithelium. The lower esophageal sphincter (LES) prevents reflux of gastric acid from entering the distal esophagus. With gastroesophageal reflux disease (GERD), decreased lower esophageal sphincter tone can lead to acid exposure of the distal esophagus. Through a poorly understood mechanism, the **lower esophagus changes (metaplasia) from squamous to columnar epithelium, so-called Barrett esophagus.** In fact, the presence **of goblet cells in the columnar epithelium is a hallmark of the disease.** Barrett esophagus appears **reddish and friable** on endoscopy and carries an increased risk for developing into **adenocarcinoma.**

APPROACH TO ESOPHAGEAL PATHOLOGY

Objectives

- Describe the mechanism of GERD and the long-term effects of the disease.
- List the risk factors for esophageal cancer.
- List the common causes of esophageal pathology.

Definitions

Esophageal diverticulum: Outpouching of one or more layers of the esophageal wall. When it occurs near the upper esophageal sphincter, it is called a **Zenker diverticulum.**

Achalasia: Condition of esophageal dilation resulting from lack of esophageal peristalsis and constant contraction of the lower esophageal sphincter associated with a loss of myenteric plexus ganglions. Affected patients complain of dysphagia (difficulty swallowing).

Gastroesophageal reflux: Condition in which gastric acid enters the distal esophagus, usually associated with decreased lower esophageal sphincter pressure. Affected patients often complain of "heartburn" that is relieved by antacids. Long-term complications of GERD include Barrett esophagus, stricture, and ulceration.

Barrett esophagus: Columnar metaplasia of the lower esophageal epithelium, predisposing to esophageal adenocarcinoma.

Esophagitis: Inflammation of the esophagus caused by GERD, infection (*Candida,* herpes simplex virus, cytomegalovirus), radiation, or uremia.

Hiatal hernia: Gastroesophageal defect in which a part of the stomach protrudes above the diaphragm, usually adjacent to the distal esophagus, may be associated with GERD.

Esophageal carcinoma: Worldwide, squamous cell carcinoma is the most common cell type, but in Western countries, it is divided equally in frequency between adenocarcinoma and squamous cell carcinoma. Patients typically complain of **dysphagia,** weight loss, and fatigue.

DISCUSSION

Normal Esophagus

The esophagus is a muscular tube that connects the pharynx to the stomach that is lined by **squamous epithelium.** It has a well-developed submucosa, and the upper third is enveloped by striated muscle, whereas the lower two-thirds are encompassed by smooth muscle. The upper esophageal sphincter is located at approximately the level of the fifth cervical vertebra (C5) level, whereas the **lower esophageal sphincter is located below the diaphragm** and its function is to **prevent regurgitation of gastric acid.** During the swallowing process peristalsis is initiated in the striated muscle and continues down through the smooth muscle with a coordinated temporary relaxation of the LES. **Both sympathetic and parasympathetic nerve fibers** innervate the **intrinsic myenteric plexus,** which is distributed in the striated and smooth muscle.

Congenital Anomalies

Tracheoesophageal (TE) fistulae are congenital disorders that manifest in affected **newborns** as **hypersalivation and difficulty feeding with choking.** The most common type (90 percent) involves distal esophageal atresia with a connection to the trachea. Maternal **polyhydramnios** may be noted in utero, resulting from the fetal inability to swallow amniotic fluid. Less common varieties of TE fistulae may involve a fistula and patent esophagus (so-called H type) or a higher location of the fistula. **Recognition and surgical repair are critical.**

Achalasia

Achalasia is characterized by **progressive dilation of the distal esophagus** caused by **disturbance of the normal peristaltic process.** This nearly always involves a **loss of myenteric ganglion cells,** although the underlying etiology is unclear. Patients typically have **increased LES pressure** and complain of **progressive dysphagia** and **vomiting of partially digested or undigested food.** The diagnosis is established by endoscopy or upper gastrointestinal barium swallow imaging (so-called "bird's beak" finding; see Figure 1-1)

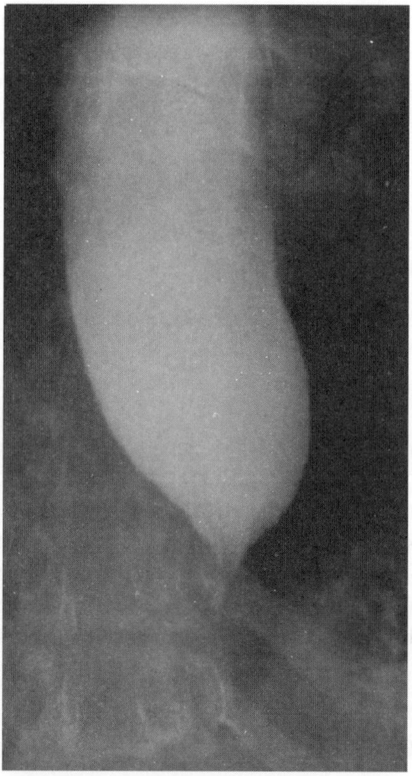

Figure 1-1. Barium esophagogram showing a markedly dilated esophagus and characteristic "bird's beak" in achalasia. (*Reproduced, with permission, from Waters PF, DeMeester TR.* Foregut motor disorders and their surgical management. *Med Clin North Am1981:65;1235.*)

GERD and Barrett Esophagus

Esophagitis, or inflammation of the esophagus, has multiple etiologies and often is associated with **chest pain, dysphagia, and painful swallowing.** By far, the **most common cause of esophagitis is gastroesophageal reflux,** which may be associated with a hiatal hernia. With chronic acid exposure, the distal esophagus may become hyperemic and ulcerated and develop scars or strictures. **Persistent GERD** may lead to a benign epithelial change (metaplasia) of the distal esophagus; the normal **squamous cell epithelium becomes columnar with the presence of intestinal goblet cells, so-called Barrett esophagus.** Barrett esophagus appears **reddish and friable on endoscopy** and is **diagnosed by biopsy; endoscopic surveillance** is important because of the **increased risk for developing adenocarcinoma.**

Esophageal Carcinoma

Esophageal cancers account for about 10 percent of all gastrointestinal cancers in the United States and are **largely asymptomatic.** Familial influences are not as important as environmental exposures. **Chronic alcohol and tobacco** exposures significantly increase the risk of esophageal cancer. Other factors may include ingestion of nitrosamine-containing foods, chronic hot and spicy foods, and lye with stricture formation. The **most common cell type worldwide is squamous cell carcinoma, usually affecting the upper and middle thirds of the esophagus.** In the **United States,** as a result of decreased tobacco use and an increased prevalence of GERD, **adenocarcinoma of the distal esophagus is encountered commonly.** Periodic endoscopic surveillance with biopsy for patients with chronic GERD may identify the cancer at an early stage. Regardless of cell type, affected patients generally have few symptoms until late in the course, with those symptoms being **progressive dysphagia, weight loss, and fatigue.** Because the cancers are **usually very large at diagnosis, surgical resection is difficult,** and **up to 80 percent of affected individuals die within 1 year of diagnosis.**

COMPREHENSION QUESTIONS

[1.1] A 55-year-old salesman is noted to have a cancer of the lower third of the esophagus. He is a nonsmoker and occasionally drinks alcohol. Which of the following is the most likely cell type?

A. Adenocarcinoma
B. Melanoma
C. Metastatic cancer
D. Sarcoma
E. Squamous cell carcinoma

[1.2] An 18-year-old man presents with difficulty swallowing over the last 3 days. He denies ingestion of unusual substances and complains of pain even when swallowing liquids. He is an intravenous (IV) drug user and has been taking several medications to "help his immunity." Which of the following is the most likely finding on esophageal endoscopy?

A. Brown blotches scattered throughout the esophagus
B. Normal-appearing esophagus
C. Red patches in the distal esophagus
D. Reddish streaks throughout the pharynx and upper esophagus
E. White patches adherent to the esophagus

[1.3] A newborn male is noted to have difficulty feeding and "turns blue and chokes when drinking formula." The prenatal records reveal that the amniotic fluid appeared normal on ultrasound. A pediatric feeding tube is passed orally to 20 cm without difficulty, with gastric secretions aspirated. Which of the following is the most likely diagnosis?

A. Congenital heart disease
B. Floppy epiglottis
C. Respiratory distress syndrome
D. Tracheoesophageal fistula
E. Zenker diverticulum

Answers

[1.1] **A.** Adenocarcinoma is the most common malignancy of the lower third of the esophagus and is strongly associated with Barrett esophagus. Squamous cell carcinoma is the most common type of cancer of the esophagus worldwide and usually affects the upper or middle region of the esophagus.

[1.2] **E.** This patient probably has HIV, and the clinical syndrome of painful and difficult swallowing is consistent with *Candida* esophagitis. Endoscopy probably would reveal white plaques adherent to the esophagus. Other causes of esophagitis include herpes simplex infection, cytomegalovirus (CMV) infection, and chemical-induced conditions such as those resulting from lye (suicide attempt).

[1.3] **D.** The vast majority newborns with TE fistulae involve a nonpatent esophagus that is diagnosed by the inability to pass a feeding tube. However, the baby in this case most likely has an unusual type of TE fistula (H type) in which the esophagus is patent but there is a connection between the esophagus and the trachea. When the baby feeds, the formula is aspirated into the tracheobronchial tree, leading to choking and cyanosis. This condition may be diagnosed with a radiologic contrast study and requires surgical correction.

PATHOLOGY PEARLS

- The normal esophagus is lined with nonkeratinized squamous epithelium.
- Gastric acid reflux into the distal esophagus may cause esophagitis, and a patient with gastroesophageal reflux disease typically complains of heartburn.
- GERD usually is treated with histamine-2 blocking agents or proton pump inhibitors, which decrease the gastric acid production.
- Long-standing GERD may lead to columnar metaplasia of the lower esophageal epithelium, so-called Barrett esophagus, which has a propensity for developing into adenocarcinoma.
- Chronic alcohol and tobacco exposures significantly increase the risk of esophageal cancer.
- Worldwide, the most common type of esophageal cancer is squamous cell carcinoma, whereas in Western countries, adenocarcinoma is increasing in incidence because of the prevalence of GERD and Barrett esophagus.

REFERENCES

Crawford JM, Liu C. The gastrointestinal tract. In: Mitchell RN, Kumar V, Abbas AK, et al., eds. Pocket Companion to Robbins and Cotran Pathologic Basis of Disease, 7th ed. Philadelphia, PA: Saunders, 2006, 410–15.

Liu C, Crawford JM. The gastrointestinal tract. In: Kumar V, Assas AK, Fausto N, eds. Robbins and Cotran Pathologic Basis of Disease, 7th ed. Philadelphia, PA: Elsevier Saunders, 2004:804–9.

Rubin E. Essential Pathology, 3rd ed. Philadelphia, PA: Lippincott Williams & Wilkins, 2001.

CASE 2

A 30-year-old male banker complains of midepigastric gnawing and boring pain for the last week. The pain is worse at night and is somewhat better immediately after he eats. He has not had any fever, nausea, or vomiting. He takes approximately one 500-mg acetaminophen tablet a week for headaches but does not take any other medications. Upper endoscopy reveals a 2-cm mucosal defect in the antrum of the stomach. There is mild edema in the adjacent mucosa, but there is no thickening of the edges of the ulcer.

- **What is the most likely diagnosis?**
- **What are complications from this condition?**
- **What is the most likely mechanism of this disorder?**

ANSWERS TO CASE 2: PEPTIC ULCER DISEASE

Summary: A 30-year-old man has acute onset of midepigastric pain somewhat relieved by eating. Upper endoscopy reveals a 2-cm gastric ulcer.

- **Most likely diagnosis:** Peptic ulcer disease.
- **Long-term complications:** Erosion or perforation with bleeding; gastric carcinoma in patients with chronic gastritis.
- **Most likely mechanism:** Most often associated with *Helicobacter pylori* organisms that produce bacterial urease and protease, damaging the mucus layer and exposing the underlying epithelium to acid-peptic injury.

CLINICAL CORRELATION

Ulcers are disruptions of the mucosa of the gastrointestinal tract that extend through the muscularis mucosa into the submucosa or deeper. Peptic ulcers occur most frequently in the stomach and duodenum. Peptic ulcers are often remitting, relapsing lesions that may be seen in young adults but more often occur in middle-aged to older adults. They are usually chronic, solitary lesions caused by the action of **gastric acid and pepsin, both of which are thought to be required for the development of peptic ulcers.** ***Helicobacter pylori* infection** of gastric mucosa is present in 90 to 100 percent of patients with a duodenal ulcer and 70 percent of those with a gastric ulcer. Damage to the protective mucus layer by bacterial urease and protease exposes the underlying epithelial cells to the influence of acid-peptic digestion and may lead to inflammation. The chronically inflamed mucosa is more susceptible to acid-peptic injury and thus more prone to ulceration.

APPROACH TO GASTRIC PATHOLOGY

Objectives

- Describe the causes of gastritis
- Know the difference between duodenal and gastric ulcers
- List the risk factors for gastric cancer

Definitions

Diaphragmatic hernia: Weakness or partial to total absence of a portion of the diaphragm, usually on the left, which may permit the abdominal contents to herniate into the thorax during in utero development. Diaphragmatic hernias differ from hiatal hernias in that the defect in the diaphragm does not involve the hiatal orifice.

Pyloric stenosis: Congenital hypertrophic pyloric stenosis is seen in infants usually during the second or third week of life. Hypertrophy of the muscularis propria of the pylorus results in a **palpable mass** and obstruction with associated regurgitation and persistent **projectile vomiting.** Male infants are affected 3 to 4 times more often than are females. Treatment consists of surgical splitting of the muscle. Pyloric stenosis may be acquired in adults with chronic antral gastritis or peptic ulcers near the pylorus. Other causes of acquired pyloric stenosis include gastric carcinomas, lymphomas, and adjacent carcinomas of the pancreas.

Gastritis: Inflammation of the gastric mucosa. The inflammation may be predominantly acute, with neutrophilic infiltration, or chronic, with a predominance of lymphocytes and plasma cells. The classification and pathogenesis of acute and chronic gastritis are discussed below.

Ulcer: A disruption of the mucosa extending through the muscularis mucosa into the submucosa or deeper. Ulcers may occur anywhere in the gastrointestinal tract but are seen most often in the stomach and duodenum, associated with peptic ulcer disease.

Peptic ulcer disease: Peptic ulcers are chronic, usually solitary lesions of the gastrointestinal mucosa caused by the action of acid-peptic juices. Both acid and pepsin are necessary for peptic ulcer disease to develop.

Hypertrophic gastropathy: A group of uncommon conditions characterized by enlargement of the rugal folds of the gastric mucosa caused by hyperplasia of the mucosal epithelial cells. The three variants are (1) **Ménétrier** disease with marked hyperplasia of the surface mucous cells with atrophy of the gastric glands that may lead to severe loss of plasma proteins, (2) **Zollinger-Ellison syndrome** with gastric gland hyperplasia secondary to **excessive gastrin secretion by a tumor (gastrinoma),** and (3) **hypertrophic-hypersecretory** gastropathy with hyperplasia of the parietal and chief cells within the gastric glands. These three conditions may mimic gastric cancer on radiographic studies. The excessive amount of acid secretion in the second and third conditions predisposes patients to peptic ulceration.

DISCUSSION

Normal Stomach

The stomach is divided into four anatomic regions: the **cardia, fundus, body or corpus, and antrum.** The pyloric sphincter demarcates the antrum from the duodenum. Infoldings of mucosa and submucosa, or **rugae,** extend longitudinally and are most prominent in the proximal stomach. Several types of cells are found in the stomach: **parietal cells** produce gastric hydrochloric acid and **intrinsic factor** involved in the absorption of vitamin B_{12}, **chief cells** secrete the proteolytic enzymes pepsinogen I and II, **surface and mucous neck cells** secrete mucus involved in the protection of the mucosa from gastric acid, and **G cells** found in the antral, pyloric, and duodenal mucosa produce **gastrin.**

The secretion of gastric acid is proportional to the total number of parietal cells in the glands of the body and fundus of the stomach. The secretory process may be divided into three phases: cephalic, gastric, and intestinal. **Gastrin, which is released in response to vagal stimulation, is the most important mediator of gastric acid secretion.** Histamine also stimulates acid secretion. Thus, surgical interruption of vagal stimulation and inhibition of histamine stimulation by blocking the H2 receptor on the parietal cell membrane are effective maneuvers for reducing gastric acid production. Several factors act together to protect the stomach from digestion by gastric acid. Mucus secretion, bicarbonate secretion, the epithelial barrier formed by tight intercellular junctions, a rich mucosal blood flow that removes back-diffused acid, and reflex vasodilation in response to toxins or acid breach of the epithelial layer all contribute to the mucosal barrier.

Gastritis

Inflammation of the gastric mucosa occurs in a variety of clinical situations and may be acute or chronic. Acute gastritis varies in severity; it may be asymptomatic, cause epigastric pain with nausea and vomiting, or present with massive hematemesis. **Acute erosive gastritis** (see Table 2-1) **is an important cause of**

Table 2-1
SELECTED ETIOLOGIES OF ACUTE GASTRITIS

Heavy use of nonsteroidal anti-inflammatory drugs (NSAIDs), particularly aspirin
Excessive alcohol consumption
Heavy smoking
Uremia
Cancer chemotherapy
Severe stress: burns (Curling ulcer), trauma, or surgery with increased intracranial pressure leading to increased vagal tone (Cushing ulcer)
Ischemia and shock
Suicide attempts with acids and alkali
Mechanical trauma (nasogastric intubation)
After distal gastrectomy

Table 2-2
SELECTED ETIOLOGIES OF CHRONIC GASTRITIS

Chronic infection, such as *Helicobacter pylori*
Immunologic, associated with pernicious anemia
Toxic, such as alcohol and cigarette use
Postsurgical, especially after antrectomy
Obstruction, such as bezoars
Radiation
Granulomatous conditions, such as Crohn disease
Other conditions, such as graft versus host disease, amyloidosis, uremia

acute gastrointestinal bleeding. In chronic gastritis, there are chronic mucosal inflammatory changes, usually without erosions, that may lead to **mucosal atrophy and dysplastic epithelium, predisposing the patient to the development of carcinoma** (see Table 2-2).

Most cases of chronic gastritis are thought to be associated with chronic ***H. pylori*** infection. Chronic gastritis that results from *H. pylori* infection most often involves the antrum and is not associated with pernicious anemia. Most patients improve with antibiotic treatment, and relapses of chronic gastritis are associated with a recurrence of infection. Patients are at risk for developing peptic ulcer disease and gastric cancer, including adenocarcinoma and lymphoma.

Patients with **autoimmune gastritis** (diffuse atrophic gastritis) may have nausea, vomiting, and upper abdominal pain. Patients usually have autoantibodies to gastric parietal cells or intrinsic factor. Destruction of gastric glands of the fundus leads to **loss of acid production (achlorhydria) and hypergastrinemia.** Loss of intrinsic factor leads to **pernicious anemia.** Thus, patients with autoimmune gastritis may initially present with peripheral neuropathy symptoms from B_{12} deficiency in addition to their abdominal symptoms. Patients may also have other autoimmune disorders, such as Hashimoto thyroiditis or Addison disease.

Peptic Ulcer Disease

Peptic ulcers are usually solitary, arising from exposure of the mucosal epithelium to acid-peptic secretions. Peptic ulcer disease (PUD) occurs most often in middle-aged to older adults. The most common anatomic sites are the duodenum and the stomach, in a ratio of 4:1 (see Table 2-3). *Helicobacter pylori*

Table 2-3
PEPTIC ULCER DISEASE

	GASTRIC	DUODENAL
Symptoms	**G**reater pain with meals	**D**ecreased pain with meals
Acid secretion	Low/normal acid secretion (associated with decreased mucosal protection)	Increased acid secretion
***Helicobacter pylori* infection**	Seen in 70% of patients	Seen in nearly all patients

infection is present in virtually all patients with duodenal ulcers and 70 percent of patients with PUD involving the stomach. *Helicobacter pylori* can cause damage by (1) secreting urease, protease, and phospholipases, (2) attracting neutrophils that release myeloperoxidase, and (3) promoting thrombotic occlusion of capillaries, leading to ischemic damage of the epithelium. **Complications of PUD include anemia, hemorrhage, perforation, and obstruction.** Malignant transformation is rare and is related to underlying chronic gastritis.

Gastric Cancer

Most (90 to 95 percent) gastric malignancies are **adenocarcinomas,** with a smaller number of lymphomas, carcinoids, and spindle cell tumors. Although the incidence of gastric carcinoma has been decreasing in Western countries over the last 50 years, the prognosis is still poor, with a 20 percent 5-year survival. Risk factors for gastric carcinoma include nitrates; smoked, salted, or pickled foods; lack of fresh fruits and vegetables; chronic atrophic gastritis; *H. pylori* infection; partial gastrectomy; gastric adenomas; blood group A; and close relatives with gastric cancer. Two types of gastric carcinoma are recognized: the **intestinal type** and the **diffuse type** (see Table 2-4).

These may represent two distinct forms of gastric carcinoma. Dissemination of gastric carcinoma, as well as other primary abdominal adenocarcinomas, to the ovaries is known as **Krukenberg tumors.** The hallmark is the **"signet ring cell"** on microscopy, which is indicative of large cells with mucin that push the nuclei to the periphery of the cell.

Table 2-4
GASTRIC CARCINOMA SUBTYPES

	INTESTINAL TYPE	DIFFUSE TYPE
Incidence	Decreasing	No change
Average age	55 years	48 years
Male:female ratio	2:1	1:1
Chronic gastritis	Frequently associated	No particular association
Macroscopic growth pattern	Exophytic, polypoid, fungating	Ulcerative and/or diffusely infiltrative resulting in a rigid thickened wall, linitis plastica
Microscopic growth pattern	Gland-forming columnar epithelium; associated with intestinal metaplasia; usually mucin-producing	Infiltrative growth; noncohesive; poorly differentiated, often **signet ring cells;** mucin-producing

COMPREHENSION QUESTIONS

[2.1] A 59-year-old woman presents with occasional nausea and vague upper abdominal discomfort. Upper endoscopy reveals chronic gastritis of the fundus with flattened gastric mucosa but no acute ulceration. Which of the following is most likely to be associated with this finding?

A. Autoantibodies to parietal cells
B. Diet high in nitrites
C. Hyperchlorhydria
D. Hypoparathyroidism
E. Ménétrier disease

[2.2] A 55-year-old man presents with upper gastrointestinal bleeding and is found to have multiple ulcers in the duodenum. Workup finds his serum gastrin levels to be markedly elevated, and an abdominal CT scan finds a large mass in the tail of the pancreas. A biopsy from this pancreatic mass finds an islet-cell adenoma that secretes gastrin. Which of the following is the best diagnosis?

A. Hypertrophic-hypersecretory gastropathy
B. Linitis plastica
C. Ménétrier disease
D. Verner-Morrison syndrome
E. Zollinger-Ellison syndrome

[2.3] A 55-year-old woman seeks medical attention for fatigue and malaise that have been worsening over the last 2 months. She also has noticed loss of appetite and early satiety. Evaluation reveals an ulcerative mass located along the lesser curvature, and a biopsy shows an infiltrating adenocarcinoma. Further evaluation by abdominal CT imaging shows bilateral ovarian masses. Which of the following is this patient most likely to have?

A. Barrett mucosa
B. Krukenberg tumor
C. Primary ovarian neoplasm
D. Uterine cancer

Answers

[2.1] **A.** Chronic atropic gastritis often is associated with autoantibodies to parietal cells. Loss of these cells leads to decreased gastric acid (hypochlorhydria) and decreased intrinsic factor. Lack of intrinsic factor results in deceased or absent vitamin B_{12} absorption (pernicious anemia).

[2.2] **E.** Zollinger-Ellison syndrome refers to gastric gland hyperplasia secondary to excessive gastrin secretion by a tumor (gastrinoma), usually found in the pancreas. The excess gastrin increases the thickness of the gastric mucosa and increases the acid production by the stomach. This results in the formation of recurrent peptic ulcers, especially within the duodenum and jejunum. As a result, the classic clinical triad associated with the Zollinger-Ellison syndrome is the combination of increased acid production by the stomach, peptic ulcers of the duodenum and jejunum, and an islet-cell tumor of the pancreas.

[2.3] **B.** The findings suggest that the patient's gastric cancer has metastasized to the ovaries; this is known as a Krukenberg tumor. Histology typically shows "signet ring cells."

PATHOLOGY PEARLS

❖ *Helicobacter pylori* is a common etiology of peptic ulcer disease.
❖ Pain from **d**uodenal ulcers **d**ecreases with food.
❖ Pain from **g**astric ulcers is **g**reater with food.
❖ Most gastric malignancies are adenocarcinomas.

REFERENCES

Crawford JM, Liu C. The gastrointestinal tract. In: Mitchell RN, Kumar V, Abbas AK, et al., eds. Pocket Companion to Robbins and Cotran Pathologic Basis of Disease, 7th ed. Philadelphia, PA: Saunders, 2006, 416–21.

Del Valle J. Peptic ulcer disease and related disorders. In: Kasper DL, Fauci AS, Longo DL, et al., eds. Harrison's Principles of Internal Medicine, 16th ed. New York: McGraw-Hill, 2004:1746–62.

Liu C, Crawford JM. The gastrointestinal tract. In: Kumar V, Assas AK, Fausto N, eds. Robbins and Cotran Pathologic Basis of Disease, 7th ed. Philadelphia, PA: Elsevier Saunders, 2004:804–9, 816–27.

CASE 3

A 57-year-old man presents with fatigue for several months and has noticed recently that the waistbands of his pants are tight in spite of a 15-lb weight loss. He has not had diarrhea, nausea, vomiting, or other gastrointestinal symptoms. He does not take any medications and denies using illegal drugs. He underwent a blood transfusion with several units in 1982 after an automobile accident. Physical examination reveals generalized jaundice, a firm nodular liver edge just below the right costal margin, and a mildly protuberant abdomen with a fluid wave. Initial laboratory studies show the following:

	Patient's Value	Reference Range
Alanine aminotransferase (ALT):	80 U/L	8–20 U/L
Alkaline phosphatase:	60 U/L	20–70 U/L
Aspartate aminotransferase (AST):	50 U/L	8–20 U/L
Albumin:	2.0 g/dL	3.5–5.5 g/dL
Bilirubin, serum, total:	5 mg/dL	0.1–1.0 mg/dL
Bilirubin, serum, direct:	4.2 mg/dL	0.0–0.3 mg/dL
Prothrombin time (PT):	28 s	11–15 s
Partial thromboplastin time (PTT):	50 s	28–40 s

- **What is the most likely diagnosis?**
- **What are the possible etiologies of this disorder?**
- **What other tests would be appropriate?**
- **What are the possible complications?**

ANSWERS TO CASE 3: HEPATITIS

Summary: A 57-year-old man with a prior history of blood transfusion presents with jaundice and ascites, along with mildly elevated transaminases as well as evidence of impaired hepatic synthetic function (hypoalbuminemia and coagulopathy).

- **Most likely diagnosis:** Chronic hepatitis/cirrhosis.
- **Possible etiologies of this disorder:** Most commonly caused by chronic toxin exposure (alcohol) or chronic viral infection; sometimes chronic hepatitis may be caused by inherited metabolic disorders such as hemochromatosis.
- **Other appropriate tests:** Hepatitis virus serologies and possibly a liver biopsy.
- **Possible complications:** Hepatic failure, gastrointestinal bleeding, hepatocellular carcinoma.

CLINICAL CORRELATION

This patient had a blood transfusion in the early 1980s, before the discovery of and the institution of screening for hepatitis C virus. He had a long asymptomatic period and now has signs of advanced liver disease. His **firm nodular liver** probably represents cirrhosis, with scarring of the liver parenchyma along with regenerative nodules. His transaminases (ALT and AST) are only mildly elevated but these tests may be within normal limits, particularly early in the course of disease. The fact that he has **impaired hepatic synthesis** of albumin and coagulation factors indicates that he has very advanced disease, especially in light of the enormous reserve and regenerative capacity of the liver. The accumulation of ascitic fluid in the peritoneum usually represents **portal hypertension,** an increase in pressure in the portal venous system that typically results from increased intrahepatic resistance to portal blood flow because of perisinusoidal deposition of collagen.

APPROACH TO LIVER PATHOLOGY

Objectives

- Know the differences between the viral hepatitis subgroups.
- Describe the serology markers used to diagnose viral hepatitis infection.
- Describe the nonviral causes of chronic hepatitis.

Definitions

Cirrhosis: Although often used as a clinical description, cirrhosis is really a **pathologic diagnosis** that is characterized by disruption of normal liver architecture by **interconnecting fibrous scars** and the creation of **parenchymal nodules** by regenerative activity and the network of scars. This pathologic process can be thought of as the final common pathway of many causes of chronic hepatic injury. The inciting factor causes hepatocyte necrosis and deposition of collagen. At some point the fibrosis becomes irreversible, and cirrhosis then develops. Cirrhosis can be classified according to morphologic features (**micronodular,** most often caused by alcohol, or **macronodular,** most often resulting from viral hepatitis) or according to the etiology: alcoholic, cardiac, biliary, or drug induced. However, a single cause of hepatic injury can produce a variety of pathologic patterns, and any given morphology can result from a variety of causes. See Figure 3-1.

Acute hepatitis: The influx of acute inflammatory cells, which may follow or precede hepatocyte necrosis. The morphologic changes in both acute and chronic hepatitis are common to the hepatitis viruses and can be mimicked by drug reactions.

Chronic hepatitis: It can be due to numerous causes, all of which result in hepatic inflammation and necrosis for at least 6 months, but without the nodular regeneration and architectural distortion of cirrhosis.

Hepatic steatosis: Also known as "fatty liver," this entity commonly is due to alcohol ingestion but also can be due to many other causes of altered lipid metabolism (diabetes, obesity, glucocorticoid use, total parenteral nutrition, some drug reactions), resulting in the accumulation of fat first in cytoplasmic microvesicles in the hepatocyte. Later, the vacuoles coalesce into macrovesicles, compressing and displacing the nucleus so that the hepatocyte resembles a lipocyte. Grossly, the liver becomes enlarged with a yellow, greasy appearance. Steatosis is usually **reversible** with discontinuation of the underlying cause, but it may lead to the development of fibrosis around the central veins and sinusoids and ultimately to cirrhosis.

DISCUSSION

APPROACH TO LIVER DISEASE

Normal Anatomy and Function

The liver receives two-thirds of its blood supply from the portal vein and one-third from the hepatic artery, and its venous drainage via the hepatic vein flows into the inferior vena cava. Its microarchitecture is arranged around this vascular supply and the biliary ducts, which join to form the hepatic duct, which leads to the common bile duct and into the duodenum. The liver is organized into 1- to 2-mm hexagonal **lobules,** with cords or plates of hepatocytes radiating out from the **central vein,** the terminal venules of the hepatic vein. At each corner of the hexagon are the **portal tracts,** composed of the terminal branches of the portal vein and the hepatic artery, as well as the bile duct. Arterial and portal venous blood flows through **sinusoids,** between the cords of hepatocytes, giving them a rich vascular supply (25 percent of cardiac output) before draining into the central vein. Bile is secreted into **bile canaliculi** between adjacent hepatocytes and flows into the canals of Herring and then to the **lobular bile ducts.** The organization of a lobule is shown in Figure 3-1.

The liver serves many functions, including maintenance of carbohydrate, lipid, and amino acid metabolism; synthesis of nearly all serum proteins; and detoxification and excretion of noxious substances in the bile. One such substance is bilirubin, a waste product that is the metabolite of the breakdown of heme from senescent red blood cells. In its initial form, **unconjugated or "indirect" bilirubin,** it is insoluble in aqueous solution, circulates highly bound to albumin, and is toxic to tissues. It undergoes conjugation with glucuronic acid in the hepatocyte to form **conjugated or direct bilirubin,** which is water-soluble and nontoxic, and then is excreted into the bile canaliculus. When liver disease causes jaundice, affected individuals usually have reflux of conjugated bilirubin into the blood, which causes the visible icterus when deposited in tissues, as well as the dark urine resulting from urinary excretion of elevated levels of water-soluble conjugated bilirubin.

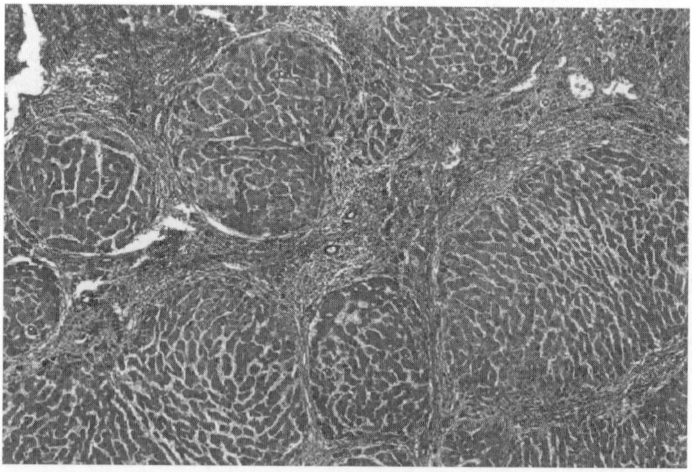

Figure 3-1. Microscopic image of liver cirrhosis.

APPROACH TO VIRAL HEPATITIS

Because of its rich vascular supply, the liver may be involved in any systemic blood-borne infection, but the most common and clinically significant infections are those with one of **five hepatotropic viruses: hepatitis A, B, C, D, and E.** Each virus can produce virtually indistinguishable clinical syndromes. Affected individuals often present with a prodrome of nonspecific constitutional symptoms, including fever, nausea, fatigue, arthralgias, myalgias, headache, and sometimes pharyngitis and coryza. This is followed by the onset of visible **jaundice** caused by hyperbilirubinemia, tenderness and enlargement of the liver, and **dark urine caused by bilirubinuria.** The clinical course, outcomes, and possible complications vary with the type of virus causing the hepatitis. A comparison of features of these five viruses is shown in Table 3-1.

Hepatitis A and **hepatitis E** are very contagious and are transmitted by the **fecal-oral route,** usually by contaminated food or water in areas where sanitation is poor, and in day-care situations by children. **Hepatitis A** is found worldwide and is the **most common cause of acute viral hepatitis** in the United States. **Hepatitis E** is much **less common** and is found in Asia, Africa, and Central America. Both hepatitis A and hepatitis E infections usually lead to self-limited illnesses and generally resolve within weeks. Almost all patients with hepatitis A recover completely and have no long-term complications. Most patients with **hepatitis E** also have uncomplicated courses, but some patients, **particularly pregnant women**, have been reported to develop severe hepatic necrosis and fatal liver failure.

Hepatitis B is the **second most common** type of viral hepatitis in the United States, and it is **usually sexually transmitted.** It **also may be acquired parenterally,** for example, through intravenous drug use, and during birth, from chronically infected mothers. The outcome then depends on the age at which the infection was acquired. Up to 90 percent of infected newborns develop chronic hepatitis B infection, which places an affected infant at significant risk of hepatocellular carcinoma later in adulthood. Among individuals infected later in life, approximately 95 percent recover completely without sequelae. Between 5 and 10 percent of patients will develop chronic hepatitis and may progress to cirrhosis. Also, a chronic carrier state may be seen in which the virus continues to replicate but does not cause hepatic damage in the host.

Hepatitis C is **transmitted parenterally by blood transfusions** or **intravenous drug use** and rarely by sexual contact. It uncommonly is diagnosed as a cause of acute hepatitis, often producing subclinical infection, but frequently is diagnosed later as a cause of chronic hepatitis. The natural history of infection is not completely understood, but **50 to 85 percent of patients with hepatitis C will develop chronic infection.**

Hepatitis D is a defective RNA virus that **requires the presence of the hepatitis B virus to replicate.** It can be acquired as a coinfection simultaneously with acute hepatitis B or as a later superinfection in a person with a chronic hepatitis B infection. Patients with chronic hepatitis B virus who then

Table 3-1
CLINICAL AND VIROLOGIC CHARACTERISTICS
OF THE HEPATITIS VIRUSES

	VIRUS TYPE	TRANSMISSION	INCUBATION	SEROLOGIC MARKERS	CARRIER STATE	CHRONIC HEPATITIS
Hepatitis A	RNA	Enteral (fecal-oral)	15–45 days (mean 30 days)	Anti-hepatitis A IgM	No	No
Hepatitis B	DNA	Parenteral	30–180 days (mean 60–90 days)	HBsAg, anti-HBsAb, or anti-HBcAb IgM (acute)	Yes	Yes
Hepatitis C	RNA	Parenteral	15–160 days (mean 50 days)	Anti-hepatitis C virus HCV RNA	Yes	Yes
Hepatitis D	Defective DNA	Parenteral	Same as hepatitis B	Anti-hepatitis D virus IgM	Yes	Yes
Hepatitis E	RNA	Enteral (fecal-oral)	14–60 days (mean 40 days)	Anti-hepatitis E virus	No	No

become infected with hepatitis D may suffer clinical deterioration; in 10 to 20 percent of these cases, the infected individuals develop severe fatal hepatic failure.

Hepatitis Serologies

Clinical presentation does not reliably establish the viral etiology, and so serologic studies are used to establish a diagnosis. **Anti-hepatitis A immunoglobulin M (IgM)** establishes an **acute** hepatitis A infection. If **anti-hepatitis C antibody** is present, acute hepatitis C is diagnosed, but the test may be negative for several months. The hepatitis C polymerase chain reaction (PCR) assay, which becomes positive earlier in the disease course, often aids in the diagnosis. Acute hepatitis B infection is diagnosed by the presence of hepatitis B surface antigen (HBsAg) in the clinical context of elevated serum transaminase levels and jaundice. HBsAg later disappears when the antibody (anti-HBs) is produced (see Figure 3-2).

There is often an interval of a few weeks between the disappearance of HBsAg and the appearance of anti-HBsAb, which is referred to as the window period. During this interval, the presence of anti-hepatitis B core antigen IgM (anti-HBc IgM) will indicate an acute hepatitis B infection. Hepatitis B precore antigen (HBeAg) represents a high level of viral replication. It is almost always present during acute infection, but its persistence after 6 weeks of illness is a sign of chronic infection and high infectivity. Persistence of HBsAg or HBeAg is a marker for chronic hepatitis or a chronic carrier state; elevated or normal serum transaminase levels distinguish these two entities (see Table 3-2).

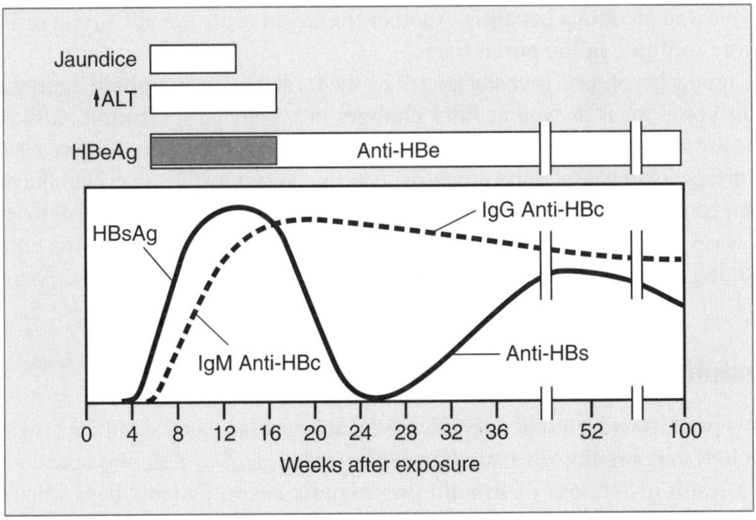

Figure 3-2. Hepatitis B serology.

Table 3-2
HEPATITIS B SEROLOGIC MARKERS

	HBsAg	HBsAb	HBcAb	HBeAg
Key Feature	Indicates presence of viral replication and infectivity	Provides immunity	Only marker positive during "window period"	Indicates high transmissibility
Stage of Disease	Acute disease; Chronic active disease; chronic carrier	Complete recovery	Acute disease (IgM); Chronic/ recovered disease (IgG)	Active disease

Pathologic Changes in Hepatitis

As was mentioned before, the pathologic findings in **acute hepatitis** can be caused by various insults, such as viral infection and toxic injury, and are not pathognomic for any particular cause. There may be hepatocyte swelling called **ballooning degeneration,** as well as liver cell necrosis, including fragmentation and condensation of hepatocytes, forming **intensely eosinophilic Councilman bodies,** which are **characteristic of viral hepatitis.** Formation of ropelike eosinophilic structures within hepatocytes, called **Mallory bodies,** is typical of alcoholic hepatitis. Another finding in acute hepatitis is an inflammatory infiltrate in the portal tracts.

Chronic hepatitis C is characterized by the formation of **lymphoid aggregates** in the portal tracts as well as **fatty changes** in hepatocytes. **Ground glass cells** often are seen in chronic hepatitis B. If inflammation is limited to the portal tracts, the disease is milder and the prognosis is better. When it spills over into the periportal parenchyma, destroying the limiting plate **(piecemeal necrosis)** or extending across lobules, such as the portal area to the central vein, which is termed **bridging necrosis,** the disease is more progressive and the prognosis is poorer.

Complications of Chronic Hepatitis

Many patients with chronic hepatitis have stable disease, but a significant fraction develops ongoing fibrosis and ultimately cirrhosis, as was described previously. As a result of the **loss of functioning hepatic mass,** patients have impaired synthesis of albumin and consequent edema, as well as diminished production of coagulation factors, leading to a coagulopathy. The fibrosis causes increased intrahepatic resistance to portal venous blood flow and thus increased pressure in this venous system. **Portal hypertension** in turn leads to the development of **ascites,** or the accumulation of intraperitoneal fluid, and the formation of collateral venous circulation, such as **esophageal varices,** which often produce life-threatening hemorrhages. Finally, patients with chronic hepatitis and cirrhosis of almost any cause, especially hepatitis B or hepatitis C, are at increased risk for developing **hepatocellular carcinoma.**

APPROACH TO TOXIC LIVER DISEASE

Alcoholic Liver Disease

Alcohol-related liver disease occurs in three overlapping forms: **hepatic steatosis** (fatty liver), **alcoholic hepatitis,** and **cirrhosis.** The pathologic features of these conditions were described previously. The major points to note here are that fat begins to accumulate within hepatocytes after even a moderate intake of alcohol and, with continued exposure, continues to accumulate until the liver may be 3 to 4 times its normal mass. Up to the point where fibrosis appears, the **fatty change is reversible** with abstention from alcohol. Alcoholic hepatitis is characterized by acute hepatocyte necrosis, particularly after bouts of heavy drinking, and is usually reversible. It typically includes some **sinusoidal and perivenular fibrosis** and, if superimposed on fatty liver, often progresses to **cirrhosis. Patients with alcoholic hepatitis often have an AST/ALT ratio greater than 2.**

Acetaminophen Toxicity

A relatively common and treatable form of hepatotoxic exposure that otherwise may lead to hepatic failure and death is acetaminophen poisoning. A minor metabolite of acetaminophen is produced by cytochrome P-450 2E1 in the form of a hepatotoxin, which normally is detoxified by binding to glutathione. Hepatotoxicity is most likely to develop in patients with single very large ingestions (such as suicide attempts) or patients with enhanced activity of this cytochrome, as well as those with depleted levels of glutathione, such as chronic alcoholics. **Blood levels of acetaminophen** correlate with the severity of hepatic injury. Patients with toxic levels of acetaminophen may be treated with doses of ***N*-acetylcysteine,** which replaces glutathione stores, allowing detoxification of the metabolite.

APPROACH TO METABOLIC DISORDERS

Hemochromatosis

Hereditary hemochromatosis, a disorder caused by the inheritance of a mutant *HFE* gene, is a common disorder of iron storage that most often is found in persons of northern European descent. The disease classically was referred to as **bronze diabetes** because of the deposition of iron causing skin pigmentation, diabetes, as well as micronodular cirrhosis, with increased levels of ferritin and hemosiderin within hepatocytes. It now can be diagnosed before the occurrence of end-organ damage resulting from iron deposition by screening for **transferrin saturation greater than 45 percent** and confirmed by ***HFE* genotyping.**

α_1-Antitrypsin Deficiency

α_1-Antitrypsin (A1AT) deficiency is an inherited disorder in which there is an abnormally low level of this serum protease inhibitor. In some patients, the abnormal A1AT is synthesized in the liver but cannot be secreted, and so it accumulates in cytoplasmic globules. The spectrum of liver diseases ranges from neonatal hepatitis, to childhood cirrhosis, to adult cirrhosis. Thus, patients with **A1AT deficiency** will often develop **emphysema** due to increased levels of **elastase** in the lungs in addition to **cirrhosis**. Diagnosis is achieved by finding low levels of serum A1AT activity and by A1AT phenotyping.

Wilson Disease

Wilson disease is an inherited disorder of copper metabolism in which there is accumulation of copper in multiple tissues, including liver, brain, and eye. Clinical manifestations may include acute or chronic hepatitis, fatty liver, and cirrhosis, along with extrapyramidal movement disorders or psychiatric disturbances. Diagnosis is made by finding **Kayser-Fleischer rings** in the cornea, which are pathognomonic, or by **low levels of serum ceruloplasmin** (a serum copper-transport protein), as well as increased levels of hepatic or urinary copper.

COMPREHENSION QUESTIONS

[3.1] Which of the following statements best describes infection with hepatitis B virus?

A. Acute infection can be diagnosed by the presence of anti-HBsAb IgM or anti-HBc IgM.
B. It is nearly always a self-limited infection without a chronic or carrier state.
C. It is an RNA virus that usually is acquired from contaminated food and water.
D. It typically is associated with the formation of Mallory bodies on biopsy.
E. When it is acquired in adulthood, more than 85 percent of patients develop chronic hepatitis.

[3.2] A 25-year-old woman develops tender hepatomegaly and hemiballism when walking. Her liver biopsy shows hepatocyte necrosis and inflammatory portal tract infiltrate. Which of the following tests is most likely to yield the diagnosis?

A. Staining of liver specimen with Prussian blue
B. Measurement of serum α_1-antitrypsin activity
C. Hepatitis C PCR
D. Ophthalmologic slit-lamp examination
E. Serum acetaminophen level

[3.3] A 26-year-old woman presents with fever, malaise, signs of jaundice, clay-colored stool, and dark urine. A liver biopsy reveals liver cell drop-out along with focal inflammation and ballooning degeneration of hepatocytes. A few intensely eosinophilic oval bodies are found. What are these microscopic bodies called?

A. Councilman bodies
B. Cowdry A bodies
C. Mallory bodies
D. Psammoma bodies
E. Russell bodies

Answers

[3.1] **A.** Acute hepatitis B infection is characterized by the presence or shedding of HbsAg, followed by a rise in anti-Hbc IgM. Adult infection has a much better prognosis (only 5 to 10 percent of patients develop chronic hepatitis) compared with perinatal infection (more than 90 percent develop chronic infection). Councilman bodies can be seen in viral hepatitis; Mallory bodies are characteristic of alcoholic hepatitis.

[3.2] **D.** The pathologic findings of acute hepatitis are nonspecific. The distinguishing feature in this case is the presence of hemiballism, an extrapyramidal movement disorder, suggesting Wilson disease. Kayser-Fleischer rings are green to brown deposits of copper in the Descemet membrane near the corneal limbus and are diagnostic.

[3.3] **A.** Councilman bodies are intensely eosinophilic bodies that may be seen in liver biopsy specimens from individuals with viral hepatitis. These Councilman bodies are in fact necrotic hepatocytes that have undergone T-cell induced apoptosis. These apoptotic cells are cleared rapidly, and there may not be as many present in a liver biopsy specimen as were originally present.

PATHOLOGY PEARLS

- Most hepatitis viruses are RNA in etiology; hepatitis B is the only DNA hepatitis virus.
- Patients infected with hepatitis B **rarely** develop chronic hepatitis (only 5 to 10 percent of the time).
- Patients with hepatitis C **often** develop chronic hepatitis (50 to 85 percent of the time).
- In viral hepatitis alanine aminotransferase (ALT) is higher than aspartate aminotransferase (AST).
- Patients with alcoholic hepatitis usually have an AST/ALT ratio above 2.
- Patients with A1AT deficiency have both cirrhosis and emphysema.

REFERENCES

Crawford JM. The liver and biliary tract. In: Kumar V, Assas AK, Fausto N, eds. Robbins and Cotran Pathologic Basis of Disease, 7th ed. Philadelphia, PA: Elsevier Saunders, 2004:878–927.

Crawford JM. The liver and biliary tract. In: Mitchell RN, Kumar V, Abbas AK, et al., eds. Pocket Companion to Robbins and Cotran Pathologic Basis of Disease, 7th ed. Philadelphia, PA: Saunders, 2006, 446–63.

Dienstag JL, Isselbacher KJ. Acute viral hepatitis. In: Braunwald E., Fauci AS, Kasper DL, et al., eds. Harrison's Principles of Internal Medicine, 16th ed. New York: McGraw-Hill, 2004:1822–37.

Ishak KG, Markin RS. Liver. In: Damjanov I, Linder J, eds. Anderson's Pathology, 10th ed. New York: Mosby, 1996:1779–858.

CASE 4

A 45-year-old man with a family history of colon cancer undergoes a screening colonoscopy. No invasive carcinomas are identified, but two small pedunculated tubular adenomas are removed and one villous adenoma measuring 5 mm in diameter is biopsied.

- **What is the most likely diagnosis?**
- **What are the syndromes that could predispose this individual to colon cancer?**
- **What other dietary factors could play a role in the development of colon cancer?**

ANSWERS TO CASE 4: COLON ADENOMA

Summary: A 45-year-old man with a family history of colon cancer underwent colonoscopy for rectal bleeding. Colonoscopic findings included several small pedunculated polyps in the right colon, all measuring less than 5 mm.

- **Most likely diagnosis:** Hyperplastic polyps or tubular adenomas.
- **Syndromes predisposing to colon cancer:** Familial adenomatous polyposis (FAP) and hereditary nonpolyposis colon cancer (HNPCC) are two common inherited colon cancer syndromes.
- **Dietary factors that play a role in the development of colon cancer:** Diets rich in fat and red meat and low in fiber may contribute to the development of colon cancer.

CLINICAL CORRELATION

Colon cancer is the third most common malignant neoplasm worldwide and the second leading cause of cancer death in the United States. The peak incidence is in the seventh decade of life. **Recommended screening for colon cancer for patients without increased risk starts at age 50, but for at-risk patients with a positive family history, screening should start at age 40 (some recommend 10 years earlier than the age at which the youngest index case presents).** Annual fecal occult blood tests should be performed as well as digital rectal examination and flexible sigmoidoscopy every 5 years. Additional screening can be done by colonoscopy every 10 years, or a double-contrast barium enema can be done every 5 to 10 years. These recommended screening intervals may be maintained after a negative examination. For patients at high risk for cancer or with polyps, rescreening by colonoscopy at 3-year intervals is recommended. New technologies such as virtual colonography and genetic testing of stool specimens are being examined for their appropriate clinical settings. In this patient, the colonic polyps showed proliferation of tubular glands, arising from a fibromuscular base with normal colonic epithelium consistent with a polyp stalk. The polyps showed no evidence of malignant transformation (i.e., carcinoma). The diagnosis was multiple tubular adenomas of the colon.

APPROACH TO COLON ADENOMAS

Objectives

- Describe the adenoma-dysplasia-carcinoma sequence.
- List the risk factors for colon cancer.
- Describe the hereditary polyp disorders.

Definitions

Adenoma: Neoplastic proliferation of colonic epithelium that results in the formation of a polyp.

Neoplasia: Usually implies abnormal, often clonal proliferation of cells that results in the formation of a tumor.

Dysplasia: Usually the result of additional genetic abnormalities in cells that lead to further dysfunction or abnormal cell maturation.

Adenoma-dysplasia-carcinoma sequence: Model for colon cancer development that outlines the genetic pathway involved in the progression from a benign neoplastic polyp (adenoma) to frankly invasive cancer (carcinoma).

Familial adenomatous polyposis syndrome: The prototypic inherited colon cancer phenotype; affected patients have hundreds to thousands of polyps and are at high risk for cancer development.

Hereditary nonpolyposis colorectal cancer: Also known as Lynch syndrome. Often presents as **right-sided colon cancer** and involves mutation in mismatch repair genes. It is inherited in an **autosomal dominant** fashion, and affected individuals are also at high risk for **extracolonic malignancies** such as **endometrial carcinomas.**

DISCUSSION

Polyps of the colon can be classified broadly into **inflammatory/reactive, hyperplastic,** and **neoplastic.** Inflammatory polyps can be seen in chronic colitides such as ulcerative colitis and Crohn disease. Hyperplastic polyps are some of the more frequently encountered polyps and are thought to represent nonneoplastic proliferation of colonic epithelium. There is accumulating evidence that some hyperplastic polyps may transform to adenomas through a serrated adenoma pathway. **Adenomas are truly neoplastic proliferations** and have the potential to transform and progress to carcinomas (see Figure 4-1). With increasing age, there is an increased incidence of adenoma formation. Approximately 50 percent of patients who have one adenoma have additional synchronous adenomas present. Most polyps are present in the rectosigmoid colon, but with increasing age, there is a tendency to see more **right-sided involvement** by polyps.

Types of Adenomas

Adenomas can be classified on the basis of the pattern of growth: whether they are flat, sessile, and broad without a stalk, or pedunculated and on a stalk. Histologically, depending on the extent of tubular gland formation versus fingerlike villous projections, they are classified as **tubular adenomas, villous adenomas,** or **tubulovillous adenomas.**

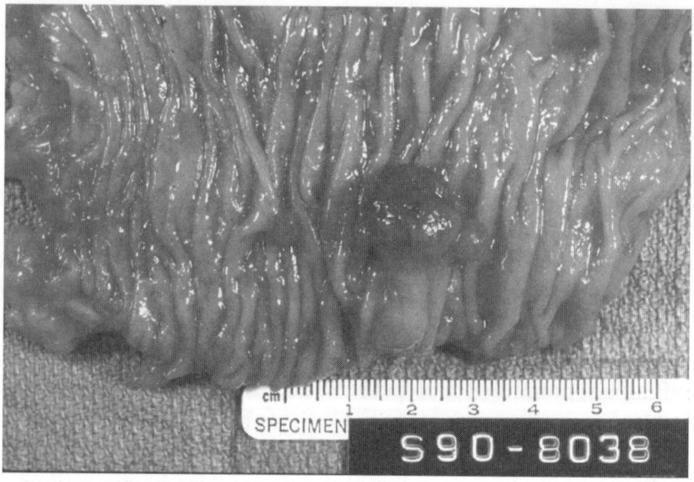

Figure 4-1. Colonic polyp: gross pictograph.

Polyposis and Inherited Colon Cancer Syndromes

Syndromes that involve the formation of multiple gastrointestinal polyps occur infrequently. Some, such as **Peutz-Jeghers syndrome** and **Cowden disease,** are **autosomal dominant,** resulting in the formation of **nonneoplastic hamartomatous polyps;** others, such as Canada-Cronkhite syndrome, are not hereditary and result in multiple juvenile polyps. Other clinically significant polyposis or colon cancer syndromes include **familial adenomatous polyposis** and **hereditary nonpolyposis colorectal cancer.**

The **autosomal dominant** ***FAP*** **gene** on **chromosome 5q21** contains the tumor suppressor gene ***APC*** (adenomatous polyposis coli). Affected individuals have hundreds to **thousands of polyps,** typically presenting in the **left colon. Almost all individuals with** ***APC*** **gene mutations eventually develop colon cancer.** Hence, carriers usually are candidates for **prophylactic colectomy.** Recent studies have shown that **cyclooxygenase inhibitors can suppress polyp formation** and possibly carcinoma development in patients with FAP.

Adenoma-Dysplasia-Carcinoma Sequence

A **variant of FAP** is **Gardner syndrome,** which involves the formation of **osteomas** of the bone, **desmoid fibromatosis. HNPCC** also is known as **Lynch syndrome,** named after the gastroenterologist Dr. Henry Lynch. The **autosomal dominant** inherited disease presents early in life, often with **right-sided cancer,** and can be associated with **polyps,** although much **less numerous** (usually fewer than 10) than what is seen in FAP. Patients with HNPCC are also at risk for **extra–gastrointestinal tract tumors.**

There are also less-well-defined familial cancer syndromes involving glandular elements (adenocarcinomas) that are associated with a family history or personal history of **breast, ovarian, endometrial, or colon cancer.**

The **development of colon cancer** is a **multifactorial** process involving not only predisposition genes but also factors such as **diet** (low-fiber foods, red meat, and refined carbohydrates are nonfavorable), **obesity,** and **inactivity.** Genetically, it is known that **adenomas** can progress and **transform** through additional mutations (i.e., genetic "hits") and progressively grow in size, increase in the degree of dysplasia, and acquire full malignant potential (carcinoma). **Additional genes** that have been shown to be involved in this process include the ***K-ras*** **oncogene,** the ***DCC*** (*d*eleted in *c*olon *c*ancer) adhesion molecule gene, and the **p53 tumor suppressor gene.**

COMPREHENSION QUESTIONS

[4.1] A 25-year-old man is discovered to have colon cancer. It is noted that several members of his family also developed colon cancer at relatively young ages. Which of the following genes is most likely to be involved?

A. Hereditary nonpolyposis colorectal cancer gene
B. Mismatch repair gene
C. p53 gene
D. *K-ras* oncogene

[4.2] Routine screening colonoscopy is performed on an asymptomatic 50-year-old man and finds a 5-mm lesion in the sigmoid colon. The lesion is removed and histologic examination reveals a polyp composed of dysplastic stratified epithelial cells having hyperchromatic nuclei and decreased mucin production. Fingerlike villous projections are not seen. Which of the following is the most likely diagnosis?

A. Hyperplastic polyp
B. Inflammatory polyp
C. Retention polyp
D. Tubular adenoma
E. Villous adenoma

[4.3] Which of the following autosomal dominant disorders is characterized by the formation of multiple gastrointestinal polyps along with pigmented lesions around the oral cavity?

A. Cowden disease
B. Gardner syndrome
C. Peutz-Jeghers syndrome
D. Rotor syndrome
E. Still disease

Answers

[4.1] **A.** Hereditary nonpolyposis colorectal carcinoma, also known as Lynch syndrome, presents as an autosomal dominant disorder characterized by the formation of colon cancer, usually early in life. The disorder is associated with the hereditary nonpolyposis colorectal cancer gene and with the formation of multiple colonic polyps, although fewer than seen in the family adenomatous polyposis syndrome.

[4.2] **D.** The presence of dysplastic epithelium within a colonic polyp defines adenomas of the colon, the three types of which are tubular adenomas, mixed tubulovillous (villoglandular) adenomas, and villous adenomas. Tubular adenomas are the smallest adenomatous polyps of the colon and have the least malignant potential. Microscopically these polyps are composed of dysplastic epithelium that forms tubules and glandular structures. If abundant finger-like (papillary) structures are present, then the polyp is classified as villous adenomas. These polyps are the largest types of colonic adenomas and have the greatest malignant potential.

[4.3] **C.** The Peutz-Jeghers syndrome is an autosomal-dominant disorder that is characterized by the combination of hamartomatous polyps of the small intestine and pigmented lesions around the oral cavity. The most common site for the hamartomatous polyps is the jejunum. This syndrome is associated with a slight increased risk for the development of colon cancer.

PATHOLOGY PEARLS

- ❖ Colonic adenomas are neoplastic proliferations with the potential for malignant transformation.
- ❖ Inherited syndromes such as FAP and HNPCC can predispose people to developing polyps and colon cancer. One pathway is the adenoma-dysplasia-carcinoma sequence.
- ❖ Additional factors, such as diet, obesity, and activity, can affect one's risk for developing colon cancer.
- ❖ Hereditary nonpolyposis colorectal cancer (HNPCC) is associated with extracolonic malignancies **such as endometrial carcinomas.**

REFERENCES

Crawford JM, Liu C. The gastrointestinal tract. In: Mitchell RN, Kumar V, Abbas AK, Fausto N. eds. Pocket Companion to Robbins and Cotran Pathologic Basis of Disease, 7th ed. Philadelphia, PA: Saunders, 2006, 437–43.

Fenoglio-Preiser C, Noffsinger AE, Stemmermann GN, et al. Gastrointestinal Pathology, 2nd ed. Philadelphia: Lippincott-Raven, 1999.

Liu C, Crawford JM. The gastrointestinal tract. In: Kumar V, Assas AK, Fausto N, eds. Robbins and Cotran Pathologic Basis of Disease, 7th ed. Philadelphia, PA: Elsevier Saunders, 2004:856–70.

❖ CASE 5

A 57-year-old man complains of severe upper abdominal pain extending to his midback. He also has had fatigue and a loss in appetite over the past several weeks. Physical examination reveals generalized jaundice but no other significant findings. An upper endoscopy does not identify any mucosal ulcerations or masses. A CT scan of the abdomen shows a large mass in the head and body of the pancreas.

◆ **What is the most likely diagnosis?**

◆ **What is the likely prognosis of this condition?**

ANSWERS TO CASE 5: PANCREATIC CARCINOMA

Summary: A 57-year-old man has severe upper abdominal pain radiating to his midback, fatigue, loss of appetite, and generalized jaundice. A large mass in the head and body of the pancreas is noted on CT imaging.

- **Most likely diagnosis:** Pancreatic carcinoma
- **Likely prognosis of this condition:** Poor prognosis with 5-year survival less than 5 percent

CLINICAL CORRELATION

The vast majority of pancreatic carcinomas involve exocrine glands and are known as adenocarcinomas. The etiology is largely unknown. However, point mutations of **the *K-ras* gene have been observed in over 90 percent of the pancreatic tumors**, suggesting abnormalities at the genetic level. Pain and nonspecific systemic symptoms such as weakness and weight loss are the usual first signs of malignancy. Obstructive jaundice is seen commonly because of the preference for tumors to occur in the head of the pancreas. The symptomatic course of pancreatic carcinoma is typically brief and progressive. Radiologic workups, including abdominal CT and ultrasound, are diagnostic for the cancer and are used for staging. No specific biological tests are available for screening or early detection. Cancer of the pancreas is now the fifth most common cause of cancer-related death in the United States. The median survival period from the time of diagnosis to demise is arguably the worst of any of the cancers. The median survival for untreated advanced cases is approximately 3.5 months; with good treatment this increases to approximately 6 months. **The 5-year relative survival rate of patients with this cancer is only 3 to 5 percent.** Even though a Whipple operation is considered the treatment of choice for localized and early disease, fewer than 15 percent of pancreatic tumors overall are resectable at the time of diagnosis. The prognosis of pancreatic carcinoma is one of the most dismal among any malignancies ever known.

APPROACH TO PANCREATIC CANCER

Objectives

- List the risk factors for pancreatic cancer.
- Describe the different neuroendocrine tumors of the pancreas.
- Describe the serum markers used for pancreatic cancer.

Definitions

Jaundice: A yellow discoloring of the skin, mucous membranes, and eyes caused by excess bilirubin in the blood. Common causes of jaundice in adults include prehepatic causes such as intravascular hemolysis, hepatic causes such as hepatitis A and hepatic tumors, and posthepatic causes, including obstruction of the bile duct as a result of infection, tumor, or gallstones.

Exocrine gland: A gland that secretes its products through ducts or canals, such as sweat glands or mammary glands. The secretion products produce their biologic effects locally.

Endocrine gland: A gland, such as the pituitary or thyroid, that secretes its products, called hormones, directly into the bloodstream. Hormones generate their biologic effects at distant locations.

Pancreatic cancer and adenocarcinoma of the pancreas: By definition, pancreatic cancer includes all malignant neoplasms of the pancreas. It includes the tumors arising from the exocrine portion of pancreas such as gland-forming adenocarcinoma of the pancreas, those of ductal origin, and tumors from endocrine components. Adenocarcinoma is the most common form of cancer, accounting for over 75 percent of all pancreatic cancers.

DISCUSSION

Normal Pancreatic Histology

The pancreas is a small, spongy gland that lies just under the curvature of the stomach and deep within the abdomen. The majority of the pancreas is composed of **exocrine glands,** which produce enzymes necessary for food digestion. The **secretions from acinar cells,** the structural unit throughout the pancreas, containing salts and enzymes, are called pancreatic fluid, which eventually drains into the pancreatic duct. The pancreatic duct usually joins the bile duct and empties its combined digestive contents into the duodenum. Additionally, the pancreas has an **endocrine,** or hormonal, function. Inside specialized groupings of cells called the **islets of Langerhans,** the pancreas produces hormones such as **insulin and glucagons,** among other hormones. These molecules are secreted directly into the bloodstream, eliciting numerous biologic effects throughout the body.

Epidemiology

Each year approximately 30,000 people in the United States are diagnosed with adenocarcinoma of the pancreas. Most of them will have passed away by the end of the first year. Most patients are between the ages of 60 and 80. Men tend to be affected more often than women. The median survival period from the time of diagnosis until demise is extremely short, with a mean of 3.5 months. It has been approximated that approximately 30 percent of the changes that initiate cancer of the pancreas are caused by smoking and that approximately 8 percent are "secondary" to a hereditary genetic predisposition. There does not appear to be a strong correlation between the onset of pancreatic adenocarcinoma and the drinking of alcohol or coffee.

Biochemical Tests

Laboratory results often reveal nonspecific elevated bilirubin and elevated liver function enzymes as a result of biliary obstruction. The **CA 19-9 marker,** a Lewis blood group–related mucin, frequently is elevated in adenocarcinoma of the pancreas, but its use in screening for or diagnosis of the cancer is not accepted in general practice. High CA 19-9 levels may be associated with but do not always indicate larger tumors and with a decreased likelihood of surgical resectability. The use of this marker is accepted more widely as a running measure in a particular individual to help reflect the stability or progression of the cancer. **Point mutation of *K-ras*** is observed in **90 percent of pancreatic cancer patients.** However, the utility of a screening test for *K-ras* mutation is not proven clinically.

Adenocarcinoma of the Pancreas

In up to **95 percent of cases,** pancreatic cancer arises from the **exocrine portion of the organ.** Most of the exocrine tumors (approximately 90 percent) are from ductal cells—those which line the pancreatic ducts. Further, under the microscope, the appearance and arrangement of these carcinoma cells can appear duct like (or "adeno"), giving the term adenocarcinoma to this most common form of pancreatic cancer. Approximately **three-quarters of exocrine tumors** of the pancreas arise in the **head and neck of the pancreas.** It is believed that cancer is caused by the mutations of a gene, which confer increased abnormal growth potential to cells. Among other abnormalities, an oncogene called *K-ras* is found to be altered in up to 95 percent of ductal adenocarcinomas of the pancreas. The Whipple operation (pancreaticoduodenectomy) typically is performed in patients with tumors localized in the head of the pancreas.

Other Malignant Tumors of the Pancreas

Neuroendocrine tumors of the pancreas (islet-cell tumors) are **much less common** than tumors arising from the exocrine pancreas. Approximately **75 percent of these tumors are "functioning,"** meaning that they are found to be producing symptoms related to one or more of the hormone peptides they secrete. The predominant peptide secreted gives the functioning islet-cell tumor its name. The hormones produced by neuroendocrine tumors include **insulin, gastrin, glucagon, somatostatin, neurotensin, pancreatic polypeptide** (PP), **vasoactive intestinal peptide** (VIP), **growth hormone-releasing factor** (GRF), and **adrenocorticotropic hormone (ACTH),** among others.

Typically, the symptoms produced by the excess secretion of the predominant hormone in a functioning endocrine tumor lead to the eventual diagnosis. It is not possible to determine malignancy from the histologic appearance. Malignancy is determined by finding additional metastatic sites. The natural history of neuroendocrine carcinoma tends to be favorable compared with that of pancreatic adenocarcinoma. For example, the median survival duration from the time of diagnosis for patients with nonfunctioning metastatic neuroendocrine tumors approaches 5 years. Immediate treatment of the symptomatic conditions created by the oversecretion of the hormone may be appropriate. Surgery is generally curative.

COMPREHENSION QUESTIONS

[5.1] A 51-year-old man presents with slowly progressive jaundice, weight loss, and upper abdominal pain that radiates to his midback. Physical examination finds an enlarged gallbladder in the right upper quadrant of his abdomen, and a CT scan shows an irregular mass involving the head of the pancreas. Histologic sections from this mass are most likely to reveal which of the following abnormalities?

A. Adenocarcinoma
B. Clear cell carcinoma
C. Medullary carcinoma
D. Signet ring carcinoma
E. Squamous cell carcinoma

[5.2] Which of the tumor markers listed below is most likely to be used by a clinician who is following a 64-year-old man to look for possible recurrence of pancreatic cancer after surgery?

A. CA 15-3
B. CA 19-9
C. CA 27-29
D. CA-50
E. CA-125

[5.3] A 44-year-old woman presents with worsening episodes of feeling "light-headed and dizzy." She says that her symptoms are relieved if she quickly eats a candy bar. Laboratory evaluation finds that during one of these episodes her serum glucose level is decreased and her serum insulin level is increased. Which of the following is the most likely cause of her symptoms?

A. Carcinoid tumor
B. Functional hamartoma
C. Islet cell adenoma
D. Microcystic adenoma
E. Tubulovillous adenoma

Answers

[5.1] **A.** Adenocarcinoma is the most common type of pancreatic malignancy arising from the pancreatic ducts. In contrast, squamous cell carcinomas usually originate from stratified squamous epithelium, such as the esophagus. Clear cell carcinomas can be found in the kidneys, and signet cell carcinomas can be found in the stomach. A medullary carcinoma is a type of carcinoma of the thyroid gland.

[5.2] **B.** CA 19-9 is currently the best available tumor marker used clinically to look for possible recurrence of pancreatic cancer after surgery. Other markers have been studied in patients with pancreatic cancer, including CA-50, SPAN-1, and DUPAN-1, but these markers have not been as useful as CA 19-9. In contrast, CA-125 is associated with ovarian cancer, whereas CA 15-3 and CA 27-29 are associated with breast cancer, particularly advanced breast cancer.

[5.3] **C.** Elevated serum levels of insulin that result in hypoglycemia can be caused by a tumor that secretes insulin; an insulinoma is a type of islet cell tumor of the pancreas. In contrast, carcinoid tumors, which are found in the appendix and small intestine, may secrete vasoactive substances such as serotonin. A microcystic adenoma is a rare type of benign tumor of the pancreas, and a tubulovillous adenoma is a type of neoplastic polyp of the colon.

PATHOLOGY PEARLS

- Pancreatic cancer usually has a very poor prognosis.
- Adenocarcinoma is the most common type of primary pancreatic cancer, usually arising from the exocrine glands.
- Neuroendocrine tumors of the pancreas tend to have a better prognosis than do adenocarcinomas.
- Painless obstructive jaundice is a common presentation of pancreatic cancer.
- Depression can herald an occult pancreatic cancer.
- **Point mutation of *K-ras*** is observed in **90 percent of pancreatic cancer patients.**

REFERENCES

Hruban RH. The pancreas. In: Mitchell RN, Kumar V, Abbas AK, et al., eds. Pocket Companion to Robbins and Cotran Pathologic Basis of Disease, 7th ed. Philadelphia, PA: Saunders, 2006, 476–82.

Hruban RH, Wilentza RE. The pancreas. In: Kumar V, Assas AK, Fausto N, eds. Robbins and Cotran Pathologic Basis of Disease, 7th ed. Philadelphia, PA: Elsevier Saunders, 2004:939–53.

Mayer RJ. Pancreatic cancer. In: Kasper DL, Fauci AS, Longo DL, et al., eds. Harrison's Principles of Internal Medicine, 16th ed. New York: McGraw-Hill, 2004:537–8.

CASE 6

A 22-year-old woman has had recurrent episodes of diarrhea, crampy abdominal pain, and slight fever over the last 2 years. At first the episodes, which usually last 1 or 2 weeks, were several months apart, but recently they have occurred more frequently. Other symptoms have included mild joint pain and sometimes red skin lesions. On at least one occasion, her stool has been guaiac-positive, indicating the presence of occult blood. Colonoscopy reveals several sharply delineated areas with thickening of the bowel wall and mucosal ulceration. Areas adjacent to these lesions appear normal. Biopsies of the affected areas show full-thickness inflammation of the bowel wall and several noncaseating granulomas.

- **What is the most likely diagnosis?**

- **What are the common complications of this disease?**

ANSWERS TO CASE 6: CROHN DISEASE

Summary: A 22-year-old woman has a 2-year history of recurrent diarrhea, abdominal pain, slight fever, joint pain, and red skin lesions. Colonoscopy reveals several sharply delineated areas with thickening of the bowel wall and mucosal ulceration, which on biopsy show full-thickness inflammation of the bowel wall and several noncaseating granulomas.

- **Most likely diagnosis:** Crohn disease
- **Common complications of this disease:** Malabsorption and malnutrition, fibrous strictures of the intestine, and fistulae to other organs, such as from bowel to skin or bowel to bladder

CLINICAL CORRELATION

The patient's presentation is very characteristic for inflammatory bowel disease, that is, a several-year history of diarrhea and abdominal pain. Additionally, the colonoscopy revealing full-thickness inflammation with noncaseating granulomas is consistent with Crohn disease. Crohn disease is a chronic inflammatory condition that is ubiquitous in its distribution in the gastrointestinal tract. It most commonly manifests in the small intestine, in particular the terminal ileum. The disease exhibits aggressive activity of the gastrointestinal immune system, but the exact cause is unknown. Published studies in the United States report incidence rates that vary between 1.2 and 8.8 per 100,000 population; the prevalence is 44 to 106 per 100,000. The condition is more common in the cold climates of the northeastern United States than in the south. Those of Jewish ethnicity have a high incidence. The disorder, which is slightly more common in females, has a bimodal age distribution, peaking in the early twenties and again emerging in the mid-sixties. Theories regarding pathogenesis have referred to genetics, infection, autoimmune or allergic processes, thromboembolic disorders, and dietary disorders.

APPROACH TO INFLAMMATORY BOWEL DISEASE

Objectives

- Describe the differences between ulcerative colitis and Crohn disease.
- Describe the comorbidities of inflammatory bowel disease.
- Describe the future risk of developing cancer in patients with inflammatory bowel disease.

DISCUSSION

The **predominant symptoms** of Crohn disease are **diarrhea, abdominal pain, and weight loss**. These symptoms may be widely variable, depending on the distribution of the inflammatory lesions in the patient's intestines. The principal stimulus for diarrhea is the mucosal immune response in association with cytokine release. If the **colon** is involved, **diarrhea** may be more marked and **tenesmus** may occur. Abdominal pain may be due to local inflammation or obstruction if it is experienced in the central abdomen or right lower quadrant. **Abscesses or fistulae** also may produce pain. Secondary causes of abdominal pain in relation to Crohn disease are **gallstones** and **renal colic. Malabsorption** leading to weight loss and failure to thrive may occur in children. Fat, protein, mineral, and vitamin deficiencies may be associated with extensive or recurrent disease. About one-third of patients develop perineal symptoms or signs such as anal fistulae or fissures.

Nongastrointestinal symptoms of Crohn disease involve the **skin, joints, or eyes.** Skin lesions include **erythema nodosum, pyoderma gangrenosa, aphthous stomatitis, and finger clubbing.** The rheumatologic manifestations often present as a large joint polyarthropathy resembling ankylosing spondylitis or a small joint fleeting polyarthropathy that is like rheumatoid arthritis. The human lymphocyte antigen B-27 (HLA-B27) may be present. Inflammatory eye lesions are confined to the anterior chamber, such as uveitis, iritis, episcleritis, and conjunctivitis. A **chronic active hepatitis** may develop; more seriously, **sclerosing cholangitis** can progress to cirrhosis. There is a predisposition to **gallstones** when **terminal ileal disease** is present.

Physical Examination

Physical examination may reveal a nutritional deficiency. The extraintestinal manifestations may be apparent. Abdominal examination may suggest partial bowel obstruction, **inflammatory mass, focal areas of tenderness, or enterocutaneous fistulae.** Perineal examination may reveal **fistulae or abscesses.** Perianal skin tags with bluish discoloration may be present. On rectal examination there may be a stricture, a palpable ulcer, or perirectal abscesses. Bloody diarrhea may be detectable. Clinical features compatible with **anemia or hypoalbuminemia** may be present. Hypoalbuminemia may manifest with peripheral edema.

APPROACH

Plain abdominal radiographs provide important information in the acute presentation of symptoms, as they may demonstrate intestinal obstruction or evidence of perforation. Biliary or renal calculi, arthropathy, or osteoporosis also may be detected. Endoscopy of the lower and upper gastrointestinal tract is used to identify disease and provide biopsy evidence. Barium follow-through examination or small bowel enteroclysis may demonstrate discrete lesions in the small intestine. Fistulograms are helpful to surgeons by providing information about the site of the fistula and the presence of obstruction or abscess cavity in association with it.

Computerized tomography is the mainstay in terms of providing information about thickened loops of bowel, abscesses, and fistulous tracts. Magnetic resonance imaging, including cholangiography, may be helpful. Ultrasound may reveal thickened terminal ileum, abscesses, and evidence of biliary tract disease. Ultrasound examination of the renal tract may reveal obstruction or stone formation. Endoscopic ultrasound may be useful in assessing bowel wall involvement and the extent of the disease process. Studies of bone density may be required.

Endoscopy allows detailed examination of the mucosa of the upper and lower intestines, with the added advantage of allowing biopsies of abnormal areas to be taken (see Figure 6-1). Capsule endoscopy is an innovation that permits detailed photography of the small intestinal lumen. There may be electrolyte abnormalities in Crohn disease. The erythrocyte sedimentation rate (ESR) frequently is elevated above 30 mm/h, and the serum vitamin B_{12} level may be reduced.

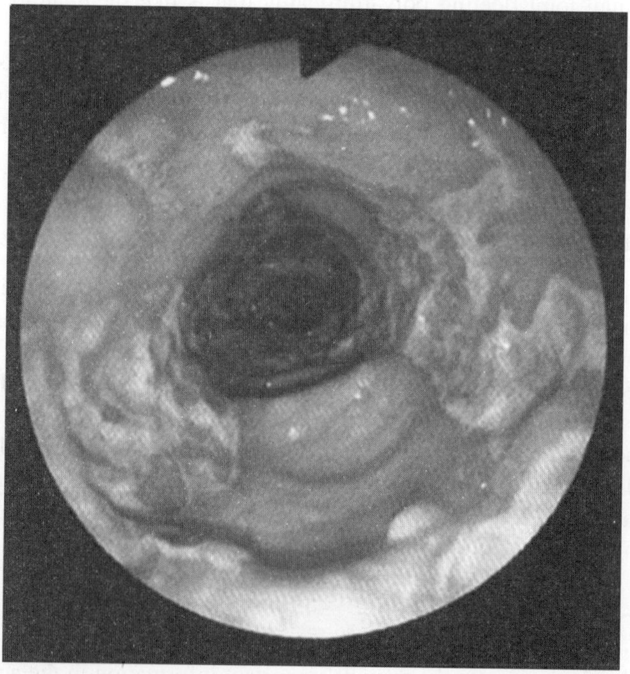

Figure 6-1. Colonoscopic view of Crohn's colitis with linear, serpiginous, white-based ulcers surrounded by colonic mucosa which is relatively normal. *(Reproduced, with permission, from Kasper DL, Braunwald E, Fauci AS, et al.* Harrison's Principles of Internal Medicine. 16th ed. *New York: McGraw-Hill, 2005.)*

Crohn Disease versus Ulcerative Colitis

These inflammatory bowel diseases share certain features, but there are fundamental and often distinguishing features. On occasion it may be very difficult to determine whether a patient has Crohn disease or ulcerative colitis, and in these circumstances the condition often is designated indeterminate colitis. The fundamental differences between Crohn disease and ulcerative colitis are that **Crohn disease** begins in the **submucosa** and **ulcerative colitis begins in the mucosa** of the gut. (See Table 6-1.) Ulcerative colitis, as its name suggests, is a disease confined to the colon and rectum, whereas, as was stated above, **Crohn** disease is **ubiquitous throughout the bowel. Full-thickness involvement** of the bowel, although more common in Crohn disease, may occur in both disorders. **Fibrosis cicatrization and fistula formation** are confined almost exclusively to patients with **Crohn disease.** The histopathologic feature that differentiates the two conditions is the presence of **granulomas in Crohn disease. Aphthoid ulcers** are more likely to occur in patients with Crohn disease. Both conditions are associated with an increased incidence of **colon cancer,** which, however, is **more likely to develop in long-standing ulcerative colitis** than in Crohn disease. The incidence of **malignant change**

Table 6-1
INFLAMMATORY BOWEL DISEASE

	CROHN DISEASE	ULCERATIVE COLITIS
Portion of GI tract	Diffuse; often rectal sparing	Rectum and colon
Route of Spread	Skip lesions	Continuous
Malignant Potential	Low	High
Macroscopic Features	Transmural inflammation, cobblestoning, creeping fat, aphthoid ulcers, "string sign," perianal fissures, fistulas	Mucosal and submucosal inflammation, friability, pseudopolyps
Microscopic Features	Noncaseating granulomas	No granulomas
Extraintestinal Manifestations	Uveitis, erythema nodosum, ankylosing spondylitis, migratory polyarthritis	Primary sclerosing cholangitis, pyoderma gangrenosum
Treatment	Corticosteroids, 5-ASA (more effective in ulcerative colitis), immunomodulating agents	5-ASA, corticosteroids, immunomodulating agents; total colectomy is curative

in the colon or rectum of ulcerative colitis is approximately 20 percent after 25 years of disease activity. Many patients develop ulcerative colitis at a young age and therefore may develop cancerous changes in the colon in their forties or fifties. A further important consideration is that patients with inflammatory bowel disease live with episodes of diarrhea and occasional rectal bleeding so that the heralding features of malignancy may be observed by referring to the underlying inflammatory disease.

Treatment

Pain Control and Anti-Inflammatory Agents

The **treatment of Crohn disease** can be divided into four areas of management: dealing with **symptoms,** treating **mucosal inflammation, nutritional management,** and **surgery.** Abdominal pain and diarrhea are dealt mostly by addressing intestinal inflammation. Pain may be due to the stretching of nerve endings as a result of distention from obstruction or inflammation. Nonsteroidal anti-inflammatory drugs (NSAIDs) should be avoided, and narcotics lead to addiction in this chronic condition. Acetaminophen, Tramadol, and Darvocet are used most frequently for pain control. 5-Aminosalicylic acid derivatives such as Azulfidine, Asacol, Pentasa, and Rowasa are used widely and have some effect. They are more effective in ulcerative colitis than in Crohn disease.

Steroids

Corticosteroids have been the mainstay in the acute treatment of Crohn disease for many years. Steroids should be used only when more conservative measures fail. The strategy employed is to induce remission by using high doses (prednisolone 60 mg per day) in the short term, followed by a temporary regime as soon as remission is induced. Maintenance therapy should employ the lowest dose possible. Approximately 20 percent of patients require long-term steroids.

Second-Line Agents

Steroid sparing in long-term management can be achieved with 6-mercaptopurine. This drug is slow to act and unpredictable in terms of achieving a therapeutic response. In doses of 50 to 125 mg daily, bone marrow suppression and other side effects are rare. The antibiotic metronidazole is also used as second-line therapy with a degree of success, particularly in treating fistulae. In addition to its properties as an antibiotic, the drug has an effect on the immune system. Other antibiotics that have been used to some effect are ciprofloxacin and clarithromycin.

Immune Suppressants

The immune suppressants methotrexate and cyclosporine have been shown to confer some benefit in the short term. The latest, still experimental, strategy in the treatment of Crohn disease involves the role of cytokines. Antitumor necrosis factor has been shown to be effective. Other cytokine therapies, such as the use of interleukin-11 (IL-11) and IL-10, have been reported to be efficacious in approximately 30 percent of cases.

Surgery

The **cumulative risk of undergoing surgery** sometime in the lives for patients with Crohn disease is **approximately 90 percent,** and the cumulative risk of recurrent disease at 20 years is 70 percent. Many recurrences may be asymptomatic, however. The major indication for surgery is failed medical therapy, usually in the presence of obstruction, fistula formation, and electrolyte or nutritional problems.

Controversy still exists over how radical the surgeon should be in treating Crohn disease. Some studies show that the more disease-free the margins are after the resection, the less likely there is to be recurrent disease. Conversely, there is a danger that overly radical resections will leave the patient with the short bowel syndrome and its nutritional consequences. Conservative surgery in the form of stricturoplasty for short stenotic lesions that are producing obstructions can be helpful without the loss of any bowel. For longer diseased segments, resection is preferred to bypass. For colonic Crohn disease with severe rectal and anal involvement, a proctocolectomy with ileostomy may be required. Meticulous care is required in performing anastomoses in patients with Crohn disease, as healing is often impaired and the risk of anastomotic leakage therefore is increased.

COMPREHENSION QUESTIONS

[6.1] A 44-year-old man presents with multiple episodes of bloody diarrhea accompanied by cramping abdominal pain. A colonoscopy reveals the rectum and distal colon to be unremarkable, but x-ray studies find areas of focal thickening of the wall of the proximal colon, producing a characteristic "string sign." Biopsies from the abnormal portions of the colon revealed histologic features that were diagnostic of Crohn disease. Which of the following histologic features is most characteristic of Crohn disease?

A. Dilated submucosal blood vessels with focal thrombosis
B. Increased thickness of the subepithelial collagen layer
C. Noncaseating granulomas with scattered giant cells
D. Numerous eosinophils within the lamina propria
E. Small curved bacteria identified with special silver stains

[6.2] Which of the therapies listed below is used most often to treat an individual with a history of Crohn disease who acutely develops abdominal pain and bloody diarrhea but has no clinical evidence of obstruction or fistula formation?

A. Aspirin
B. Interleukin-10
C. Metronidazole
D. Prednisolone
E. Surgery

[6.3] Which of the following findings is more characteristic of ulcerative colitis rather than Crohn disease?

A. Inflammation beginning in the rectum and extending proximally without "skip lesions"
B. Pericolonic fibrosis forming "creeping fat" around the outside of the gut
C. Intestinal obstruction resulting from a pericolonic abscess
D. Superficial noncaseating granulomas forming hamartomatous polyps
E. Transmural inflammation producing fissures and fistulas

Answers

[6.1] **C.** Microscopic examination of the abnormal bowel from an individual with Crohn disease will reveal transmural inflammation with fibrosis, but the histologic feature that is most diagnostic of Crohn disease is the presence of noncaseating granulomas. This characteristic histologic feature, however, may be present in only approximately 50 percent of patients; however, the diagnosis of Crohn disease can still be made without finding granulomas by the characteristic clinical presentation, which includes the production of fissures, fistulae, and bowel obstruction by the transmural inflammation.

[6.2] **D.** In the absence of bowel obstruction or fistula formation, several types of medical therapies have been used to treat the acute inflammation associated with Crohn disease. Corticosteroids, such as high-dose prednisolone, have been used commonly to treat the acute symptoms and induce remissions. In contrast, the antibiotic metronidazole may be used to treat patients with fistula formation, whereas the use of cytokines such as interleukin-10 is experimental. Surgical resection of bowel usually is done to treat problems such as obstruction.

[6.3] **A.** Crohn disease and ulcerative colitis are both inflammatory bowel diseases characterized by marked acute inflammation, but the inflammation in ulcerative colitis begins in the rectum and distal portions of the colon and precedes proximally without "skip lesions," whereas the inflammation in Crohn disease can be found throughout the gastrointestinal tract (hence the alternate name "regional enteritis"). Another major difference between these two disorders is that with Crohn disease the inflammation, which may form noncaseating granulomas, begins in the submucosa and may involve the entire bowel wall, whereas ulcerative colitis begins in the mucosa and the inflammatory response remains superficial in location and does not involve the full thickness of the wall of the colon. The inflammation along with repair may form inflammatory polyps with both of these disorders.

PATHOLOGY PEARLS

- Crohn disease is transmural (full thickness) and can occur anywhere along the gastrointestinal tract.
- Intestinal strictures and fistulae are complications of Crohn disease.
- Individuals with Crohn disease have an increased risk of colon cancer, but the risk is lower than that with ulcerative colitis.
- **Nongastrointestinal symptoms** of Crohn disease involve the **skin, joints, and eyes.** Skin lesions include **erythema nodosum, pyoderma gangrenosa, aphthous stomatitis, and finger clubbing.**

REFERENCES

Crawford JM, Liu C. The gastrointestinal tract. In: Mitchell RN, Kumar V, Abbas AK, et al., eds. Pocket Companion to Robbins and Cotran Pathologic Basis of Disease, 7th ed. Philadelphia, PA: Saunders, 2006, 431–3.

Friedman S, Blumberg RS. Inflammatory bowel disease. In: Kasper DL, Fauci AS, Longo DL, et al., eds. Harrison's Principles of Internal Medicine, 16th ed. New York: McGraw-Hill, 2004:1776–88.

Liu C, Crawford JM. The gastrointestinal tract. In: Kumar V, Assas AK, Fausto N, eds. Robbins and Cotran Pathologic Basis of Disease, 7th ed. Philadelphia, PA: Elsevier Saunders, 2004:846–9.

❖ CASE 7

A 62-year-old man returns home from playing bingo, complaining of midline abdominal pain. He denies being hit or suffering any other trauma. Over the next few hours the pain does not remit but becomes more severe and is localized to the lower right quadrant. He also develops nausea and vomiting. He denies diarrhea and has not had similar episodes. The patient lies down in bed, and over the next 24 hours, the pain worsens and he develops fever and chills and is brought to the emergency center. On examination, he has a temperature of 38.8°C (102°F) and appears ill. His abdomen is mildly distended and has hypoactive bowel sounds. The abdomen is diffusely tender to palpation, particularly in the right lower quadrant.

- **What is the most likely diagnosis?**
- **What additional tests would help in making an accurate diagnosis?**

ANSWERS TO CASE 7: APPENDICITIS

Summary: A 62-year-old man complains of midline abdominal pain. He denies being hit or suffering any other trauma. Over the next few hours, the pain worsens and is localized to the lower right quadrant. He also develops nausea and vomiting and, after 24 hours, develops fever and chills and an acute abdominal pain.

- **Most likely diagnosis:** Acute appendicitis
- **Additional diagnostic tests:** CT scan of the abdomen and pelvis

CLINICAL CORRELATION

This older man has a typical picture of a ruptured appendicitis with sepsis. He originally had mild right lower quadrant abdominal pain, but it worsened, and after 24 hours he developed fever and chills. Perhaps the most worrisome finding on physical examination is that he "appears ill." He probably has sepsis, which is a systemic condition of infection-mediated illness. The chills probably reflect bacteremia. The emergency physician should expeditiously manage this situation, because delay could lead to morbidity or mortality, particularly in a geriatric patient. The blood pressure is not mentioned, but the patient could be in septic shock. Treatment should be addressed in a systematic manner: airway, breathing, and circulation (ABC) with oxygen administered, two large-bore intravenous lines (IV), volume repletion for the probable volume depletion and sepsis, blood cultures, urine culture, and antibiotic therapy aimed at gram-negative bacilli and anaerobic bacteria. Blood work to be obtained includes a complete blood count and a chemistry panel to assess electrolytes and serum creatinine for kidney function. After stabilization, the patient should be taken to the operating room. If the diagnosis is unclear, a CT scan of the abdomen sometimes can help distinguish other abdominal pathologies, such as diverticulitis.

APPROACH TO APPENDICITIS AND DIVERTICULITIS

Objectives

- Describe the differences in the clinical presentation of appendicitis versus diverticulitis.
- Describe the mechanism of diverticulitis.
- Know the treatment of diverticulitis.

Definitions

Appendicitis: Inflammation of the vermiform appendix.
Diverticulitis: Inflammation of an outpouching of the diverticulum.
Diverticulosis: A condition of outpouching of the large bowel near the taeniae coli where the blood vessels penetrate. Complications include hemorrhage (lower gastrointestinal bleeding) and inflammation.

DISCUSSION

Appendicitis

Acute appendicitis is a common disease in Western countries and is uncommon in Africa and Asia. The incidence of the disease in the United States has fallen considerably over the last 30 years; however, it remains the **most common abdominal emergency in childhood, adolescence, and early adult life.** Fewer than 5 percent of cases of acute appendicitis occur in patients over age 60 years.

The pathologic process begins on the **mucosal surface of the appendix,** and there is often an element of obstruction of the appendicular lumen by a fecalith. This may lead to pressure necrosis of the mucosa and invasion of the appendicular wall by bacteria. Common causes of obstruction include elongation or kinking of the appendix, adhesions, and neoplasias such as carcinoma and carcinoid tumors, both of which are rare. Some cases spontaneously resolve, but more commonly, infection of the wall of the appendix progresses, leading to impairment of its blood supply. When the **pathologic process** has **extended throughout the wall of the appendix to involve the parietal peritoneum,** the **pain and tenderness are classically over the McBurney point** at the site of the appendix. The pathologic process may continue and produce gangrene, perforation, and more generalized peritonitis. Once perforation has occurred, the advancing bacteria may be controlled by the ability of the omentum to wall off the inflammation; alternatively, the peritonitis may become more widespread. In advanced appendicitis, a mass may develop; alternatively, generalized peritonitis may lead to the **septic inflammatory response syndrome** (SIRS), ultimately with the development of **multiple organ failure and death.**

The site of the pain in appendicitis may vary. When the appendix is **retrocecal** in position, somatic pain may be perceived in the **flank and loin** rather than in the right lower quadrant. **Anorexia** is an almost invariable symptom in association with appendicitis. The presence of hunger usually eliminates this diagnosis. In association with anorexia, nausea is common and tends to proceed to vomiting. Diarrhea sometimes occurs and may be a result of the appendix lying in a pelvic position.

Laboratory investigations commonly performed include the peripheral white blood cell count, which may be elevated with a predominance of polymorphonuclear leukocytes. The urinalysis is usually normal. A CT scan of the abdomen may show thickening of the appendix with periappendicular inflammation and the presence of intraperitoneal fluid.

The **differential diagnosis** includes **acute gastroenteritis,** which typically has vomiting and diarrhea as prominent symptoms and abdominal pain that is less well defined. **Intestinal obstruction** must be considered and typically presents with vomiting and abdominal distention. **Mesenteric adenitis** may mimic appendicitis closely but is associated with a generalized viral illness and causes less severe pain. Inflammation of **Meckel diverticulum** may produce symptoms remarkably similar to those of appendicitis, and laparoscopy or laparotomy may be needed for the diagnosis. **Crohn disease** may closely simulate appendicitis; affected patients generally have intestinal obstruction, and usually conservative management is the best therapy. Gynecologic disorders such as **pelvic inflammatory disease** with cervical motion tenderness and adnexal tenderness may present similarly to appendicitis. **Ureteral colic** is associated with pain and tenderness of the flank area, radiating to the groin region. Other conditions include **acute diverticulitis, colonic carcinoma, acute cholecystitis,** and **pancreatitis.**

Appendicitis in the **elderly** may have a more rapid course. **Gangrene and perforation are more common in those over age 60 years,** and this may be due to a delay in diagnosis. A classic picture of the appendicitis may be lacking, and the pain may be a less prominent feature. Overall, although there has been a decline in the incidence of peritonitis, paradoxically, it has increased among the elderly. Thus, appendicitis should be at the forefront of the differential diagnosis in males with right lower quadrant pain and tenderness.

The treatment of uncomplicated appendicitis is surgical, consisting of an **appendectomy.** The abdomen is opened, and if the appendix is found to be normal in the absence of any other pathology, it should be removed prophylactically. At the present time, most appendixes are removed laparoscopically rather than in an open operation.

Diverticulitis

Diverticula are blind pouches involving the bowel. They result from **herniation of the mucosa through the circular muscle** at the site of small penetrating blood vessels. Their walls consist of an outer layer of serosa and an inner mucosa. There is **no muscle in the wall of the diverticulum.** Diverticular disease is associated with increased intraluminal pressure in the large intestine with hypertrophy of both circular and longitudinal muscle layers. Diverticula can occur anywhere in the large bowel and small bowel but are found most commonly in the **sigmoid colon.** Muscle hypertrophy predates the development of diverticula and results in a narrowing of the bowel and, consequently, an increase in the intraluminal pressure. (See Figure 7-1.)

Diverticular disease may produce central or left lower quadrant abdominal pain together with an alteration in bowel habit with occasional rectal bleeding. The diagnosis is **confirmed by barium enema or colonoscopy,** which will show muscle thickening and multiple diverticula with small orifices emerging through the colonic wall. Diverticular disease of the colon is common in Western countries and rare in central Africa, the Middle East, the Far East, and the Pacific islands. The incidence of the disease in Japan is increasing, possibly because of the adoption of a more westernized diet. African Americans

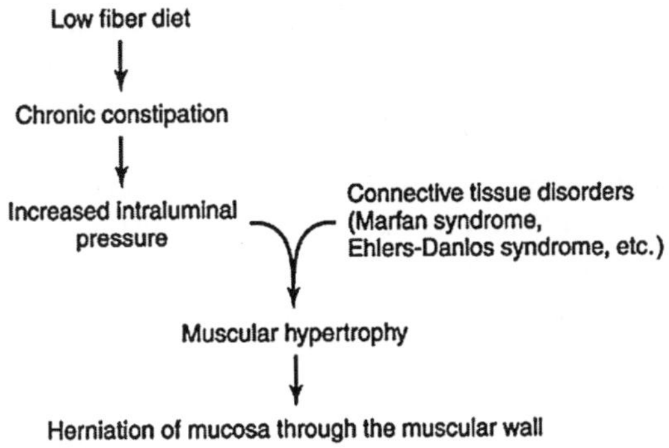

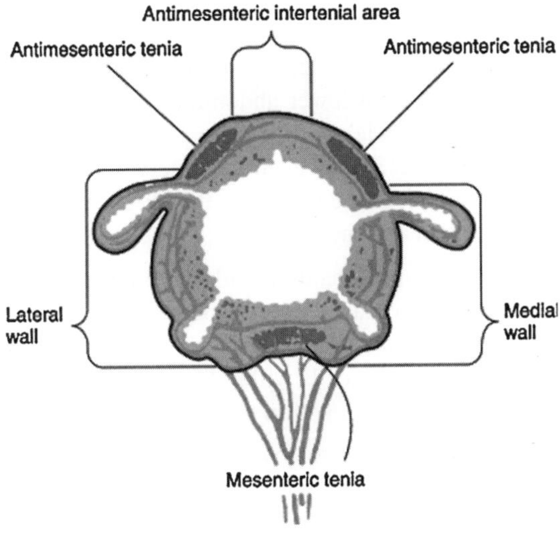

Figure 7-1. Top: Pathophysiology of diverticular disease. **Bottom:** Cross-sectional drawing of the colon, showing principal points of diverticula formation between mesenteric and antimesenteric teniae.

residing in the United States now have an incidence of the disease equal to that of the white population. Epidemiologic studies support the concept that the disease is not racially determined but is related to changes in the environment and to dietary factors. Postmortem studies in the Western countries report an incidence of approximately 40 percent overall and one as high as 60 percent in those over age 60 years.

Acute or chronic inflammation within a diverticulum is designated **diverticulitis.** It is estimated that the approximately 20 percent of patients with diverticulosis will manifest diverticulitis. Localized inflammation, or even perforation and peritonitis, may occur. **Pneumaturia, resulting from a**

colovesical fistula, may occur, and on occasion, fecal material may be passed in the urine. CT imaging of the abdomen remains the primary method of diagnosing the acute process, whereas barium enema and endoscopic examinations are relatively contraindicated during acute infection.

Known **complications** of diverticulitis include **bleeding, abscess formation, peritonitis, and fistula formation.** Colonic **obstruction** can also occur. The **treatment** of diverticulitis includes **broad-spectrum antibiotics, intravenous fluids, and nothing by mouth** until the condition settles. Frank peritonitis or abscess formation usually requires surgical intervention, commonly involving excision of the affected area, such as a sigmoid colectomy. Postoperatively, patients should be instructed to eat a high-residue diet and drink plenty of liquids.

COMPREHENSION QUESTIONS

[7.1] A 20-year-old woman presents with the sudden development of nausea, vomiting, and right lower abdominal pain. Physical examination finds a mild fever, and laboratory evaluation finds an increased peripheral leukocyte count. She is taken to surgery, where an appendectomy is performed. Which of the following histologic changes is most likely to be present in her appendix?

A. Amorphic mucinous material within the lumen
B. Caseating granulomas within the periappendiceal fat
C. Hyperplastic lymphoid follicles within the lamina propria
D. Multinucleated giant cells within the epithelium
E. Numerous neutrophils within the muscular wall

[7.2] A 61-year-old woman presents with nausea, vomiting, and the sudden onset of left-sided abdominal pain. Physical examination finds a low-grade fever, and laboratory evaluation finds increased numbers of neutrophils in her peripheral blood. Which of the following is the most likely diagnosis?

A. Appendicitis
B. Cholecystitis
C. Colitis
D. Diverticulitis
E. Pancreatitis

[7.3] Which of the clinical findings listed below is most likely to be present in an older individual with diverticulosis?

A. Abdominal colic caused by intestinal obstruction
B. Iron deficiency anemia caused by chronic blood loss
C. Megaloblastic anemia caused by vitamin B_{12} deficiency
D. Steatorrhea caused by malabsorption of fat
E. Chronic diarrhea caused by decreased absorption of protein

Answers

[7.1] **E.** The histologic hallmark of acute inflammation, such as that seen with acute appendicitis, is the presence of numerous acute inflammatory cells, namely, neutrophils. Therefore, histologic sections of an appendix surgically removed from an individual with acute appendicitis will reveal numerous neutrophils within the muscular wall. The inflammation can be so marked that it causes complete destruction of the muscular wall, which can lead to perforation and peritonitis.

[7.2] **D.** Acute inflammation of diverticula (diverticulitis) will produce the sudden onset of left-sided abdominal pain accompanied by fever and peripheral leukocytosis (mainly neutrophils). These clinical signs are essentially the same as those seen with acute appendicitis except that the abdominal pain is on the left side rather than the right side. As such, diverticulitis sometimes is referred to as left-sided appendicitis.

[7.3] **B.** Diverticulosis refers to the presence of numerous diverticula in the colon. The diverticula usually are located in the sigmoid colon in older individuals. Although they may become inflamed and produce signs of acute diverticulitis, more often they produce chronic blood loss as a result of chronic bleeding, which will lead to heme-positive stools and iron deficiency anemia.

PATHOLOGY PEARLS

- ❖ Appendicitis usually is a 24-hour disease with periumbilical pain localizing to the right lower quadrant.
- ❖ The primary treatment of appendicitis is surgical.
- ❖ Appendicitis continues to have high morbidity and mortality in older patients.
- ❖ Diverticula usually involve the left colon, particularly the sigmoid colon.
- ❖ Diverticulitis presents as left lower abdominal pain, fever, and nausea and vomiting.
- ❖ CT imaging is helpful in diagnosing both acute appendicitis and diverticulitis.

REFERENCES

Crawford JM, Liu C. The gastrointestinal tract. In: Mitchell RN, Kumar V, Abbas AK, et al., eds. Pocket Companion to Robbins and Cotran Pathologic Basis of Disease, 7th ed. Philadelphia, PA: Saunders, 2006:435, 443–4.

Liu C, Crawford JM. The gastrointestinal tract. In: Kumar V, Assas AK, Fausto N, eds. Robbins and Cotran Pathologic Basis of Disease, 7th ed. Philadelphia, PA: Elsevier Saunders, 2004:854–6, 870–2.

Silen AW. Acute appendicitis and peritonitis. In: Kasper DL, Fauci AS, Longo DL, et al., eds. Harrison's Principles of Internal Medicine, 16th ed. New York: McGraw-Hill, 2004:1805–6.

CASE 8

A 55-year-old woman presents to the emergency department with profuse bright red bleeding with emesis diagnosed as bleeding esophageal varices. She also is icteric and is suspected of having cirrhosis. She has been followed for several years for Sjögren syndrome and Raynaud syndrome. Investigation into the cause of her cirrhosis reveals negative hepatitis antibodies but elevated antimitochondrial antibodies.

- **What is the most likely underlying etiology for her liver disease?**
- **What is the most likely mechanism?**

ANSWERS TO CASE 8: PRIMARY BILIARY CIRRHOSIS

Summary: A 55-year-old woman has cirrhosis and elevated antimitochondrial antibodies.

- **Most likely diagnosis:** Primary biliary cirrhosis.
- **Most likely mechanism:** The etiology of primary biliary cirrhosis is not known; however, evidence points toward an autoimmune basis to the disease.

CLINICAL CORRELATION

This 55-year-old woman presents with bleeding esophageal varices and cirrhosis. The first priorities in her management include ABC: airway, breathing, and circulation. She should receive oxygen by a nasal cannula, and two large-bore intravenous lines should be established. Her blood pressure and heart rate should be monitored to assess for volume loss and replacement with blood as needed. Because of her liver disease, she may have a coagulopathy caused by depletion of vitamin K–dependent factors (factors II, VII, IX, and X). Transfusion with coagulation factors and initiation of vitamin K may be indicated. Endoscopic examination to determine the etiology of the upper gastrointestinal bleeding is paramount. Bleeding esophageal varices may be treated with sclerotherapy injected into the bleeding vessels. Also, a tamponade may be attempted with special esophageal devices.

After the acute situation has been addressed, attention should be directed to the etiology of her liver disease. A careful history and physical examination and selected laboratories usually yield the diagnosis. Toxic effects such as with alcohol use and infections such as with hepatitis viruses are the most common causes of cirrhosis. This patient's hepatitis serology studies are negative, but she does have a history of Sjögren syndrome, Raynaud syndrome, and antimicrosomal antibodies. These findings are consistent with primary biliary cirrhosis. Careful history may reveal pruritus years before frank cirrhosis.

APPROACH TO CHRONIC LIVER DISEASE

Objectives

- Describe the laboratory findings seen in primary biliary cirrhosis.
- Describe other causes of chronic hepatitis.
- Describe the link between cirrhosis and emphysema in patients with α_1-antitrypsin deficiency.

Definitions

Primary biliary cirrhosis (PBC): A chronic progressive cholestatic liver disease associated with intrahepatic biliary tree destruction and finally cirrhosis.

Chronic liver disease: Liver disease that lasts for 6 months or more and includes chronic hepatitis and cirrhosis.

Cirrhosis: Progressive and irreversible condition of the liver in which hepatocyte damage and destruction occur. Regenerating hepatocytes form nodules.

DISCUSSION

Primary Biliary Cirrhosis

The etiology of primary biliary cirrhosis is not known; however, evidence points toward an **autoimmune** basis of the disease. Other autoimmune diseases are associated with this condition and include Sjögren syndrome, scleroderma, rheumatoid arthritis, and thyroiditis. Aberrant human lymphocyte antigen (HLA) class II molecules are expressed in the biliary epithelium of patients with PBC; this might be responsible for the triggering of an inflammatory response. Defective immunoregulation allows cytotoxic T cells to damage bile ducts. A liver biopsy usually shows a **portal tract infiltrate composed of mainly lymphocytes and plasma cells** (see Figure 8-1). In approximately half

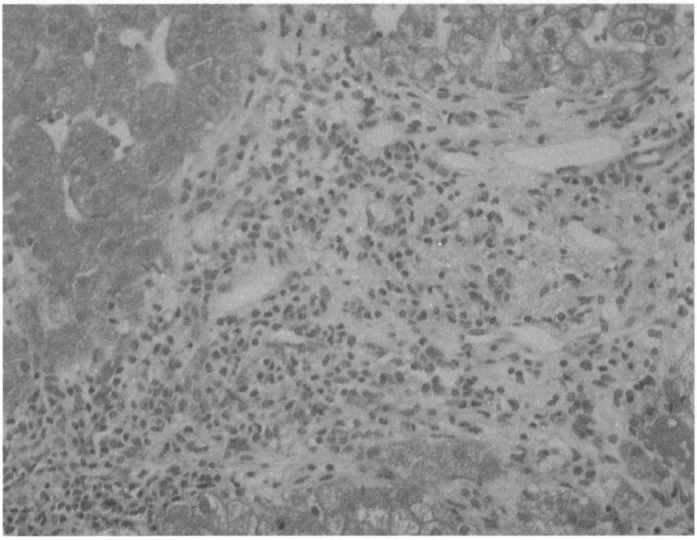

Figure 8-1. Microscopic pictograph of primary biliary cirrhosis. *(Courtesy of Dr. Aaron Han, Reading, PA.)*

the patients, **granulomas** may be seen. **Destruction of medium-sized bile ducts with bile ductular proliferation** will be evident. With time, hepatocyte necrosis and fibrosis are apparent. After years to decades, the clinical features of cirrhosis will be present. There is an **increased synthesis of IgM** because of failure to switch from immunoglobulin M (IgM) to IgG antibody synthesis. Most patients have **antimitochondrial antibodies** in their serum, with the antigen M2 being specific to PBC. The role of this antibody in the pathogenesis of PBC is not clear.

Features of **cholestatic liver disease** dominate the initial clinical picture. This includes **pruritus,** which may precede jaundice by years. **High serum alkaline phosphatase** with normal or nearly normal alanine aminotransferase (ALT) and aspartate aminotransferase (AST) is characteristic in the early part of the disease. **Secondary hypercholesteremia** with features such as xanthelasma may be seen. After a variable amount of time (usually years), the features of cirrhosis, such as icterus, bleeding, and ascites, may become apparent. Table 8-1 shows the laboratory findings that are consistent with a diagnosis of PBC.

Management

Treatment addresses the symptoms and disease course of the patient. Because the disease is thought to be autoimmune, corticosteroids have been tried. These agents improve the biochemical and histologic picture of the disease but lead to significant osteoporosis. Patients with primary biliary cirrhosis are prone to osteoporosis caused by cholestasis and subsequent impaired malabsorption of vitamin D. Complications associated with cirrhosis requires management. **Liver transplantation** remains the specific treatment and has a 5-year survival of at least 80 percent.

Table 8-1
LABORATORY FINDINGS CONSISTENT WITH PRIMARY BILIARY CIRRHOSIS

1. High serum alkaline phosphatase
2. High serum cholesterol
3. High serum IgM
4. High antimitochondrial antibodies; M2 antibody is specific
5. Liver biopsy; portal infiltrate with lymphocytes and plasma cells; granulomas; bile duct damage with ductular proliferation; eventual cirrhosis

Cirrhosis and Chronic Hepatitis

Chronic liver disease includes chronic hepatitis and cirrhosis (see Table 8-2). In **chronic hepatitis, inflammatory cells consisting of lymphocytes, macrophages, and plasma cells are present in the portal tract. Interface hepatitis and bridging necrosis** are signs of active liver damage. **Lymphoid aggregates** are seen in cases caused by **hepatitis C** virus. The hallmark of irreversible liver damage is deposition of fibrous tissue. This brings about the onset of cirrhosis. Initially, the fibrosis is periportal. With time, bridging fibrosis between lobules is seen. **Regenerating nodules** from surviving hepatocytes complete the picture of cirrhosis. Based on the size of the nodules, there are two types of cirrhosis: micronodular (nodules less than 3 mm) and macronodular. **Micronodular cirrhosis** is seen in **alcoholics,** whereas **macronodular cirrhosis is seen after hepatitis.**

Table 8-2
CAUSES OF CHRONIC HEPATITIS

Viruses Hepatitis B and C
Autoimmune
Hereditary α_1-Antitrypsin deficiency, Wilson disease
Drugs Methyldopa, isonicotine hydrazine, ketoconazole
Causes of cirrhosis Alcohol (common) Viral hepatitis caused by B or C (common) Autoimmune hepatitis Primary biliary cirrhosis Wilson disease Hemochromatosis α_1-Antitrypsin deficiency Drugs: methotrexate
Complications of cirrhosis Portal hypertension and gastrointestinal hemorrhage Ascites

Autoimmune Liver Disease

Autoimmune liver disease is seen most frequently in females and is associated with other autoimmune diseases. Autoantibodies such as antinuclear, anti-smooth muscle and anti-liver kidney microsomal antibodies (anti-LKM) are frequently present. Serum IgG levels may be elevated.

α_1-Antitrypsin Deficiency

α_1-Antitrypsin deficiency is inherited as an **autosomal recessive condition.** α_1-Antitrypsin is a glycoprotein whose main role is to inhibit the proteolytic enzyme neutrophil elastase. Deficiency results in **liver damage and emphysema,** especially in smokers. Serum levels are low, and liver biopsy shows periodic acid-Schiff (PAS) positive diastase-resistant globules within the hepatocytes.

Wilson Disease

Wilson disease is inherited as an **autosomal recessive** condition. The copper-transporting protein **ceruloplasmin** is reduced in amount because of poor synthesis. There is also failure of biliary excretion of copper. As a result, free copper is deposited in various sites, including liver basal ganglia and cornea (with resultant **Kayser-Fleischer rings**), resulting in damage to those organs. Urinary excretion of free copper also is increased. **Acute hepatitis, chronic hepatitis, cirrhosis, and extrapyramidal features** (caused by basal ganglia damage) are the usual clinical features.

Hereditary Hemochromatosis

Hereditary hemochromatosis also is inherited as an autosomal recessive condition. There is an association with HLA-A3. Excessive iron absorption results in iron deposition and damage to various organs including liver, pancreas, heart, joints, and pituitary gland. At the same time excess iron deposition is observed in the skin. This results in **bronze discoloration of skin.** This, along with diabetes resulting from pancreatic damage, explains the synonym of hemochromatosis, bronze diabetes. Other features include **cirrhosis, cardiomyopathy, hypogonadism, and arthropathy.** As females lose iron through blood loss from menstruation, the features are milder or are seen later in them.

Alcoholic Liver Disease

The spectrum of alcoholic liver disease includes **fatty liver, acute hepatitis, and cirrhosis. Fatty liver (hepatic steatosis)** consists of **microvesicular** lipid droplets in the liver cells, **displacing the nucleus to the periphery.** On gross inspection, the liver appears yellow and greasy. Refraining from alcohol generally leads to reversal of these changes. In **acute hepatitis,** there is **infiltration with polymorphonucleocytes and hepatocyte necrosis.** Cytoplasmic inclusions resulting from intermediate filaments known as **Mallory bodies** are seen. Eventually, fibrosis ensues. Finally, **cirrhosis** develops as an end-stage result of chronic alcohol use. The **liver is small and shrunken.** Microscopy reveals **fibrous septae that create a micronodular and macronodular pattern** with regeneration. Clinically, the patient may develop portal hypertension, ascites, jaundice, and peripheral edema.

COMPREHENSION QUESTIONS

[8.1] A 37-year-old woman presents with fatigue and pruritus. Laboratory evaluation finds the presence of antimitochondrial antibodies in her serum, but the tests for viral hepatitis antibodies were negative. A biopsy of her liver reveals numerous lymphocytes in the portal tracts, along with occasional granulomas. Which of the substances listed below is most likely to have markedly elevated serum levels in this individual?

A. Acid phosphatase
B. Alanine aminotransferase
C. Alkaline phosphatase
D. Aspartate aminotransferase
E. Conjugated bilirubin

[8.2] A 42-year-old woman presents with signs of jaundice and hepatic failure. Physical examination finds that she has uncontrolled choreiform movements of the arms, and a rust-colored ring is seen at the periphery of both corneas. Laboratory examination finds increased serum and urine levels of copper with decreased levels of ceruloplasmin. Which of the following is the most likely diagnosis?

A. α_1-Antitrypsin deficiency
B. Budd-Chiari syndrome
C. Primary biliary cirrhosis
D. Whipple disease
E. Wilson disease

[8.3] Which of the abnormalities listed below is most likely to be found in an individual with hereditary hemochromatosis?

A. Black cartilage
B. Blue sclera
C. Bronze skin
D. Red pupils
E. White hair

Answers

[8.1] **C.** The presence of antimitochondrial serum antibodies, particularly to the M2 antigen, in an individual with liver disease is highly suggestive of primary biliary cirrhosis. Individuals with this autoimmune disorder, which is more common in women, develop clinical signs of cholestatic liver disease with pruritus. Before the development of jaundice, however, patients will have high serum levels of alkaline phosphatase with normal or nearly normal levels of ALT and AST.

[8.2] **E.** Increased serum levels of copper with decreased levels of ceruloplasmin in a patient with liver disease are diagnostic of Wilson disease. This autosomal recessive disorder is characterized by the deposition of copper in multiple sites, which include the liver, the basal ganglia, and the cornea of the eye. Destruction of the basal ganglia leads to extrapyramidal signs such as choreiform movements, whereas deposition of copper at the periphery of the cornea produces characteristic Kayser-Fleischer rings.

[8.3] **C.** Patients with hereditary hemochromatosis develop clinical signs because of the deposition of excess iron in many organs. The classic triad of clinical signs includes a bronze skin color, diabetes mellitus, and cirrhosis. The combination of the bronze skin color and diabetes mellitus sometimes is referred to as bronze diabetes. Deposition of iron in the islets of Langerhans in the pancreas leads to the destruction of the β-cells, and subsequent decreased levels of insulin lead to diabetes mellitus. The abnormal skin color results from the deposition of iron in the skin. In addition, deposition of iron in the adrenal cortex leads to decreased cortisol levels. This in turn will increase levels of proopiomelanocortin (POMC) and lead to increased melanin-stimulating hormone (MSH) activity.

PATHOLOGY PEARLS

- Primary biliary cirrhosis is thought to be an autoimmune disease seen predominantly in middle-aged women.
- In PBC patients, serum IgM is elevated and antimitochondrial antibody (M2 is specific) is found.
- Cirrhosis is a progressive and irreversible condition of the liver in which there occurs hepatocyte damage and destruction. Regenerating hepatocytes form nodules.
- Complications of cirrhosis include portal hypertension, gastrointestinal hemorrhage, ascites, portosystemic encephalopathy, hepatorenal syndrome, and hepatocellular carcinoma.
- α_1-Antitrypsin deficiency is an autosomal recessive condition in which liver damage and emphysema are the main features.
- Wilson disease is an autosomal recessive condition characterized by liver and basal ganglia damage.
- Hereditary hemochromatosis, or bronze diabetes, also is inherited in an autosomal recessive fashion. Deposition of iron and organ damage occurs in liver, pancreas, heart, joints, and pituitary gland.
- In alcoholic hepatitis there occurs infiltration with polymorphonucleocytes and hepatocyte necrosis. Cytoplasmic inclusions caused by intermediate filaments known as Mallory bodies are seen.

REFERENCES

Chung RT, Podolsky DK. Cirrhosis and its complications. In: Kasper DL, Fauci AS, Longo DL, et al., eds. Harrison's Principles of Internal Medicine, 16th ed. New York: McGraw-Hill, 2004:1860–2.

Crawford JM, Liu C. The gastrointestinal tract. In: Mitchell RN, Kumar V, Abbas AK, et al., eds. Pocket Companion to Robbins and Cotran Pathologic Basis of Disease, 7th ed. Philadelphia, PA: Saunders, 2006:410–45.

Crawford JM. The gastrointestinal tract. In: Kumar V, Assas AK, Fausto N, eds. Robbins and Cotran Pathologic Basis of Disease, 7th ed. Philadelphia, PA: Elsevier Saunders, 2004:914–5.

CASE 9

A 54-year-old woman notes a 6-month history of progressive vaginal discharge with an odor. She also has noted vaginal spotting after intercourse. She had gone through menopause 2 years earlier and took an oral contraceptive for 10 years. She has smoked one pack of cigarettes per day for 20 years. She denies a cough or dyspnea. She complains of right back pain and right leg swelling. The speculum examination shows a 4-cm irregular fungating mass arising from the cervix.

- **What is the most likely diagnosis?**
- **What is the next step?**
- **What is the likely pathophysiology for this condition?**

ANSWERS TO CASE 9: CERVICAL CANCER

Summary: A 54-year-old postmenopausal woman has a 6-month history of an odiferous vaginal discharge and postcoital spotting. She has smoked one pack of cigarettes per day for 20 years. She also complains of right back pain and right leg swelling. The speculum examination shows a 4-cm irregular fungating mass arising from the cervix.

- **Most likely diagnosis:** Cervical cancer
- **Next step:** Biopsy of the lesion to confirm the diagnosis, followed by staging to assess the extent of the disease
- **Likely pathophysiology:** Human papillomavirus

CLINICAL CORRELATION

This patient most likely has cervical cancer. Indications leading the clinician to the diagnosis in this case include the patient's risk factors and presenting symptoms. Her risk factors for cervical cancer include age, a history of oral contraceptive use, and a history of smoking. The presenting symptoms of **malodorous vaginal discharge** and **postcoital bleeding** are characteristic of **cervical cancer.** The history should guide the clinician to examine the cervix. In this case, a grossly visible lesion was seen on the cervix during speculum examination. The next step in management is to biopsy the lesion for a definitive diagnosis.

APPROACH TO CERVICAL DYSPLASIA AND CANCER

Objectives

- Describe how to diagnose cervical cancer.
- Know the cause of cervical cancer.
- Describe the difference between carcinoma in situ and invasive squamous cell carcinoma.

Definitions

Cervical intraepithelial neoplasia (CIN): Dysplastic growth and development of the epithelial cells of the cervix. Lesions may be defined by mild, moderate, or severe, or CIN I, CIN II, or CIN III (see Figure 9-1).

Human papillomavirus (HPV): A double-stranded DNA virus associated with condyloma, cervical intraepithelial lesions, and cervical cancer. Cellular changes seen in HPV infection include an expanded parabasal cell layer and koilocytes but normal maturation and mitoses. There are over 70 types of HPV, which have varying oncogenic capacities. High-risk HPV types are those most often associated with high-grade lesions and invasive cancer. These types include 16, 18, 31, 39, 45, 56, 58, and 68.

Koilocyte: A viral expression of E4 protein that disrupts cytoplasmic keratin matrix in squamous cells and causes pleomorphism, hyperchromasia, perinuclear halos, and nuclear changes, including enlarged nuclei with abnormal edges, multinucleation, and variations in nuclear size.

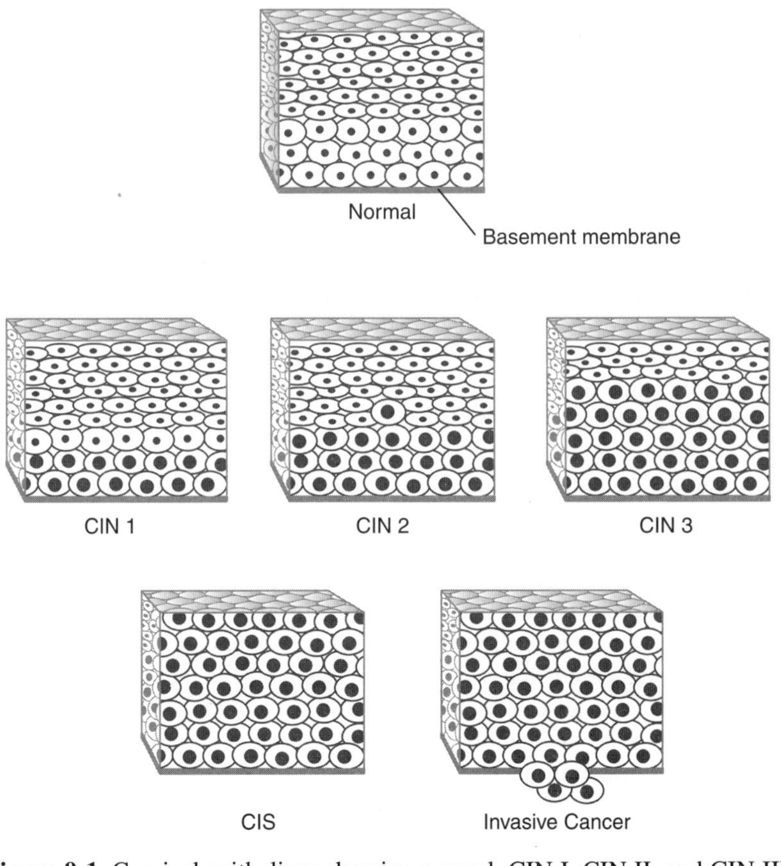

Figure 9-1. Cervical epithelium showing normal, CIN I, CIN II, and CIN III.

DISCUSSION

Cervical cancer is the **third most common cancer of the female lower reproductive system.** More than 80 percent of cervical dysplasias and more than 90 percent of cervical cancers are associated with **HPV infection.** Because HPV is transmitted through **sexual contact,** many of the risk factors for cervical cancer involve behaviors that increase the risk of all sexually transmitted diseases. These risk factors include early intercourse, many sexual partners, high-risk sexual partners, infection with other sexually transmitted diseases, and immunosuppression by HIV infection. Relative risk factors may include oral contraceptive use, tobacco use, and immunodeficiency. Other possible risk factors are under investigation.

Cervical dysplasia is found most often in females in their twenties, whereas **cervical cancers** usually become evident in the fifth decade of life. The classic presentation of cervical malignancies includes **abnormal bleeding and leukorrhea.** The bleeding can range from blood streaking in a discharge or spotting to heavy bright red blood. Foul-smelling purulent leukorrhea is often present. Other symptoms, such as pelvic or leg pain, urinary or fecal material in the vagina, weight loss, and generalized weakness, are suggestive of advanced disease.

The **squamocolumnar junction** is where the squamous ectocervix abuts the columnar endocervix. Just distal to this junction there is an area of squamous metaplasia that is influenced by factors such menarche, pregnancy, local hormonal influences, infection, and trauma. As columnar epithelium is replaced by squamous cells, a new squamocolumnar junction is formed. The area between the old junction and the new junction is called the **transformation zone. It is in this transformation zone that most cervical cancers arise.**

Cervical cancer begins with infection of cervical epithelium by human papillomavirus. Most infections resolve spontaneously without progression to cancer. This suggests that viral infection alone is not responsible for cervical cancer and that other, undefined factors are involved in the pathogenesis. Additionally, there are many types of HPV that vary in oncogenic potential, with **subtypes 16 and 18** being found most commonly in cervical caner.

Progression to dysplasia will occur if the viral genome is integrated into the nucleus of the cell under the influence of other factors that contribute to a favorable environment. Distinct cellular changes will occur, representing malignant transformation to low-grade cervical intraepithelial neoplasia (CIN I). A typical lesion will appear slightly raised or thickened with **koilocytes** in the upper and middle epithelial layers. Koilocytes are cells that have undergone cellular changes because of the presence of a virus. These cells are pleomorphic, hyperchromic, and multinucleated and have perinuclear halos. There are **few if any mitotic figures and no atypical mitotic figures in CIN I, usually involving the lower third of the epithelium.**

These low-grade CIN I lesions may regress spontaneously without treatment but may progress to higher-grade lesions. When atypical cells spread to between the lower one-third and two-thirds of the epithelium or the majority of the cells of the keratinizing layers, the lesion is defined as **CIN II.** These lesions demonstrate some areas of maturation but have areas of immature atypical koilocytic cells with a decreased nuclear to cytoplasmic ratio and increased numbers of mitotic figures (see Figure 9-2). **Progression to CIN III** involves the upper one-third of the epithelium by atypical cells with loss of maturation, an increase in hyperchromasia, and more mitotic figures with atypical mitoses. As the lesion progresses to squamous carcinoma in situ, the dysplastic cells may lose their cell walls and form syncytial-like groups. Many small round nuclei with scant cytoplasm can be seen. The majority of cells are atypical and are more hyperchromatic with coarse chromatin, a higher degree of pleomorphism, and increased atypical mitoses. **Carcinoma in situ** becomes **invasive** squamous cell carcinoma when atypical cells **invade the basement membrane.** Invasive carcinoma has wide variations of irregularly shaped cells and may have **keratin pearls.** There may also be evidence of necrosis, hemorrhage, and inflammatory cells.

The progression from CIN to cervical cancer is a slow process that usually occurs over several years. This allows many opportunities for screening before advanced-stage disease is evident. Most cases of cervical dysplasia are asymptomatic, and the diagnosis is made when a Pap smear reveals **abnormal cytology.** Good screening of asymptomatic patients, including a thorough history and physical and routine Pap smears have led to a decreased incidence of cervical cancer. The role of the **Pap smear** is paramount in early detection of cervical dysplasia to afford timely treatment and avoid progression to invasive cervical cancer. Even after the development of cervical cancer, a Pap smear has an important role in detection because diagnosis early in the disease process may offer a better prognosis. Treatment of early cervical cancer offers a 95 percent cure rate, whereas more advanced stages often lead to death in more than a third of cases. This underscores the importance of diligent efforts by the physician in counseling patients to receive an annual Pap smear.

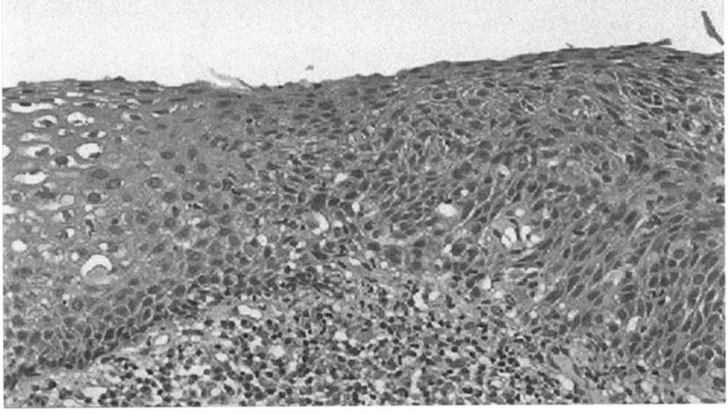

Figure 9-2. Microscopy of cervical dysplasia.

COMPREHENSION QUESTIONS

[9.1] A 24-year-old woman is noted to have atypical cells on a Pap smear that are consistent with infection by human papillomavirus (HPV). Which of the listed abnormalities describes the characteristic cytopathic effect caused by infection with HPV?

A. Acanthosis
B. Apoptosis
C. Hyperkeratosis
D. Koilocytosis
E. Parakeratosis

[9.2] A hysterectomy specimen is performed on a 38-year-old woman for resection of a large intramural leiomyoma, and the cervix is examined histologically by the pathologist. Microscopic sections of the cervix reveal atypical dysplastic squamous epithelial cells in the lower one-third of the epithelium. These cells have condensed nuclei with perinuclear clearing. No papillary structures are found. Mitoses are present only in the basal one-third of the epithelium. No invasion into the underlying tissue is noted. Which of the following is the best pathologic diagnosis for this cervical biopsy specimen?

A. Condyloma acuminatum
B. Cervical intraepithelial neoplasia grade I
C. Cervical intraepithelial neoplasia grade II
D. Carcinoma in situ
E. Invasive carcinoma

[9.3] A 32-year-old woman with a previous history of abnormal Pap smears is lost to follow-up but presents with vaginal bleeding. Physical examination finds a 3-cm fungating lesion of the cervix. Histologic examination of this lesion is most likely to reveal which of the following abnormalities?

A. Adenocarcinoma
B. Clear cell carcinoma
C. Small cell carcinoma
D. Squamous cell carcinoma
E. Verrucous carcinoma

Answers

[9.1] **D.** Koilocytes are squamous epithelial cells that have nuclei with dense, hyperchromatic, condensed chromatin surround by a clear space. These cells have been described as having the appearance of a raisin. Koilocytes are the characteristic cytopathic effect of HPV. These changes are present in biopsy specimens from the cervix, but they can also be seen in Pap smears from the cervix where these abnormal dysplastic cells have a characteristic increased nuclear/cytoplasmic ratio.

[9.2] **B.** Cervical intraepithelial neoplasia (CIN) I entails mild squamous dysplasia that involves the lower third of the epithelium of the cervix. Because the basal cells (those closest to the basement membrane) are the actively dividing cells, especially in an area of squamous metaplasia (transformation zone), they are the ones affected by HPV. This infection forms koilocytes, which are characteristic of HPV.

[9.3] **D.** The most common histologic type of invasive malignancy of the cervix is squamous cell carcinoma. Microscopy may reveal wide variations (pleomorphism) of irregularly shaped squamous epithelial cells which may have intracytoplasmic keratin. Keratin pearls may also be present. Necrosis, hemorrhage, and inflammatory cells are also typically seen. Cervical squamous cell carcinoma arises from previous squamous dysplasia of the cervix that has progressed from mild dysplasia to moderate dysplasia to severe dysplasia and finally to involve the full thickness of the cervical epithelium (carcinoma in situ). The latter then becomes invasive squamous cell carcinoma when atypical cells invade through the basement membrane. Cervical squamous cell carcinoma is then classified as being either microinvasive or invasive.

PATHOLOGY PEARLS

- Cervical intraepithelial neoplasia is a precursor to cervical cancer.
- The vast majority of cases of cervical dysplasia and cancer are associated with human papillomavirus, particularly subtypes 16 and 18.
- The best method for analyzing a visible cervical lesion is biopsy, not a Pap smear.
- The Pap smear has decreased the incidence of cervical cancer in the United States dramatically.
- The Bethesda classification for Pap smears reports atypical squamous cells of uncertain significance (ASCUS), low grade squamous intraepithelial lesion (LSIL), high grade squamous intraepithelial lesion (HSIL), and invasive cancer.
- LSIL includes human papilloma viral changes and CIN I.
- HSIL includes CIN II and CIN III and carcinoma in situ.

REFERENCES

Crum CP. The female genital tract. In: Kumar V, Assas AK, Fausto N, eds. Robbins and Cotran Pathologic Basis of Disease, 7th ed. Philadelphia, PA: Elsevier Saunders, 2004:1072–9.

Crum CP. The female genital tract. In: Mitchell RN, Kumar V, Abbas AK, et al., eds. Pocket Companion to Robbins and Cotran Pathologic Basis of Disease, 7th ed. Philadelphia, PA: Saunders, 2006:532–50.

DeCherney A, Lauren N. Current Obstetric & Gynecologic Diagnosis and Treatment, 9th ed. Chicago, IL: McGraw-Hill, 2003.

Stenchever M, Droegemueller W, Herbst AL, et al. Comprehensive Gynecology, 4th ed. St. Louis, MO: Mosby, 2001.

CASE 10

A 21-year-old nulliparous woman complains of lower abdominal "heaviness." She takes an oral contraceptive and is in a monogamous relationship. On examination, she has a normal-sized, nontender uterus, and a 9-cm right adnexal mass is palpated. Her pregnancy test is negative. On sonography, the mass appears cystic and solid.

- **What is the most likely diagnosis?**

- **What are some of the histologic findings expected in this mass?**

ANSWERS TO CASE 10: OVARIAN TERATOMA

Summary: A 21-year-old nulliparous woman has a 9-cm right adnexal mass that on sonography appears cystic and solid.

- **Most likely diagnosis:** Benign cystic teratoma of the ovary
- **Expected histologic findings in this mass:** Any tissue may be found, but the most common are sebum, skin, hair, teeth, thyroid, and neurologic tissues

CLINICAL CORRELATION

This young woman has an ovarian mass that on ultrasound has cystic and solid components, a classic presentation of a benign cystic teratoma (dermoid cyst) of the ovary. Although benign cystic teratomas are often asymptomatic, larger dermoids (as in this case) can present with pelvic pain, pressure, fullness, or dyspareunia. The patient's pregnancy test was reported as negative; however, in rare cases, degenerating ectopic pregnancies can be missed with urine human chorionic gonadotropin (hCG) assays because of the low sensitivity of urine pregnancy tests in the presence of very low (<25 mIU/mL) serum hCG levels. The fact that the patient is engaged in a monogamous relationship should decrease the risks of her contracting gonorrhea or *Chlamydia,* hence decreasing the possibility of pelvic inflammatory disease and tuboovarian abscess (TOA). The patient also gives a history of oral contraceptive (OC) use, which also serves to decrease the risk of pelvic inflammatory disease and/or TOA. Oral contraceptives also greatly decrease the likelihood of the mass being a physiologic ovarian mass (follicular cyst, hemorrhagic corpus luteum cyst, etc.). The ultrasound shows a complex (both cystic and solid) ovarian mass, which also is not consistent with an abscess or a physiologic ovarian or paraovarian cyst.

Although some disagreement exists over the timing and indications for surgery in complex masses under 6 cm or simple cysts of any size, a 9-cm complex ovarian mass almost always needs to be explored surgically. This is due primarily to the small but not insignificant risk of malignancy. Upon confirmation of benign intraoperative findings, efforts should be directed at salvaging all normal tissue from the affected ovary and removing only that tissue which has undergone neoplastic degeneration.

APPROACH TO OVARIAN NEOPLASM

Objectives

- Describe the classifications of ovarian neoplasms.
- Describe the serum marker used to evaluate ovarian neoplasms.
- Describe the differential for a pelvic mass.

Definitions

Tuboovarian abscess: An abscess formed within the adnexal space consisting of ovary, fallopian tube, and matted bowel caused by untreated or inadequately treated pelvic inflammatory disease.

Endometrioma: A large (6- to 8-cm) loculated collection of endometrial tissue that can develop in the pelvis in females with endometriosis. As this tissue degenerates, it turns brownish in color and is known as a "chocolate cyst."

Struma ovarii: A benign teratoma in which functional thyroid tissue is the predominant histologic finding. Approximately 2 to 3 percent of teratomas are classified as struma ovarii. Thyrotoxicosis is clinically apparent in 5 percent of these cases.

Ovarian torsion: A condition in which the ovary twists on its attachment to the infundibulopelvic ligament, thus interrupting ovarian blood supply. This usually is seen in conjunction with pathologic enlargement of the ovary and can be dynamic (intermittent) in nature or complete; the latter results in infarction and necrosis of the affected ovary.

DISCUSSION

Although they may present in any decade of life, **benign cystic teratomas** are the most common ovarian neoplasm found in females under age 35 (excluding physiologic follicular and corpus luteum cysts) and are also the most common ovarian neoplasm found in pregnancy. Approximately 10 to 15 percent of all cases involve both ovaries. Table 10-1 lists the differential diagnoses of a pelvic mass, and Table 10-2 lists the categories of ovarian neoplasms.

Benign cystic teratomas arise from a single germ cell in the ovary and have a normal female karyotype (46,XX). Because of the pluripotent nature of germ cells, teratomas can differentiate into tissues derived from all three embryologic cell lines (endoderm, ectoderm, and mesoderm). Thus, a **"mature" teratoma** often contains **skin, fat, sebaceous glands, sweat glands, hair, smooth and striated muscle, cartilage, bone, teeth, neural tissue, and gastrointestinal tissue** (see Figure 10-1). Functional **thyroid tissue** is found in approximately 12 percent of benign cystic teratomas, and rarely this tissue will proliferate into the predominant cellular element in the teratoma. This unique teratoma hence is referred to as struma ovarii and will secrete enough functional thyroid hormone to cause acute thyrotoxicosis in approximately 5 percent of cases.

Benign cystic teratomas are usually asymptomatic and are found most commonly during routine gynecologic screening or incidentally during unassociated surgical or radiographic procedures. Larger teratomas give rise to acute adnexal torsion in approximately 11 percent of cases. The increased risk of torsion with teratomas compared with other causes of ovarian enlargement is thought to be due to fat content, allowing the teratoma to "float" in the

Table 10-1
DIFFERENTIAL DIAGNOSES OF A PELVIC MASS

Full bladder
Intrauterine or extrauterine pregnancy
Functional ovarian cysts (follicular or corpus luteum)
Tuboovarian abscess
Diverticular abscess
Appendiceal abscess
Matted bowel and/or omentum
Paratubal or paraovarian cyst
Stool in sigmoid colon
Leiomyomas (submucosal, subserosal, pedunculated, or intraligamentous)
Pelvic kidney
Müllerian abnormality (e.g., bicornuate uterus)
Benign or malignant ovarian tumors

abdominal cavity instead of lodging against other structures. Other significant complications include secondary infection and acute hemorrhage with the potential for septic and/or hypovolemic shock. Rupture or perforation is seen in less than 5 percent of cases and occurs more frequently in association with pregnancy. When acute rupture occurs, spillage of the contents of the teratoma into the abdominal cavity often precipitates a surgical emergency, whereas more chronic leakage of contents can produce a severe chemical peritonitis that also requires surgical intervention. Malignant degeneration occurs in less than 2 percent of all recognized teratomas.

Other germ cell tumors include dysgerminomas, endodermal sinus tumors, and choriocarcinomas. These neoplasms usually occur in females under age 30 years. Dysgerminomas are rapidly growing and very radiosensitive and chemosensitive. Endodermal sinus tumors often secrete α-fetoprotein, whereas choriocarcinomas secrete human chorionic gonadotropin.

Table 10-2
OVARIAN NEOPLASMS

Benign epithelial ovarian tumors Serous cystadenoma Mucinous cystadenoma
Brenner tumor
Malignant epithelial ovarian tumors Serous cystadenocarcinoma Mucinous cystadenocarcinoma Endometrioid adenocarcinoma Transitional cell carcinoma
Malignant germ cell tumors Dysgerminoma Endodermal sinus tumor Embryonal carcinoma
Polyembryonal carcinoma Choriocarcinoma Teratoma (immature)
Benign germ cell tumors Benign cystic teratoma (dermoid)
Sex cord–stromal tumors Thecoma Sertoli-Leydig cell tumor Granulosa-theca cell tumor

Epithelial tumors of the ovary most commonly affect females over age 30 years, particularly **postmenopausal women.** Malignant **serous cystadenocarcinomas** are the most common, usually presenting with **ascites.** Treatment includes surgical excision followed by combination chemotherapy. **Mucinous** tumors may become very large, sometimes exceeding 30 lb in weight; their rupture can lead to chronic bouts of bowel obstruction **(pseudomyxoma peritonei).**

Stromal tumors of the ovary are often functional, secreting **estrogen (granulosa-theca cell tumors) or androgens (Sertoli-Leydig cell tumors).** These neoplasms can present as precocious puberty, postmenopausal bleeding, or hirsutism. They are usually solid tumors that are slow growing and rarely metastasize early. Surgery is the best treatment for these tumors.

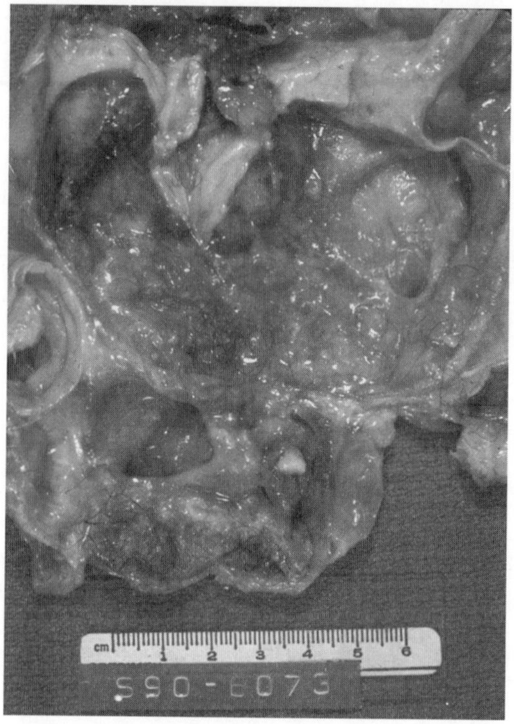

Figure 10-1. Gross photograph of an ovarian teratoma. Note the hair. *(Courtesy of Dr. Aaron Han, Reading, PA.)*

COMPREHENSION QUESTIONS

[10.1] Pseudomyxoma peritonei is a complication that is most commonly associated with which histologic subtype of ovarian tumor?

A. Brenner
B. Clear cell
C. Endometrioid
D. Mucinous
E. Serous

[10.2] A 25-year-old woman is noted to have a solid and cystic right ovarian mass measuring 10 cm in diameter by ultrasound. The mass is resected surgically and after examining histologic sections the diagnosis of benign teratoma (dermoid cyst) is made. Which of the listed microscopic descriptions is characteristic of this tumor?

A. A tumor mass composed of a uniform proliferation of blood vessels and fibroblasts
B. A tumor mass composed of islands of transitional-like epithelial cells
C. A tumor mass composed of malignant cytotrophoblast and syncytiotrophoblasts
D. A tumor mass composed of multiple cysts lined by ciliated columnar epithelial cells
E. A tumor mass composed of structures derived from all three germ lines

[10.3] A 4-year-old girl is noted to have breast enlargement and vaginal bleeding. On physical examination, she is noted to have a 9-cm pelvic mass. Which of the following is the most likely etiology?

A. Cystic teratoma
B. Dysgerminoma
C. Endodermal sinus tumor
D. Granulosa cell tumor
E. Mucinous tumor

[10.4] A 55-year-old woman presents with fatigue and malaise that have been worsening over the last 2 months. She has also noticed loss of appetite and early satiety. Evaluation finds an ulcerative mass located along the lesser curvature of the stomach along with bilateral ovarian masses. Which of the following is this patient most likely to have?

A. Barrett mucosa
B. Gastric leiomyosarcoma
C. Krukenberg tumor
D. Meig syndrome
E. Ovarian dysgerminoma

Answers

[10.1] **D.** Mucinous tumors of the ovary, the histology of which reveals the presence of nonciliated mucinous columnar epithelial cells similar to the endocervix, can rupture and cause widespread abdominal dissemination of the mucinous material. This condition, which is called pseudomyxoma peritonei, may cause compression of abdominal organs, such as the bowel or kidneys.

[10.2] **E.** The benign cystic teratoma or dermoid cyst is the most common type of ovarian tumor in females younger than age 30 years. Dermoid cysts, which usually have solid and cystic components when found in the ovary, are composed of elements from multiple embryonic layers, such as mature skin, bone, cartilage, and teeth.

[10.3] **D.** This young girl has signs of precocious puberty. Thus, the adnexal mass is likely to be an estrogen-secreting granulosa-theca cell tumor. These low-grade malignancies are slow-growing so-called stromal cell tumors. The androgen-secreting tumors are usually Sertoli-Leydig cell tumors and may cause virilism.

[10.4] **C.** The presence of a ulcerated gastric mass along with bilateral ovarian masses suggests that the patient's gastric cancer has metastasized to the ovaries; this is known as a Krukenberg tumor. Histology typically shows "signet ring" cells, in which intracytoplasmic mucin fills the cell and pushes the nucleus to the periphery of the cell, leading to the histologic appearance of a signet ring.

PATHOLOGY PEARLS

- Benign cystic teratomas are the most common nonphysiologic ovarian tumor in females under age 30.
- Ten to fifteen percent of all teratomas are bilateral.
- Ovarian torsion occurs frequently with teratomas.
- The most common ovarian cancers are epithelial in origin and usually occur in postmenopausal women.
- Surgical excision followed by combination chemotherapy is the best treatment for ovarian carcinoma.
- Ovarian cancer is associated with ascites.
- Granulosa-theca cell tumors often secrete estrogen, and Sertoli-Leydig cell tumors often secrete androgens.
- Metastatic tumors to the ovary may have a "signet ring" appearance on microscopy and are called Krukenberg tumors.

REFERENCES

Crum CP. The female genital tract. In: Kumar V, Assas AK, Fausto N, eds. Robbins and Cotran Pathologic Basis of Disease, 7th ed. Philadelphia, PA: Elsevier Saunders, 2004:1092–104.

Crum CP. The female genital tract. In: Mitchell RN, Kumar V, Abbas AK, et al., eds. Pocket Companion to Robbins and Cotran Pathologic Basis of Disease, 7th ed. Philadelphia, PA: Saunders, 2006:532–50.

Novak E, Hillard PA, Berek J. Novak's Gynecology, 13th ed. Philadelphia, PA: Lippincott Williams & Wilkins, 2002.

Stenchever MA, Droegmueller W, Herbst HR, et al. Comprehensive Gynecology, 4th ed. Philadelphia, PA: Mosby, 2002.

❖ CASE 11

A 30-year-old man complains of "heaviness" in the scrotal area, which he has noted for approximately 1 month. He denies any trauma to the area and has no medical problems. He denies the use of tobacco and drinks alcohol occasionally on weekends. On examination, there is a 5-cm firm, nontender area inside the right scrotum. There is no lymphadenopathy.

◆ **What is the most likely diagnosis?**

◆ **What is the most likely histologic finding?**

ANSWERS TO CASE 11: TESTICULAR CANCER

Summary: A 30-year-old male has a 1-month history of right scrotal "heaviness." Examination reveals a 5-cm firm, nontender area inside the right scrotum. There is no adenopathy.

- **Most likely diagnosis:** Testicular cancer.
- **Most likely histologic finding:** One or more germ cell tumor types, including seminoma, embryonal carcinoma, choriocarcinoma, yolk sac tumor, and teratoma.

CLINICAL CORRELATION

This patient, a young man with "scrotal heaviness," represents a very typical presentation of a testicular mass. Not all masses in the scrotum are testicular in nature. Physical examination and ultrasound of the scrotum often help differentiate a solid testicular mass from benign entities such as hydrocele (water sac around the testicle), varicocele (dilated testicular veins), and epididymoorchitis (infection and/or inflammation of the epididymis and testis).

A hard painless mass within the testicle should be considered testicular cancer until proved otherwise. Such a mass often is overlooked by the patient until it is discovered accidentally or brought to his attention by an unrelated regional occurrence such as minor trauma to the scrotum. Germ cell tumors of the testis peak in men between ages 15 and 40 years. Seminoma, embryonal carcinoma, choriocarcinoma, yolk sac tumor, and teratoma can appear in a pure or, more often, mixed form. Characterizing the tumor awaits review of the surgical specimen and is not possible before orchiectomy (surgical removal of the testicle). Although cure of testicular tumors now occurs in the high 90 percent range, because the malignancy affects primarily young men, issues of compromised fertility, complications of therapy, and surveillance for recurrence and second malignancies are matters of concern.

APPROACH TO TESTICULAR TUMORS

Objectives

- Describe the classifications of testicular neoplasms.
- Describe the serum markers used to evaluate testicular neoplasms.
- Discuss which testicular neoplasm is radiosensitive.

Definitions

Cryptorchidism: Congenital failure of one or both testes to descend from the abdominal (in utero) position to the scrotal postnatal position. Cryptorchid testicles have a higher incidence of malignancy, which is not reduced by surgical relocation into the scrotum. Patients who have had surgical correction of cryptorchid testes require intensive education about the importance of self-examination because of the increased risk of malignancy.

Radical orchiectomy: Removal of the testicle, epididymis, and testicular cord up to the internal inguinal ring. This operation is performed through an incision in the inguinal area that is similar to the incision made to repair inguinal hernias.

Nonseminomatous germ cell tumors: Because of the distinct difference in treatment of a pure seminoma, germ cell tumors often are divided into two categories: (1) pure seminomas and (2) nonseminomatous germ cell tumors (all other pure tumors or seminomas with a mixed component). Pure seminomas are very radiosensitive, whereas nonseminomatous tumors are radioresistant (see Table 11-1 for classification).

Tumor markers: Substances secreted by cancers that can be detected and measured to assess the presence and extent of the primary, metastatic, or recurrent disease. α-Fetoprotein and human chorionic gonadotropin–β are tumor markers for testicular cancer.

Retroperitoneal lymph node dissection (RPLND): Removal of lymph nodes that provide the primary lymphatic drainage from the testes from the bifurcation of the great vessels up to and beyond the renal hilum. This procedure may be curative in cases of low-volume metastatic disease, because most germ cell tumors progress in an orderly fashion from primary intratesticular to lymphatic before metastasis to solid organs.

Table 11-1
TESTICULAR NEOPLASMS

Germ cell tumors account for >90%
Pure Seminoma Embryonal carcinoma Choriocarcinoma Yolk sac tumor Teratoma
Mixed tumor: any combination of the above
Gonadal stromal tumors Leydig cell Sertoli cell Gonadoblastoma
Other tumors, e.g., carcinoid: metastatic from another site

DISCUSSION

Any male presenting with an intrascrotal mass requires a thorough physical examination of the genitalia. The examination should be performed with the male standing as well as lying flat. The primary goal is to determine whether the mass lies within the testicle or is extratesticular. Masses within the testes require further evaluation. **Scrotal ultrasound** is an excellent study to confirm the presence of and characterize a suspected testicular mass. If an intratesticular mass is confirmed on examination and/or ultrasound study, the diagnosis of a germ cell tumor is made by inguinal orchiectomy and pathologic analysis of the testis. Once the diagnosis of a germ cell tumor is confirmed and characterized by the histology, tumor staging is performed.

Before an inguinal orchiectomy, **serum markers** are drawn, such as **α-fetoprotein** and **human chorionic gonadotropin–β** levels, if a germ cell tumor is confirmed. A CT scan of the abdomen is obtained after the inguinal orchiectomy, looking for the presence of enlarged lymph nodes in the retroperitoneum. The use of intravascular contrast material helps outline the aorta and vena cava, on which lies the primary lymphatic drainage echelon of the testis. A chest radiograph is obtained with additional views if needed. These staging studies augment the physical examination, which assesses for abdominal masses, breast enlargement (caused by the influence of serum tumor markers), and the Virchow lymph node in the supraclavicular region.

Patients with **pure seminoma** and disease that is thought not to be metastatic are treated with a short course of **radiotherapy** to the retroperitoneal and ipsilateral iliac lymph nodes. Such simple therapy yields 90 percent 5-year disease-free survival. For patients with mixed germ cell tumors, treatment depends on the presence and extent of metastatic disease. Retroperitoneal lymph node dissection may be chosen as a therapy when there is no evidence of gross metastatic involvement. Surgery will define the extent of disease and in some cases may cure the malignancy.

For patients for whom chemotherapy is chosen, a variety of chemotherapeutic protocols exists that are administered using x-ray and serum studies to monitor effectiveness. Sometimes metastatic deposits will be reduced but not eliminated by the chemotherapy, requiring surgical excision.

The **five types of germ cell tumors—seminoma, embryonal carcinoma, choriocarcinoma, yolk sac tumor,** and **teratoma**—are collectively responsible for approximately 90 percent of testicular tumors. The remaining testicular tumors originate from the gonadal stroma, such as Leydig and Sertoli cells. A variety of rare tumors occur with a frequency far less than that of the more common germ cell tumors. The histologic subtype of germ cell tumors is an important distinction, because therapy is predicated on a complete examination of the entire tumor to determine whether it is of pure type or mixed in origin. **Pure seminomas** are distinct from other solid tumors of the testicle in that seminomas are **exquisitely radiosensitive.** Other germ cell tumors, whether in pure or mixed form, do not have sufficient radiosensitivity to make radiation therapy a commonly employed treatment modality.

Whatever combination of radiation, surgery, and/or chemotherapy is used, patients with testis tumor **often are cured of their malignancies.** After a diagnosis of testis cancer, the patient is warned that therapies, especially chemotherapy, can have a negative long-term impact on fertility. Some patients choose to bank sperm before the initiation of chemotherapy. All patients with testis tumor have at least a 5-year period of intensive monitoring on or off therapy. Compliance with the rigorous program of physical examinations, x-rays, and blood tests must be stressed to the patient. Radiation, surgery, and chemotherapy have their own distinct set of side effects, which, depending on the patient's age, maybe not only short-term but also long-term, revealing themselves many decades later.

COMPREHENSION QUESTIONS

[11.1] A 35-year-old man presents with the painless enlargement of one testicle. Physical examination finds a single nontender testicular mass that measures approximately 3 cm in the greatest dimension and does not transilluminate. Which of the following types of testicular tumor is most likely to be present in this individual?

A. Germ cell tumor
B. Gonadal stromal tumor
C. Mesenchymal tumor
D. Sex cord tumor
E. Surface epithelial tumor

[11.2] Which of the following types of primary testicular tumor is most radiosensitive?

A. Seminoma
B. Embryonal carcinoma
C. Yolk sac tumor
D. Choriocarcinoma
E. Immature teratoma

[11.3] A 27-year-old man has surgery for a testicular mass. Histologic sections reveal the mass to be a testicular yolk sac tumor. Which of the substances listed below is most likely to be increased in this patient's serum?

A. Acid phosphatase
B. Alkaline phosphatase
C. α-Fetoprotein
D. Human chorionic gonadotropin
E. Prostate-specific antigen

Answers

[11.1] **A.** An intratesticular mass in an adult, especially a mass that does not transilluminate, should be considered a testicular tumor until proved otherwise. The two main types of primary testicular tumors are germ cell tumors and sex cord gonadal stroma. Germ cell tumors are more common and have a peak incidence in men between 15 and 40 years of age.

[11.2] **A.** The histologic classification of testicular germ cell tumors includes seminomas, embryonal carcinomas, yolk sac tumors, choriocarcinomas, and teratomas. It is important, however, to group these testicular tumors into two general categories: those which are pure seminomas and those tumors which contain nonseminomatous elements. The reason for this classification is the fact that pure seminomas are very radiosensitive and nonseminomatous tumors are radioresistant and require the use of chemotherapy.

[11.3] **C.** Tumors sometimes secrete specific substances that appear in the serum. These tumor markers can be used clinically for diagnosis, for staging, and for following patients after surgery to look for recurrences of the tumor. Two important tumor markers associated with testicular neoplasms are α-fetoprotein (AFP) and human chorionic gonadotropin–β (hCG-β). Increased levels of AFP are associated with embryonal cell carcinoma or endodermal sinus tumor, whereas increased levels of hCG are associated with choriocarcinoma. Increased levels of both AFP and hCG are seen with mixed germ cell tumors. It is important to note that although seminomas may be associated with increased levels of hCG, pure seminomas are never associated with increased levels of AFP.

PATHOLOGY PEARLS

❖ The majority of testicular tumors are germ cell tumors.

❖ Seminomas are very radiosensitive.

❖ An intratesticular mass should be considered a testicular tumor until proved otherwise.

REFERENCES

Campbell MF, Walsh PC, Retik AB. Campbell's Textbook of Urology. Philadelphia, PA: Lippincott Williams & Wilkins, 2002.

Epstein JI. The lower urinary tract and male genital system. In: Mitchell RN, Kumar V, Abbas AK, et al., eds. Pocket Companion to Robbins and Cotran Pathologic Basis of Disease, 7th ed. Philadelphia, PA: Saunders, 2006:510–31.

Gillenwater JY, Howards SS, Grayhack JT, et al. Adult and Pediatric Urology. St. Louis, MO: Mosby, 2002.

Tanagho E, McAninch J. Smith's General Urology. Lange Medical Review Books: New York: McGraw-Hill, 2003.

CASE 12

While eating dinner with his wife, a 68-year-old man experienced loss of function of his left upper and lower extremities. Earlier in the day he had experienced several episodes of left-sided weakness lasting a few minutes, but he had recovered function after each of those episodes. Previously, he had been in good health except for occasional angina relieved by rest.

- **What are the possible causes of the left-sided weakness?**
- **What are the underlying mechanisms associated with these disorders?**
- **What are the risk factors for developing these disorders?**

ANSWERS TO CASE 12: STROKE/CEREBRAL INFARCT

Summary: A 68-year-old man with chronic stable angina experienced loss of function of his left upper and lower extremities. Earlier in the day, he had experienced several episodes of left-sided weakness lasting a few minutes, which completely resolved.

- **Possible causes of the left-sided weakness and subsequent loss of function:** Cerebrovascular accident (stroke), seizures, syncope, hypoglycemia, psychiatric disorder, cerebral infections, and drug toxicity

- **Underlying mechanisms associated with these disorders:** Thrombosis (a clot blocks a cerebral artery either by atherosclerotic plaque formation or by embolizing and lodging in the artery) or intracerebral hemorrhage

- **Risk factors for developing these disorders:** Hypertension, diabetes mellitus, hyperlipidemia, cigarette smoking, AIDS, drug abuse, heavy alcohol consumption, family history of stroke, increased serum levels of homocysteine, history of previous strokes, and cardiac diseases

CLINICAL CORRELATION

The most important first step in evaluating a patient suspected of having a stroke is to address ABCs: airway, breathing, and circulation. After a quick assessment and stabilization, treatment should be instituted. Earlier treatment offers a greater benefit to the patient. A complete history and physical should be directed at the central nervous system, the cardiac system, mental status, and a differential diagnosis. Carotid artery bruits may be a sign of arterial narrowing or stenosis. Neurologic deficits, mental status changes, and assessment of language function to detect aphasia are important. Laboratory evaluation includes obtaining a complete blood count (CBC) with platelets, a chemistry panel, a rapid plasma reagin (RPR), antiphospholipid antibodies, a cholesterol level, a triglyceride level, a urine drug screen, coagulation tests, an electrocardiogram (ECG), a CT scan of the head (without contrast) for detecting hemorrhage, and blood cultures if endocarditis is suspected. Lumbar puncture is performed if the CT scan is negative. A cerebrovascular accident (ischemic stroke) may be caused by complete occlusion of the internal carotid artery, resulting in embolization to the right middle cerebral artery. Other possible causes include intracerebral hemorrhage (ICH), subarachnoid hemorrhage (SAH), hematoma, transient ischemic attack (TIA), encephalitis, brain tumor, brain abscess, epilepsy, and trauma. The differential diagnosis for ischemic or hemorrhagic strokes includes seizures, syncope, hypoglycemia, psychiatric disorder, cerebral infections, and drug toxicity. Cardiac causes include rheumatic heart disease, mitral valve disease, cardiac arrhythmia, infective endocarditis, atrial myxoma, mural thrombi complicating myocardial infarction, atrial septal defect, and patent foramen ovale.

APPROACH TO CEREBROVASCULAR ACCIDENT

Objectives

- Describe the categories of stroke.
- Describe the presentations of stroke.
- Describe the treatments of stroke.

Definitions

Ischemia: Inadequate blood flow. Moderate is defined as a 40 to 50 percent reduction of normal cerebral blood flow. Severe is defined as a 75 percent or greater reduction.

Aphasia: An abnormal neurologic condition in which language function is defective or absent because of an injury to certain areas of the cerebral cortex.

Expressive aphasia: Difficulty producing free-flowing speech.

Hemiparesis: Muscular weakness of one-half of the body.

Hemiplegia: Paralysis of one side of the body.

Hemiparesthesia: Numbness or impaired sensation experienced on one side of the body.

Hemiplegic gait: A manner of walking in which an affected limb moves in a semicircle with each step.

Horner syndrome: Named after the Swiss ophthalmologist Johann F. Horner; a neurologic condition characterized by miotic pupils, ptosis, and facial anhidrosis.

Miosis: Contraction of thc sphinctcr musclc of the iris, causing the pupil to become smaller.

Ptosis: An abnormal condition of one or both eyelids in which the eyelids droop because of the weakness of the levator muscle or paralysis of cranial nerve III.

Anhidrosis: An abnormal condition characterized by inadequate perspiration.

Circle of Willis: A vascular network at the base of the brain. It is formed by the interconnections of seven arteries.

Amaurosis fugax: A transient episode of blindness caused by decreased blood flow to the retina.

DISCUSSION

Stroke, or a cerebrovascular accident (CVA), is the third leading cause of death in the United States. **Strokes** are divided into **two categories: ischemic infarcts and hemorrhages.** Infarcts can be thrombotic (atherosclerotic), cardioembolic, or lacunar in origin. **Lacunar infarcts are small,** less than 5 mm, and occur in short penetrating arterioles. Infarcts account for 85 percent of strokes. Hemorrhages can be either intracerebral, such as a hematoma, or aneurysmal. The **most common cause of a subarachnoid hemorrhage is an aneurysm.** Long-standing hypertension is the most common cause of intracerebral hemorrhage. Hemorrhages account for 15 percent of strokes. Patients often develop symptoms before the ischemic event. Patients with a history of atherosclerosis have a history of transient ischemic attacks 50 percent of the time. TIAs usually last less than 24 hours.

Normal Anatomy

Two sets of arteries perfuse the brain: the paired internal carotids and the paired vertebral arteries. The common carotid artery bifurcates into the internal and external carotids. The **internal carotid (ICA) supplies 80 percent of cerebral blood flow.** Twenty percent comes from the vertebral arteries. The ICA frequently is affected by atherosclerosis.

Pathophysiology

Stenosis of the internal carotid arteries leads to **ischemic stroke** by two mechanisms: **thrombus** and **embolization.** Complete occlusion of the ICA can result in embolization to the middle cerebral artery (MCA) when there is poor collateral flow through the **circle of Willis.** This leads to distal hypoperfusion and ischemic injury. A watershed area of infarction can occur in the brain and can cause clinically a contralateral proximal arm and leg weakness.

Stroke also may be caused by hemorrhage. **Nontraumatic ICH** most commonly is due to long-standing hypertension, with the **basal ganglia being the most common site involved.** The hemorrhages are caused by rupture of microscopic aneurysms that form on small arteries.

Pathology

The bulk of the brain is formed by two large paired cerebral hemispheres. Each hemisphere is divided into four lobes. The autoregulatory capacity of the brain keeps a constant average level of cerebral blood flow. Ischemic changes in the brain can be diffuse or local. Diffuse pattern of cortical injury can occur. The brain becomes edematous, and blood vessels are dilated. There is an increase in petechial hemorrhage in the cortical fibers. Focal areas of ischemia can be seen as a very bland or a white area. The brain can soften in the area of the infarct, and petechia can develop if a hemorrhage occurs after the infarct. The infarcted tissue becomes vacuolated and can become spongy. In a cerebral hemorrhage, the blood dissects and destroys brain tissue, forming a hematoma that can expand and act like a space-occupying tumor. Initially, the hematoma becomes cystic and then discolored secondary to the presence of hemosiderin macrophages. The necrotic tissue can become edematous and vacuolated.

Subarachnoid Hemorrhage

The **most common cause of significant subarachnoid hemorrhage is rupture of berry (saccular) aneurysms.** These outpouchings usually occur at the anastomosis points of the **circle of Willis.** They are usually less than 3 cm in diameter and can be as small as several millimeters. Rupture can occur at any age, but usually occur in the fourth or fifth decade of life. Bigger aneurysms have a higher chance of rupture. Valsalva or sexual orgasm is associated with rupture. Additionally, **berry aneurysms** are often seen in patients with **polycystic kidney disease.** Patients describe symptoms of aneurysm rupture as **"the worst headache of my life."** Up to half of individuals who suffer a berry aneurysm rupture will die.

Management of Ischemic Stroke

Oxygen should be administered to any stroke victim. With ischemic strokes, **tissue plasminogen activator (tPA) is a thrombolytic therapy** that may be considered, but to be effective, it must be administered within 3 hours after the onset of the ischemic event. **Contraindications to its use are blood pressure** higher than 185/110 mm Hg and evidence of a cerebral hemorrhage. Antihypertensives should be given to achieve a systolic blood pressure of 170 to 200 mm Hg within the first 2 weeks. The National Stroke Association (NSA) recommends treatment for blood pressures higher than 220/120 mm Hg on repeated measures over 1 hour. The goal is to **lower the blood pressure gradually,** not to lower the blood pressure to normal levels initially in the acute phase. After a stroke, there is loss of cerebral autoregulation, and lowering the blood pressure too quickly may compromise the circulation further. Aspirin is started daily; it can reduce the risk of recurrence. Corticosteroids are used to decrease the edema and intracranial pressure. If there is a cardiac source of embolization, anticoagulation is instituted.

Management of Hemorrhagic Stroke

The **treatment of an intracranial hemorrhage** includes **supportive measures** and **treatment of hypertension.** The prognosis depends on the level of consciousness, the size and location of the hematoma, and the underlying medical condition. The larger the hemorrhage, the poorer the prognosis. With a subarachnoid hemorrhage, patients may need **surgical clipping for aneurysms or arteriovenous malformations.** If the patient is conscious, he or she should be confined to bed with no exertion, and any anxiety should be treated. Stool softeners may help avoid straining.

COMPREHENSION QUESTIONS

[12.1] A 42-year-old woman presents to the emergency department at 8 PM, mildly somnolent and complaining of the "worst headache of her life," which began at 6 AM on the same day, awakening her. She took acetaminophen (Tylenol) twice during the day, with some relief. At noon she started to have nausea with vomiting, and by 3 PM she had developed right arm and leg weakness. She denies any head trauma. Which of the following is the most likely diagnosis?

A. Contusion
B. Epilepsy
C. Hypoglycemia
D. Subarachnoid hemorrhage
E. Transient ischemic attack

[12.2] A 50-year-old man with a history of atrial fibrillation has been taking Coumadin daily, 10 mg, over the last 5 years. He traveled to California with his wife and left his medication at home. He realized this after 5 days. While traveling as a passenger in the car, he developed sudden left-sided body weakness and loss of vision. His symptoms lasted for several weeks. Which of the following is the most likely diagnosis?

A. Brain tumor
B. Embolic stroke
C. Hematoma
D. Ischemic stroke
E. Transient ischemic attack

[12.3] A 58-year-old man with a 15-year history of hypertension, a history of smoking two packs of cigarettes a day, and diabetes mellitus experiences the acute onset of weakness and numbness on the left side of his body and an inability to walk. He admits to having a severe headache. His wife reports that during the ride to the emergency center he became lethargic. His blood pressure upon arrival was 192/105 mm Hg. Which of the following is the most likely finding on the initial CT scan of the head?

A. Hemorrhage in the cerebellum (posterior fossa)
B. Hemorrhage in the right cerebral hemisphere
C. Hemorrhage in the left cerebral hemisphere
D. Enlarged cerebral ventricles and prominent gyri
E. Ischemic changes in the right cerebral hemisphere
F. Ischemic changes in the left cerebral hemisphere
G. Normal-appearing cerebral hemispheres

Answers

[12.1] **D.** Spontaneous SAH often is due to aneurysmal rupture. These headaches are described as the worst headache of the patient's life. They frequently are misdiagnosed as migraine or tension headaches or viral illness. The clinical presentation consists of one or more of the following: decreased level of consciousness, increasing headache, or focal motor deficit.

[12.2] **B.** An important cause of cerebral ischemia is embolization arising from atrial fibrillation. Transient ischemic attacks can have a similar clinical presentation. However, the neurologic deficits last less than 24 hours.

[12.3] **B.** This patient probably has an intracerebral hemorrhage resulting from his long-standing hypertension. The right side of the brain probably is affected, because he has left-sided body weakness. Other causes of his symptoms may include ischemic stroke, subarachnoid hemorrhage, brain tumor with hemorrhage, and sepsis.

PATHOLOGY PEARLS

- Stroke is the third leading cause of death in the United States. Controlling and/or eliminating medical risk factors can reduce the chance of developing a stroke.
- Strokes are divided into two categories: ischemic infarcts and hemorrhages. Infarcts cause 85 percent of strokes, and hemorrhages account for 15 percent.
- Ischemic stroke can result from a thrombus secondary to atherosclerosis or an embolus arising from a cardiac condition.
- Intracerebral hemorrhage commonly is secondary to long-standing hypertension.
- Ruptured aneurysms frequently cause subarachnoid hemorrhage. SAH clinically presents as the worst headache of the patient's life.
- After a stroke occurs, rapid stabilization and prompt treatment of the patient improve the long-term prognosis. Initiation of treatment within 3 hours of the onset of a stroke results in a better chance for recovery.
- A ruptured berry aneurysm in the circle of Willis is a common cause of subarachnoid hemorrhage.

REFERENCES

Anthony DC, De Girolami U, Frosch MP. The central nervous system. In: Mitchell RN, Kumar V, Abbas AK, et al., eds. Pocket Companion to Robbins and Cotran Pathologic Basis of Disease, 7th ed. Philadelphia, PA: Saunders, 2006:678–83.

Curran RC, Crocker J. Curran's Atlas of Histopathology, 4th rev. ed. New York: Oxford University Press, 2000.

Garcia JH. Neuropathology: The Diagnostic Approach, 2nd ed. St. Louis, MO: Mosby-Year. Book, 1999.

McPhee SJ, Papadakis MA, Tierney LM. Current Medical Diagnosis and Treatment, 47th ed. New York: McGraw-Hill, 2008.

CASE 13

An 86-year-old man resident of a nursing home is found wandering the streets, looking for his way "home." The patient's family describes deteriorating cognitive function that has been worsening progressively over the last several years. He does not have a history of head trauma or cardiovascular disease. In addition to the disorientation, the patient has demonstrated significant language impairment.

- **What is the most likely cause of this patient's symptoms?**
- **What are the distinctive pathologic findings in these disorders?**

ANSWERS TO CASE 13: ALZHEIMER DISEASE

Summary: An 86-year-old male nursing home resident is found wandering the streets. His cognitive function has worsened progressively over several years. He does not have a history of head trauma or cardiovascular disease but has significant language impairment.

- **Most likely etiology:** Alzheimer disease
- **Distinctive pathologic findings:** Cortical atrophy, neuritic or senile plaques, neurofibrillary tangles, and amyloid angiopathy

CLINICAL CORRELATION

This 86-year-old man has dementia, which is impaired cognitive function with slow progression, as represented by forgetfulness, disorientation, alterations in mood, and difficulty with speech. He has wandered from his home, which is a common behavior among patients with dementia. He does not have a history of head trauma or neurologic symptoms, which may indicate a brain tumor, a subarachnoid hemorrhage, or an infection such as syphilis. Depression or stroke is also in the differential diagnosis. Thus, the workup of dementia includes a careful history and physical examination, an assay for vitamin B_{12} deficiency, syphilis serology, HIV serology, thyroid function testing, testing for systemic lupus erythematosus, and CT imaging of the brain. The most common cause of dementia is Alzheimer disease, which has a predilection for those of advanced age. This individual has a moderate to severe form of the disease; more advanced disease may include immobility, being mute, and being severely disabled.

APPROACH TO ALZHEIMER DISEASE

Objectives

- Describe the pathology and microscopic findings of Alzheimer disease.
- Describe the pathology and microscopic findings of Parkinson disease.
- Describe the key differences between the neurologic degenerative diseases.

Definitions

Dementia: Slow onset of loss of cognitive function such as memory loss and confusion. Usually does not change from one day to the next.

Delirium: Acute onset of mental status change, such as confusion, disorientation, and agitation; often is due to drugs, hypoxia, or metabolic condition.

DISCUSSION

Alzheimer disease (AD) is the **most common cause of dementia in the elderly.** The disease usually becomes apparent with slow impairment of higher intellectual function and alterations in behavior and mood. Later, progressive disorientation, memory loss, and aphasia indicate severe cortical dysfunction, and eventually the patient becomes noncommunicative and immobile.

Patients usually become symptomatic after 50 years of age, and the progressive increase in the incidence of the disease in recent years has given rise to major medical, social, and economic problems in countries with a growing number of elderly individuals. When considered by age groups, the rates are 3 percent for those aged 65 to 74 years, 19 percent for those aged 75 to 84 years, and 47 percent for those aged 85 years or more. **Most cases are sporadic,** but up to 10 percent of cases are familial. Pathologic changes identical to those observed in Alzheimer disease occur in almost all older patients with Down syndrome. Although histologic analysis of brain tissue is the "gold standard" for the diagnosis of Alzheimer disease, it rarely is needed in clinical practice. The combination of clinical assessment and modern imaging allows an accurate diagnosis in the vast majority of cases.

Pathologically, the brain shows a variable degree of **cortical atrophy** with **widening of the sulci** and **ventriculomegaly** because of the loss of brain tissue. The major microscopic abnormalities of Alzheimer disease are **neurofibrillary tangles, senile or neuritic plaques, and amyloid angiopathy.** All these abnormalities may be present to a lesser extent in the brains of nondemented elderly people. The diagnosis of Alzheimer disease is based on a combination of clinical and pathologic features.

Neurofibrillary tangles are filament bundles in the cytoplasm of the neurons that displace or encircle the nucleus. They often have an **elongated "flame" shape** or take on a rounded contour. They are visible as basophilic fibrillary structures. They are found commonly in cortical neurons, especially in the entorhinal cortex; in pyramidal cells of the hippocampus; and in the amygdala. Neurofibrillary tangles are insoluble, and so they remain in tissue sections as "ghost" tangles long after the death of the neuron. Neurofibrillary tangles are composed predominantly of paired helical filaments with some straight filaments that appear to have a comparable composition. A major component of paired helical filaments is abnormally hyperphosphorylated forms of the protein tau, an axonal microtubule-associated protein that enhances microtubule assembly.

Neuritic plaques can be found in the hippocampus and amygdala as well as in the neocortex. The major motor and sensory cortex regions generally are spared. These lesions have been described as spherical in shape, taking up Congo red or silver stain, and tortuous in appearance. The amyloid core, which can be stained by Congo red, contains several abnormal proteins.

Although there is some disagreement about the best histologic criteria for Alzheimer disease, **the number of neurofibrillary tangles correlates better**

with clinical impairment than does the number of neuritic plaques. Although amyloid-rich plaques correlate less well with dementia and clinical disease than do neurofibrillary tangles, most current work has focused on the role of amyloid because of its relative specificity for Alzheimer disease and because of evidence from familial Alzheimer disease.

Familial Alzheimer disease accounts for a small minority of cases of Alzheimer disease, and genetic investigations suggest a role for amyloid precursor protein (*APP*) and its processing to amyloid β-protein (Aβ) peptides in the pathogenesis of these cases. The gene that encodes *APP* is on chromosome 21, and several forms of familial Alzheimer disease have been linked to mutations in the *APP* gene. These mutations lead to increased production of Aβ.

Two other genetic loci linked to early-onset familial Alzheimer disease have been identified on chromosomes 14 and 1. They probably account for the majority of cases of early-onset familial Alzheimer disease. The genes on these two chromosomes encode highly related intracellular proteins: presenilin-1 and presenilin-2. Two mechanisms are proposed for the role of presenilins. First, mutations in the presenilins increase the production of Aβ, providing a genetic link for the deposition of amyloid. Second, the presenilins are also targets for cleavage by caspase proteases that are activated during apoptosis, suggesting a role for these proteins in neuronal cell death.

One allele, E4, of the apolipoprotein E (*ApoE*) gene on chromosome 19 increases the risk of Alzheimer disease and lowers the age of onset. The percentage of individuals with the E4 allele is high in populations of patients with Alzheimer disease compared with control populations. *ApoE* can bind Aβ and is present in plaques, but the manner in which this allele increases the risk for Alzheimer disease is unknown.

The **course of Alzheimer disease is slow but progressive,** with a symptomatic period extending beyond 10 to 15 years. The early course of AD is difficult to determine because the patient is usually a poor historian and because the early signs may be so subtle that they evade the notice of family members. These early features include impaired memory, difficulty with problem solving, preoccupation with events long past, decreased spontaneity, and an inability to respond to the environment with the patient's usual speed and accuracy. Patients may forget names, misplace household items, and forget what they were about to do. Often these individuals have insight into the memory deficits and occasionally relay their concerns to family members. Anomia, or difficulty with word finding, is common in the middle stage of Alzheimer disease. In the late stage of Alzheimer disease, physical and cognitive effects are marked. In the final stages, patients may become incontinent, mute, and unable to walk. Myoclonus with muscle tremors occasionally occurs. Mood disturbances such as depression are common. Alzheimer disease progresses at a slow pace to a state of complete helplessness. Intercurrent disease, often pneumonia, is usually the terminal event for these individuals. See Table 13-1 for comparison of etiologies for degenerative diseases.

Table 13-1
DEGENERATIVE DISEASES

DISEASE	SIGNS/SYMPTOMS	MACROSCOPIC FEATURES	MICROSCOPIC FEATURES	CHROMOSOMES
Alzheimer disease	Early: impaired memory, difficulty with problem solving, preoccupation with past events, decreased spontaneity Middle: difficulty with word finding Late: incontinence, mutism, immobility	Cortical atrophy, widening of sulci, ventriculomegaly	Neurofibrillary tangles, senile or neuritic plaques, and amyloid angiopathy	Chromosome 19 (*ApoE* gene) Chromosomes 1, 14, 21
Pick disease	Behavioral changes with personality alterations and some language disturbances	Cortical atrophy of the frontal and temporal lobes	Pick bodies; Neuronal loss in the outer layers of the cortex	
Parkinson disease	Mask-like facies, stooped posture, slowness of voluntary movement, shuffling gait, cogwheel rigidity, "pill-rolling" tremor	Pallor of the substantia nigra and locus caeruleus	Lewy bodies; Loss of the pigmented catecholaminergic neurons in the substantia nigra and locus caeruleus	
Huntington disease	Choreiform movements, dementia	Small brain with atrophy of the caudate nucleus and putamen	Loss of GABAergic neurons	Chromosome 4—expansion of CAG repeats

APPROACH TO PICK DISEASE

Pick disease is a rare, distinct progressive dementia with lobar atrophy. Clinically, the patient experiences **behavioral changes with personality** (frontal lobe signs) alterations and some **language disturbances** (temporal lobe signs). A brain with Pick disease shows **cortical atrophy of the frontal and temporal lobes.** In addition to the localized cortical atrophy, there is often bilateral atrophy of the caudate nucleus and putamen. The cortical gyri can be reduced to a thin wafer-like appearance. This pattern of lobar atrophy is often prominent enough to distinguish Pick disease from Alzheimer disease on macroscopic examination.

On microscopic examination, **neuronal loss is most severe in the outer layers of the cortex.** Some of the surviving neurons show Pick cells (with characteristic swelling) or contain **Pick bodies. Pick bodies are slightly eosinophilic, cytoplasmic, round to oval filamentous inclusions.** Pick bodies stain strongly with silver methods. They are composed of vesiculated endoplasmic reticulum, neurofilaments, and paired helical filaments that are immunocytochemically similar to those found in Alzheimer disease. Unlike the neurofibrillary tangles of Alzheimer disease, Pick bodies do not remain after the neuron dies. In some cases with typical clinical history and macroscopic findings of lobar atrophy, it is not possible to find either Pick cells or Pick bodies; nonetheless, these cases are classified as Pick disease.

APPROACH TO PARKINSON DISEASE

Parkinson disease is a syndrome characterized by **limited facial expression, stooped posture, slowness of voluntary movement, shuffling gait, rigidity, and a "pill-rolling" tremor.** These symptoms are seen in a number of conditions that include damage to the nigrostriatal pathway. Drugs that affect this system, such as dopamine antagonists and toxins, also may induce parkinsonism. Parkinson disease usually appears later in life. The diagnosis is one of exclusion in which no toxic or other underlying etiology is known. Although there is no evidence for a genetic component in most cases, the disease can show autosomal dominant inheritance. In addition to the movement disorder, there are less-well-characterized changes in mental function, including dementia.

Degeneration of the **dopaminergic neurons of the substantia nigra occurs** in Parkinson disease. The severity of the motor syndrome is proportional to the dopamine deficiency, which can be corrected to some degree by replacement therapy with L-dopa, the immediate precursor of dopamine. Treatment does not, however, reverse the morphologic changes or arrest the progress of the disease, and with progression, drug therapy tends to become less effective and symptoms become more difficult to manage.

On pathologic examination, the typical macroscopic findings are **pallor of the substantia nigra and the locus caeruleus.** Microscopically, there is loss of the **pigmented, catecholaminergic neurons** in these regions associated with gliosis. **Lewy bodies** may be found in some of the remaining neurons. Lewy bodies are single or multiple intracytoplasmic, eosinophilic, round to elongated inclusions that often have a dense core surrounded by a pale halo. Lewy bodies are composed of fine filaments that are densely packed in the core but loose at the rim.

Approximately 10 to 15 percent of patients with idiopathic Parkinson disease develop dementia, with an increasing incidence with advancing age. Although many affected individuals also have pathologic evidence of Alzheimer disease, the dementia in others is attributed to widely disseminated Lewy bodies, particularly in the cerebral cortex.

APPROACH TO HUNTINGTON DISEASE

Huntington disease (HD; Huntington chorea) is an inherited **autosomal dominant disease** characterized by **progressive movement disorders and dementia.** Motor symptoms often precede the cognitive impairment. The movement disorder of HD is **choreiform,** with increased and involuntary jerky movements of all parts of the body. **Writhing movements** of the extremities are typical. Some patients may develop parkinsonism with bradykinesia and rigidity later. Early symptoms of higher cortical dysfunction include forgetfulness and thought and affective disorders, and there is progression to a severe dementia. HD patients have an increased risk of suicide, with infection being the most common natural cause of death. The disease is progressive, with the age at onset usually in the fourth and fifth decades and with an average course of approximately 15 years to death. Histologically, it is known for neuronal degeneration of striatal neurons, especially the caudate nucleus.

The ***HD* gene,** which is located on **4p16.3,** encodes a predicted protein (huntingtin) with a molecular mass of 348 kD. The coding region of the gene contains a polymorphic CAG trinucleotide repeat in which patients with *HD* have an increased number of repeats. The normal *HD* genes contain 11 to 34 copies of the repeat. The more repeats a patient has in the gene, the earlier the onset of the disease is. This disease is an example of "triple repeat mutation" disorders. The expanded repeat appears to result in protein aggregation and the formation of intranuclear inclusions.

Pathologically, the **brain is small and shows atrophy of the caudate nucleus** and, less dramatically, the **putamen.** The lateral and third ventricles are dilated. Also, atrophy is seen frequently in the frontal lobe. HD especially affects the neurons that use γ-aminobutyric acid (GABA) as their neurotransmitters. There is a direct relationship between the degree of degeneration in the striatum and the severity of clinical symptoms.

COMPREHENSION QUESTIONS

[13.1] Which of the following situations describes a major risk factor for early-onset familial Alzheimer disease?

A. Expansion of CAG trinucleotide repeats on chromosome 4
B. Ingestion of 1-methyl-4-phenyl-tetrahydrobiopteridine
C. Mutations in the genes encoding for presenilins
D. Mutations in the superoxide dismutase 1 gene
E. The presence of the E4 isotype of apolipoprotein E

[13.2] A 62-year-old man is found to have a shuffling gait, a stooped posture, slowness of movement, muscle rigidity, and a pill-rolling tremor at rest. Physical examination finds that he has a "mask-like" facial expression. The disorder this individual most likely has is associated with the formation of intracytoplasmic eosinophilic inclusions within neurons that are located in which of the following areas of the nervous system?

A. Anterior cerebellum
B. Caudate nucleus
C. Geniculate ganglion
D. Spinal cord
E. Substantia nigra

[13.3] A 42-year-old man is being followed for worsening involuntary jerky movements. During the course of his disease, he develops depression and progressive dementia. Within several years he dies, and during an autopsy, bilateral atrophy of the caudate nuclei is found. What is the basic abnormality involved in this individual's disease process?

A. Acquired enzyme deficiency
B. DNA repair defect
C. Slow virus infection
D. Toxic chemical exposure
E. Triple repeat mutation

Answers

[13.1] **C.** Although most cases of Alzheimer disease are sporadic, up to 10 percent of cases are inherited. The more common sporadic form of Alzheimer disease is associated with the presence of the E4 isotype of *ApoE*. In contrast, many familial cases are associated with amyloid precursor protein (APP) and its processing to Aβ peptides. Additionally, two genes are associated with early-onset familial Alzheimer disease. These genes encode for presenilin-1 and presenilin-2. Mutations in these genes may increase the production of Aβ.

[13.2] **E.** The combination of a shuffling gait, stooped posture, slowness of movement (bradykinesia), muscle rigidity, and a pill-rolling tremor at rest is highly suggestive of the diagnosis of Parkinson disease. These symptoms are caused by a deficiency of dopamine that results from degeneration of the dopaminergic neurons of the substantia nigra. Within this area some of the neurons will have intracytoplasmic eosinophilic inclusions that are called Lewy bodies.

[13.3] **E.** Bilateral atrophy of the caudate nuclei is characteristic of Huntington disease, an inherited autosomal dominant disease that is characterized by the combination of choreiform movements, depression, and progressive dementia. This disorder results from increased numbers of trinucleotide repeats within the *HD* gene. Thus, this disorder is an example of a triple repeat mutation disorder, other examples of which include fragile X syndrome and myotonic dystrophy.

PATHOLOGY PEARLS

- The most common cause of dementia in the elderly is Alzheimer disease.
- The pathologic features of Alzheimer disease are cortical atrophy, neuritic or senile plaques, neurofibrillary tangles, and amyloid angiopathy.
- Pick disease is a rare cause of progressive dementia with characteristic pathologic findings of cortical atrophy of the frontal and temporal lobes and Pick bodies.
- The symptoms of Parkinson disease consist of shuffling gait, motor retardation, limited facial expression, and muscle rigidity. Pathologic changes include degeneration of the dopaminergic neurons of the substantia nigra.
- Huntington disease is an autosomal dominant disease characterized by progressive choreiform movement disorder and dementia. The histologic findings include a small brain and atrophy of the caudate nucleus and putamen.

REFERENCES

Anthony DC, De Girolami U, Frosch MP. The central nervous system. In: Mitchell RN, Kumar V, Abbas AK, et al., eds. Pocket Companion to Robbins and Cotran Pathologic Basis of Disease, 7th ed. Philadelphia, PA: Saunders, 2006:691–7.

Bird TD, Miller BL. Alzheimer's disease and other dementias. In: Kasper DL, Fauci AS, Longo DL, et al., eds. Harrison's Principles of Internal Medicine, 16th ed. New York: McGraw-Hill, 2004:2393–405.

Frosch MP, Anthony DC, DeBirolami U. The central nervous system. In: Kumar V, Assas AK, Fausto N, eds. Robbins and Cotran pathologic Basis of Disease, 7th ed. Philadelphia, PA: Elsevier Saunders, 2004:1386–400.

CASE 14

A 9-year-old girl is evaluated for headaches and clumsiness with walking (ataxia) over the last month. A CT scan reveals a midline, partially cystic cerebellar mass. The tumor is removed surgically, and microscopic examination shows elongated bipolar astrocytes with fibrillar processes and Rosenthal fibers.

- **What is the most likely diagnosis?**

- **What are the most common types of primary central nervous system (CNS) tumors in children and in adults?**

ANSWERS TO CASE 14: JUVENILE PILOCYTIC ASTROCYTOMA

Summary: A 9-year-old girl undergoes surgery for a cerebellar mass. The microscopic findings of the surgical specimen reveal elongated bipolar astrocytes with fibrillar processes and Rosenthal fibers.

- **Most likely diagnosis:** Juvenile pilocytic astrocytoma.
- **Most common primary brain tumors:** In adults, glioblastoma, multiforme, meningioma, and acoustic neuroma; in children, cerebellar astrocytoma and medulloblastoma.

CLINICAL CORRELATION

One of the most common complaints to primary care physicians is headaches, which usually have a benign etiology. The differential diagnosis includes eyestrain, stress, sinusitis, and migraine; however, indications of increased intracranial pressure such as nausea and emesis and the presence of neurologic deficits are "red flags" that necessitate much more careful evaluation. This patient presents with headache and a clumsy gait, or ataxia; this is a worrisome set of complaints. Illicit drug or alcohol use must be considered, and infection of the inner ear should be assessed, but the focus should be on a posterior fossa disorder such as a cerebellar tumor. The **most common type of primary CNS tumors** in **children** are **cerebellar astrocytoma** and **medulloblastoma.** In contrast, the most common types of primary CNS tumors in adults are glioblastoma multiforme, meningioma, and acoustic neuroma. In children the majority of primary brain tumors are infratentorial in the posterior fossa. In contrast, the majority of adults have primary CNS tumors that are supratentorial. CT imaging may not be able to visualize the posterior fossa as well, and so magnetic resonance imaging (MRI) is typically the method of choice (see Figure 14-1).

APPROACH TO CEREBRAL TUMORS

Objectives

- List the most common CNS tumors seen in children.
- Describe the most common CNS tumors seen in adults.
- Describe the location of majority of CNS tumors in adults and children.

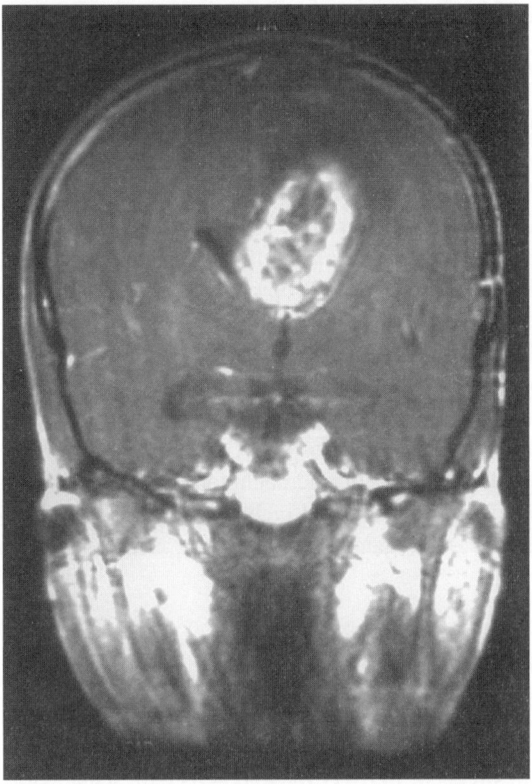

Figure 14-1. MRI of an aggressive astrocytoma. *(Reproduced, with permission, from Rudolph CD, Rudolph AM, Hostetter MK, et al., eds.* Rudolph's Pediatrics, 21st ed. *New York: McGraw-Hill, 2003:2223.)*

Definitions

Ataxia: Incoordination and unsteadiness due to the brain's failure to regulate the body's posture and regulate the strength and direction of limb movements.

Rosenthal fibers: Irregularly shaped, hyaline, eosinophilic structures formed within astrocytes

Cerebellopontine angle: Space that is superior-dorsal to the pons and superior-ventral to the cerebellum

Tinnitus: A sound in one or both ears, such as buzzing, ringing, roaring or whistling, occurring without an external stimulus

DISCUSSION

Pilocytic Astrocytoma

These tumors usually occur in children and young adults and have a typical pathologic appearance. Grossly, they consist of a cystic component and a mural nodule in the cyst wall. Sometimes they may present as solid masses that are distinct or, rarely, infiltrative. These tumors occasionally impinge into the cerebellopontine angle and mimic the symptoms of an acoustic neuroma (hearing loss and tinnitus). Microscopically, pilocytic astrocytomas are **composed of bipolar cells with long, thin "hairlike" processes. Rosenthal fibers** and **microcysts** are usually present. Often, there are increased vascular formations, but necrosis and mitosis are rare. The tumors grow very slowly and thus behave in a **benign manner.** Affected individuals usually notice symptoms that result from cerebrospinal fluid obstruction (increased intracranial pressure and headache) or encroachment on the cerebellum (ataxia and vertigo). The differential diagnosis includes fibrillary astrocytoma, pleomorphic xanthoastrocytoma, ganglion cell tumor, and dense chronic pilocytic gliosis.

Medulloblastoma

Medulloblastoma is **another common neoplasm of children and is located only** in the **cerebellum.** Microscopic examination reveals cells that are undifferentiated with **sheets of densely packed cells** with scant cytoplasm arranged in a **rosette pattern.** Located in the midline of the cerebellum, these rapidly growing tumors often occlude cerebral spinal fluid (CSF) flow and cause hydrocephalus. The **tumor is highly malignant** and can kill quickly if untreated. However, by virtue of its rapid growth, it is usually **very radiosensitive** and **chemosensitive.** The prognosis also is related to the amount of tumor resected at surgery. The 5-year survival rate with total resection and radiation may approach 75 percent.

Glioblastoma Multiforme

Glioblastoma multiforme is **the most common primary intracranial neoplasm** in adults, occurring most often in **individuals in late middle age and older.** This tumor almost always is found in the **cerebral hemispheres (supratentorial)** but occasionally is found in the cerebellum, brainstem, or spinal cord. Common presenting signs and symptoms are seizures, headaches, and focal neurologic deficits. On gross examination, glioblastomas appear as a mixture of firm white areas and softer yellow foci of necrosis, cystic change, and hemorrhage, thus the name *multiforme.* Glomeruloid structures are characteristic on microscopy. **Necrosis is also widespread,** as is "pseudopalisading."

The **prognosis of patients with glioblastoma multiforme is extremely poor,** with a mean survival after optimal treatment of only 8 to 10 months. Fewer than 10 percent of patients live for 2 years.

Meningioma

Meningiomas are **common benign tumors** that occur in **adults.** They arise from the meningothelial cells of the arachnoid cells but are closely associated with the dura. They may arise from the external surface of the brain or from the ventricular system. Commonly affected sites include the parasagittal area, the wing of the sphenoid, the olfactory groove, the sella turcica, and the foramen magnum. They are usually **slow-growing** and **solitary lesions.** Morphologically, meningiomas are rounded tumors with a well-defined base, and they commonly are somewhat easy to remove surgically. They are the **second most common** primary CNS tumor.

Acoustic Neuroma

The acoustic neuroma is a type of **schwannoma,** a benign tumor that arises from the neural crest–derived Schwann cell. **The most common location is the cerebellopontine angle,** where these cells are attached to a vestibular branch of the eighth cranial nerve. Patients can present with **tinnitus or hearing loss.** These are circumscribed, encapsulated masses that are attached to the nerve but can be separated from it. They are firm and gray but also may have cystic areas and a yellowish appearance. **Malignant change is extremely rare** in acoustic neuromas, although recurrences can follow incomplete resection.

COMPREHENSION QUESTIONS

[14.1] A 65-year-old man develops new-onset seizures and headaches. A CT scan reveals a 6-cm left-sided intracerebral mass. Which of the following is the most likely diagnosis?

A. Meningioma
B. Metastatic testicular carcinoma
C. Schwannoma
D. Glioblastoma multiforme

[14.2] A 40-year-old woman has been in good health until recently, when she developed recurrent headaches. A CT scan reveals a 2-cm mass in the foramen magnum. Which of the following is the most likely diagnosis?

A. Glioblastoma multiforme
B. Astrocytoma
C. Meningioma
D. Neurofibroma

[14.3] A 10-year-old girl develops ataxia and hydrocephalus. CT scan shows a midline cerebellar mass. Which of the following is the most likely diagnosis?

A. Astrocytoma
B. Meningioma
C. Neurofibroma
D. Medulloblastoma

Answers

[14.1] **D.** The most likely diagnosis in this patient is glioblastoma multiforme. It is the most common primary CNS tumor, especially in this age group. The intracerebral location is also typical.

[14.2] **C.** The foramen magnum is a common location for meningiomas. In addition, there is a slight female predominance for this second most common primary CNS tumor in adults.

[14.3] **D.** Medulloblastoma is a cerebellar midline tumor that presents commonly in the pediatric population. These tumors are rapidly growing and often cause hydrocephalus.

PATHOLOGY PEARLS

- ❖ CNS tumors are the second most common type of malignancy in children. Only leukemia is more common.
- ❖ The majority of CNS tumors in **children** are infratentorial.
- ❖ The most common types of primary CNS tumors in children are cerebellar astrocytoma and medulloblastoma.
- ❖ The majority of CNS tumors in **adults** are supratentorial in location.
- ❖ The most common types of primary CNS tumors in adults are glioblastoma multiforme, meningioma, and acoustic neuroma.

REFERENCES

Anthony DC, De Girolami U, Frosch MP. The central nervous system. In: Mitchell RN, Kumar V, Abbas AK, et al., eds. Pocket Companion to Robbins and Cotran Pathologic Basis of Disease, 7th ed. Philadelphia, PA: Saunders, 2006:700–8.

Burger PC, Scheithauer BW. Tumors of the CNS. Washington DC: AFIP Press, 1994.

Frosch MP, Anthony DC, DeGirolami U. The central nervous system. In: Kumar V, Assas AK, Fausto N, eds. Robbins and Cotran Pathologic Basis of Disease, 7th ed. Philadelphia, PA: Elsevier Saunders, 2004:1401–14.

❖ CASE 15

A 45-year-old woman who works as an accountant has right-sided hearing loss as well as "ringing of the ears" (tinnitus) that has begun to interfere with her work. She reports that this has been happening over a 6-month period. She denies headache or trauma. She has not had previous medical problems. A CT scan of the head reveals a 2-cm mass at the cerebellopontine angle.

- **What is the most likely diagnosis?**
- **What other types of tumors arise from peripheral nerves?**

ANSWERS TO CASE 15: SCHWANNOMA OF THE EIGHTH CRANIAL NERVE

Summary: A 45-year-old healthy accountant has right-sided hearing loss and tinnitus progressing over 8 months. A CT scan of the head reveals a 2-cm mass at the cerebellopontine angle.

◆ **Most likely diagnosis:** Acoustic neuroma/schwannoma of eighth cranial nerve.

◆ **Other types of tumors that arise from peripheral nerves:** Neurofibromas, malignant peripheral nerve sheet tumor, and neurofibromatosis types 1 and 2.

CLINICAL CORRELATION

Hearing loss is a common complaint, with up to 10 percent of adults having some deficit, usually among patients older than age 65 years. Hearing loss usually is subdivided into disorders of conduction (auricle, external auditory canal, and middle ear) and disorders relating to sensorineural conditions (inner ear or eighth cranial nerve). Excessive cerumen in the external ear canal or middle ear effusion, for instance, would be considered conduction problems. Other neurologic symptoms may suggest a central nervous system process. This patient has tinnitus, a buzzing or ringing in the ears. The slow onset of the process speaks against infections such as those caused by viruses or a cerebrovascular accident, which usually results in the acute onset of hearing loss. On physical examination, a Weber test, which entails placing a vibrating tuning fork on the patient's head in the midline, usually will help discriminate the etiology of hearing loss: With **conduction disorders,** the patient will perceive the **tone lateralizing to the affected ear,** whereas in **sensorineural disorders,** the patient will perceive the **tone as lateralizing to the unaffected ear.** Common causes of sensorineural hearing loss of gradual progression include otosclerosis, noise-induced hearing loss, vestibular schwannoma, and Ménière disease. Ménière disease usually presents with vertigo, a sensation of fullness in the ears, and hearing loss. Small schwannomas may present with unilateral hearing loss and tinnitus, but usually not with vertigo or dizziness. The diagnosis is made by imaging, usually with a magnetic resonance imaging (MRI) scan. The treatment is generally surgical excision.

APPROACH TO CENTRAL NERVOUS SYSTEM SCHWANNOMAS

Objectives

- Describe the signs and symptoms of acoustic neuromas.
- Describe the signs and symptoms of neurofibromatosis type 1.

Definitions

Myxoid: Containing or resembling mucus. Mucoid.

Kyphoscoliosis: Abnormally increased convexity in the curvature of the thoracic spine as viewed from the side (hump back) and lateral curvature of the spine as viewed from front or back.

Autosomal dominant: Form of inheritance where only one gene is required in order to manifest that trait. This gene is not located on the X or Y chromosome.

Neurofibromatosis type 1: Also known as von Recklinghausen syndrome

DISCUSSION

Individuals with neurofibromatosis tend to develop a variety of tumors, including **neurofibromas, acoustic nerve schwannomas,** and **gliomas of the optic nerve. Meningiomas, pigmented nodules of the iris (Lisch nodules),** and **hyperpigmented macules of the skin (café-au-lait spots) also may be seen.**

Schwannomas are fairly common tumors, usually arising from cranial or spinal nerve roots; infrequently, they reside within the substance of the brain itself. Schwannomas often involve cranial nerve VIII, and in this setting, they are called **acoustic neuromas** or **acoustic schwannomas.** In fact, acoustic neuromas are the **third most common primary intracranial neoplasm.** Affected individuals usually complain of **hearing loss** or **tinnitus (ringing in the ears).** These tumors may grow into the intracranial compartment to occupy the **cerebellopontine angle,** producing cerebellar dysfunction such as ataxia or other gait disorders, or may affect the fifth and seventh cranial nerves.

Schwannomas are usually well circumscribed and have a distinct capsule attached to the nerve but can be separated from it. The tumors are generally firm and have areas of yellowish coloration and cystic degeneration. Pressure of the tumor on the involved nerve leading to compression atrophy is common. Radiologically, acoustic neuromas appear as distinct contrast-enhancing masses. Large tumors are associated with enlargement of the entry of the internal auditory canal. Treatment consists of surgical excision, taking care not to injure the nerve.

Neurofibroma

Two distinct lesions have been termed neurofibromas. The cells are of diverse lineages, such as Schwann cells, perineural cells, and fibroblasts. The most common form of neurofibroma occurs in the skin **(cutaneous neurofibroma)** (see Figure 15-1) or in the peripheral nerve **(solitary neurofibroma).** These neurofibromas may occur sporadically or in association with type 1 neurofibromatosis. The skin lesions appear as nodules, sometimes with **hyperpigmentation.** The lesions may become very large and even become pedunculated. Malignant transformation is rare. Cosmetic appearance is of primary concern.

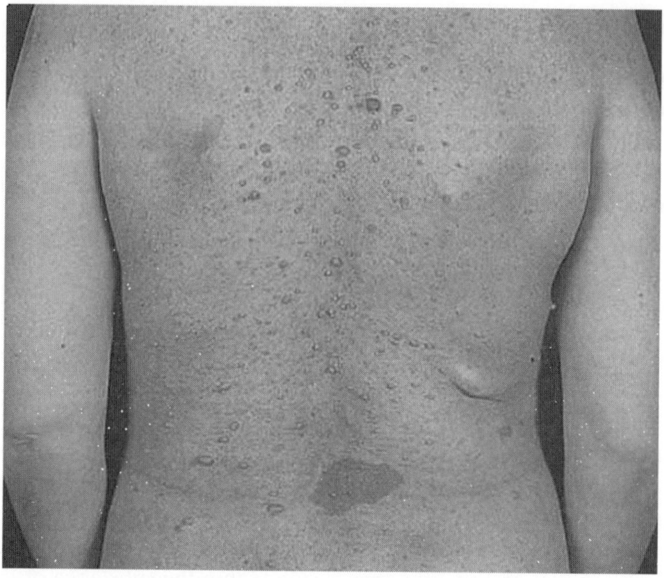

Figure 15-1. Neurofibromatosis (NF1). Skin colored and pink tan, soft papules and nodules on the back are neurofibromas. *(Reused, with permission, from Wolff K, Johnson RA, Suurmond D.* Fitzpatrick's Color Atlas and Synopsis of Clinical Dermatology, 5th ed. *New York: McGraw-Hill, 2005:465.)*

The **plexiform neurofibroma** is the other form of the tumor. It is considered by many to be the **defining lesion of type 1 neurofibromatosis.** It is not a sporadic tumor but is found only in association with neurofibromatosis. There is the potential for **malignant transformation** and also difficulty in removing the lesions when they involve major nerve trunks. These tumors may occur anywhere along the course of the nerve and may be multiple. Unlike schwannomas, they cannot be separated easily from the nerve, making surgical excision difficult. Microscopically, the lesion has a loose **myxoid appearance** with low cellularity.

Malignant Peripheral Nerve Sheath Tumor

Malignant peripheral nerve sheath tumors are **highly malignant sarcomas that arise** de novo or from malignant degeneration of a plexiform neurofibroma. They are **locally invasive** and lead frequently to recurrences, metastatic spread, and a **poor prognosis.** They also may be associated with radiation therapy. The tumors are poorly defined, with invasion of surrounding soft tissue. Necrosis is a common finding.

Neurofibromatosis Type 1

Neurofibromatosis type 1 is an **autosomal dominant disorder** characterized, as was mentioned earlier, by **several distinct lesions,** including **neurofibromas, acoustic nerve schwannomas, gliomas of the optic nerve, meningiomas, pigmented nodules of the iris (Lisch nodules),** and **hyperpigmented macules of the skin, so-called café-au-lait spots.** The tumors are histologically identical to those that occur sporadically, except for the plexiform types, which are **pathognomic of neurofibromatosis type 1.**

The clinical course is extremely varied. Some patients may be asymptomatic, and others may have a rapidly progressive course. Complications include spinal deformity, most notably, kyphoscoliosis. Lesions around the brain and spinal may have devastating consequences.

Neurofibromatosis Type 2

Neurofibromatosis type 2 is a **distinct autosomal dominant disorder** with its gene located on chromosome 22. **It is much less common than neurofibromatosis type 1.** Tumors are common, and are usually **bilateral schwannomas of the eighth cranial nerve** or **multiple meningiomas.**

COMPREHENSION QUESTIONS

[15.1] A 35-year-old woman complains of drooling from the right side of the mouth. An MRI of the brain is performed. The neurosurgeon states that the diagnosis is a schwannoma. Compression of which of the cranial nerves listed below would be most likely to produce these signs and symptoms?

A. Cranial nerve VII
B. Cranial nerve VIII
C. Cranial nerve IX
D. Cranial nerve X
E. Cranial nerve XI

[15.2] A 60-year-old woman has a history of being treated for endometrial cancer with surgery and radiation 5 years ago. She now presents with a large necrotic tumor that follows the course of the sciatic nerve. Which of the following is the most likely diagnosis?

A. Recurrent endometrial cancer
B. Solitary neurofibroma
C. Malignant peripheral nerve sheath tumor
D. Schwannoma
E. Neurofibromatosis type 2

[15.3] A 40-year-old man who works as a gardener is in good general health. Over the last several months he has noticed a "bump" under the skin of his left axilla. The bump is pigmented and has become pedunculated. Which of the following is the most likely diagnosis?

A. Cutaneous neurofibroma
B. Neurofibromatosis type 1
C. Neurofibromatosis type 2
D. Schwannoma
E. Lipoma

Answers

[15.1] **A.** Hearing loss is caused by a deficit in cranial nerve (CN) VIII, whereas the difficulty with drooling is caused by weakness of the facial muscles (CN VII).

[15.2] **C.** The development of a necrotic tumor involving a peripheral nerve in an area that was irradiated previously is characteristic of a malignant peripheral nerve sheath tumor.

[15.3] **A.** Solitary skin tumors that are pigmented and may become pedunculated are usually cutaneous neurofibromas.

PATHOLOGY PEARLS

❖ Schwannomas commonly involve the eighth cranial nerve.
❖ Hearing loss on the affected side and tinnitus are common early symptoms of acoustic neuromas.
❖ Acoustic neuromas occur at the cerebellopontine angle.
❖ Neurofibromatosis type 1 includes many types of lesions.
❖ Neurofibromas may occur sporadically or as part of the neurofibromatosis type 1 syndrome.
❖ Neurofibromatosis type 2 is a distinct autosomal dominant disorder.

REFERENCES

Anthony DC, De Girolami U, Frosch MP. The central nervous system. In: Mitchell RN, Kumar V, Abbas AK, et al., eds. Pocket Companion to Robbins and Cotran Pathologic Basis of Disease, 7th ed. Philadelphia, PA: Saunders, 2006:706–8.

Burger PC, Scheithauer BW. Tumors of the CNS. Washington DC: AFIP Press, 1994.

Frosch MP, Anthony DC, DeGirolami U. The central nervous system. In: Kumar V, Assas AK, Fausto N, eds. Robbins and Cotran Pathologic Basis of Disease, 7th ed. Philadelphia, PA: Elsevier Saunders, 2004:1401–14.

Schneider AS, Szanto PA. Pathology. Baltimore, MD: Lippincott Williams & Wilkins, 2002.

CASE 16

A 20-year-old woman notices a swelling in her neck, just to the left of the midline. Physical examination suggests a nontender 1.5-cm thyroid lesion, and thyroid function tests reveal normal serum thyroid hormone levels. A radioisotope scintiscan demonstrates very little uptake of the iodine in the nodule, consistent with a nonfunctioning nodule, or "cold" nodule.

- **What are the diagnostic considerations?**

- **What is the prognosis for these disorders?**

ANSWERS TO CASE 16: THYROID NODULE

Summary: A 20-year-old woman presents with a nontender thyroid nodule and normal thyroid function tests. No uptake is seen on radioisotope scintiscan.

- **Diagnostic consideration:** Requires a diagnostic workup for adenoma or carcinoma, such as biopsy.
- **Prognosis:** No radioisotope uptake on scintiscan increases suspicion for malignancy.

CLINICAL CORRELATION

The clinical presentation of a **young female** with a **solitary nodule** increases the likelihood of a neoplastic process. If the nodule is palpable, the risk of malignancy rises from 5 to 10 percent to 20 percent. **The incidence of thyroid cancer is greater in the young to middle-aged female population.** This association of age and gender may be due to a correlation between estrogen levels and the neoplastic epithelial expression of estrogen receptors. The negative uptake of the radioisotope scintiscan indicates the absence of excessive thyroid function, which is commonly referred to as a "cold" nodule. Approximately 10 percent of cold nodules are found to be malignant. It is rare to have thyrotoxicosis or thyroiditis with malignancy; therefore, a cold nodule typically creates suspicion for a malignancy or adenoma. The differential diagnosis of a cold nodule would include adenoma, papillary carcinoma, medullary carcinoma, follicular carcinoma, and anaplastic carcinoma (see Table 16-1). Typically the first diagnostic step would be a fine needle aspirate (FNA) of the thyroid or ultrasound, radioisotope scan, and then, if indicated, surgery with a histologic evaluation of the resected mass. **The major distinction of malignancy from a benign process is the histologic visualization of characteristic cells or invasion of the capsule or blood vessels.**

APPROACH TO THYROID NODULE

Objectives

- Describe the types of thyroid nodules.
- Describe the meaning of "hot" versus "cold" nodules on radioisotope scan.
- Describe the prognosis of the different thyroid nodules.

Table 16-1
TYPES OF THYROID NEOPLASMS

TYPE	EPIDEMIOLOGY	HISTOLOGY	PROGNOSIS
Papillary ca.	**Common** 80% children 60% adults	Papillary structure Glandular epithelium **Orphan Annie nucleus** **Psammoma bodies**	Best prognosis: good 5-year survival Spread by lymphatics
Follicular ca.	10–20% increased frequency with age >40 years	Uniform follicles Invasion of capsule indicates malignancy	Prognosis: good Metastasis usually to bone or lungs via angioinvasion
Medullary ca.	5% adults	C cells present Amyloid present in stroma Slow growth	Secretes **calcitonin;** levels can be used to follow cancer progress Can be part of MEN 2 syndrome
Anaplastic ca.	<5% Elderly	Poorly differentiated cells **Rapid growth** Usually evolves from preexisting well-differentiated neoplasm	**Poor prognosis** Metastasis via lymphatics or bloodstream
Benign follicular adenoma		**Well-defined basement membrane** Usually solitary nodule	Can occasionally cause hyperthyroidism (toxic adenoma with hot nodule)

Definitions

Carcinoma: Indicates a malignant tumor consisting of epithelial cells.

Cold nodule: Indicates a nonfunctional thyroid with no uptake of the radioisotope, usually indicative of malignancy.

Hot nodule: Indicates increased thyroid functioning with subsequent uptake of the radioisotope; can be treated with radioablation, less than 1 percent chance of malignancy.

Multiple endocrine neoplasia 2a (MEN 2a): Familial condition consisting of bilateral medullary carcinoma, pheochromocytoma, and parathyroid hyperplasia or adenoma.

Radioisotope scintiscan: Uses radioisotopes of iodine 123 or technetium pertechnetate to detect nodules greater than 5 mm in diameter. The use of iodine is a means of evaluating physiologic function. This study has a low specificity and sensitivity with respect to differentiating benign from malignant lesions; therefore, it is not recommended for initial evaluation.

DISCUSSION

Normal Thyroid

The thyroid is composed of two lobes, which contain follicles. A follicle consists of simple cuboidal epithelium surrounding a central colloid filled lumen. Between the follicles are the parafollicular cells, which produce calcitonin. The parenchyma also contains many dark staining, round cells named chief or principal cells. The larger cells with a pale cytoplasm are the oxyphil cells.

Pathogenesis of Thyroid Carcinoma

The etiology of thyroid cancers is multifactorial with both genetic and environmental influences. Genetic mutations in the *RET* protooncogene are responsible for familial medullary thyroid carcinoma, a familial papillary thyroid carcinoma, and sporadic forms. Thyroid carcinoma can also be associated with loss-of-function genes such as the *APC* gene associated with familial adenomatous polyposis. See Table 16-1 for classification.

Papillary Carcinoma

Papillary carcinoma is the **most common thyroid cancer at any age.** Metastasis is via lymphatics. Ionizing radiation exposure, especially before age 20 years, causes an increased risk for *RET* gene rearrangement leading to papillary carcinoma. It has the **best prognosis among thyroid carcinomas.** Grossly, it may be solitary or a multifocal lesion with calcification and fibrosis. It can have a well-defined capsule or infiltrate. Papillary architecture includes the "finger-like" projections that are often present but are not necessary for diagnosis, because there are variants such as the follicular variant. Definitive diagnosis is based on nuclear features such as **"Orphan Annie"** or **"ground glass" nuclei.** These terms refer to the **clear appearance of the nucleus resulting from the dispersion of the chromatin.** There also can be concentric calcified structures called **psammoma bodies.**

Follicular Carcinoma

Follicular carcinoma is the **second most common thyroid carcinoma,** with an **increased frequency after 40 years of age.** Gross examination can appear similar to the follicular adenoma if there is minimal invasion. It can be infiltrative or grossly circumscribed. Histologically, the cells can be uniform with small follicles or abnormally enlarged with deformed nuclei. Similar to classic follicular carcinoma, there is also a **Hürthle cell variant** distinguished by eosinophilic, granular cellular changes. Follicular carcinoma is more common in communities with iodine deficiency–related goiters; however, there is no evidence to suggest that an adenoma contributes to the formation of follicular carcinoma. In 20 percent of follicular thyroid carcinomas, a translocation on chromosome t(2;3)(q13:p25) gives rise to a novel protooncogenic protein. **Metastasis is usually vascular to the lungs, bone, and liver.** The treatment of choice is **surgical excision.** In rare cases, there may be a hyperfunctional well-differentiated type of follicular carcinoma presenting as a "hot" nodule that can be treated with radioactive ablation.

Medullary Carcinoma

Medullary carcinoma occurs in **less than 5 percent of the population**, affecting **mainly individuals in the fifth decade and older.** Children and younger patients may be affected if it is associated with **multiple endocrine neoplasia 2 (MEN 2).** Approximately 80 percent of medullary carcinomas are sporadic, with the remaining 20 percent having a familial origin. Medullary carcinoma is a slow-growing mass **derived from the parafollicular cells and therefore can produce calcitonin. Focal proliferation of C cells is considered a precursor to familial medullary carcinomas.** Gross examination may reveal a solitary lesion in the sporadic cases or bilobar multicentric lesions in the aggressive MEN-associated carcinomas. Microscopic identification of **amyloid deposits,** derived from the calcitonin, is characteristic of this neoplasm. Immunohistochemical methods can allow for visualization of calcitonin. Medullary carcinoma also may produce hormones such as carcinoembryonic antigen, somatostatin, serotonin, and vasoactive intestinal peptide (VIP). Clinically, a patient may present with diarrhea caused by the VIP; however, no hypocalcemia is associated with the calcitonin. **The production of calcitonin is a useful clinical tool for the diagnosis and to follow the postoperative progression of the carcinoma.** Patients in families with known *RET* mutations associated with MEN can be given elective prophylactic thyroidectomies.

Anaplastic Carcinoma

Anaplastic carcinoma occurs in less than 5 percent of the population and affects mainly the **elderly.** This neoplasm is the **most aggressive and therefore also has the worst prognosis.** Death usually occurs within a year by **lymphatic or vascular metastasis.** Gross examination reveals a large mass that invades beyond the capsule into surrounding structures. Characteristic microscopic findings include **highly anaplastic cells** appearing as **pleomorphic giant cells, spindle cells, frequent mitotic figures,** and cells with a squamoid appearance. A *TP53* gene inactivation mutation can induce anaplastic cancers and be used as a marker to diagnose tumor progression. **Treatment** mainly consists of **external radiation.**

Adenoma

An adenoma is usually a **solitary, well-encapsulated neoplasm of follicular epithelium.** It may cause clinical symptoms as a result of local mass effect such as difficulty swallowing. These tumors usually have **uniform colloid-filled follicles with well-defined cell borders.** There are many subtypes that are based on the presenting histology; however, a papillary presentation should raise suspicion for papillary carcinoma. **Hürthle cell adenoma** is characterized by oxyphil that also is known as **Hürthle cell change.** Oxyphil describes the **eosinophilic granular cytoplasm resulting from increased numbers of mitochondria** in the neoplastic cells. Benign follicular adenomas can present with **endocrine atypia,** which refers to the presence of nuclear pleomorphism, and atypia. **Because a well-differentiated follicular carcinoma can be relatively unremarkable, it is essential to look for invasion of the capsule or blood vessels to determine malignancy.**

COMPREHENSION QUESTIONS

[16.1] A 22-year-old woman is discovered to have a nontender thyroid nodule that is found to be a cold nodule on a radioisotope scan. The pathology report from a fine needle aspiration of the nodule describes a follicular neoplasm, the differential of which includes a benign follicular adenoma and a malignant follicular carcinoma. Which is the single best histologic criterion to differentiate between these two neoplasms?

A. Hyperplasia of follicles
B. Inspissation of colloid
C. Invasion into vessels
D. Number of mitoses
E. Presence of atypia

[16.2] A 25-year-old man presents because of "fullness" in his neck. Physical examination finds enlargement of the thyroid gland resulting from the presence of several small masses in both thyroid lobes. These nodules are surgically resected, and the pathology report from this surgical specimen diagnoses a papillary carcinoma. Which of the following histologic changes is most characteristic of this type of carcinoma?

A. An amyloid stroma
B. Bland microfollicles
C. Extracellular Russell bodies
D. Neoplastic C cells
E. Orphan Annie nuclei

[16.3] A 23-year-old man is being evaluated for the new development of a nodule in his neck. Physical examination finds a 3.5-cm thyroid nodule. The lesion is removed surgically, and histologic sections reveal groups of poorly differentiated tumors cells within a stroma with large areas of amyloid. This familial form of this type of malignancy is associated with abnormalities of which of the following protooncogenes?

A. *erf*
B. *myc*
C. *ras*
D. *ret*
E. *sis*

Answers

[16.1] **C.** The differential diagnosis of a cold nodule of the thyroid includes follicular adenoma, follicular carcinoma, papillary carcinoma, medullary carcinoma, and anaplastic carcinoma. The first diagnostic step is usually a fine needle aspirate of the nodule. An FNA, however, cannot differentiate between the two "follicular neoplasms": the benign follicular adenoma and the malignant follicular carcinoma. The only histologic means to differentiate between these two neoplasms is the presence of cells invading through the capsule surrounding the tumor or into blood vessels.

[16.2] **E.** The most common histologic type of thyroid carcinoma is called a papillary carcinoma. This type of malignancy, which has the best prognosis among thyroid carcinomas, may be solitary or multifocal. The term *papillary* refers to the finger-like projections formed by fronds of tumor cells with fibrovascular cores. The papillary areas sometimes are associated with the formation of concentric calcified structures called psammoma bodies. The presence of these papillary projections is not necessary for the diagnosis of papillary thyroid carcinoma. Instead, the definitive diagnosis is based on characteristic nuclear features, which include ground glass nuclei ("Orphan Annie eyes"), nuclear grooves, and intranuclear inclusions (cytoplasmic invaginations into the nucleus).

[16.3] **D.** Medullary carcinoma of the thyroid is a malignant neoplasm that originates from the parafollicular C cells of the thyroid. These cells normally secrete calcitonin. Stromal aggregates of procalcitonin are seen histologically within these tumors as amyloid, which is a type of protein that demonstrates an "apple-green" birefringence with a special Congo red stain. Although most cases of medullary thyroid carcinomas are sporadic, the familial form is associated with abnormalities of the *ret* protooncogene. This type of malignancy also is seen in multiple endocrine neoplasia types 2 and 3.

PATHOLOGY PEARLS

- A cold nodule on radioisotope scan usually indicates the presence of an adenoma or carcinoma, whereas an active hot nodule indicates a benign process.
- The most common thyroid carcinoma is papillary carcinoma, which affects people of all ages.
- Medullary carcinoma is a slow-growing tumor associated with MEN 2a; it usually affects elderly persons and can be followed clinically by calcitonin levels.
- Anaplastic carcinoma is the most aggressive tumor, with the worst prognosis.
- Treatment in each case is surgical except for anaplastic carcinoma, in which external radiation therapy is used.

REFERENCES

Burkitt HG, Stevens A, Lowe JS, et al. Wheater's Basic Histopathology. New York: Churchill Livingstone, 1996.

Chandrasoma P., Taylor CR. Concise Pathology. Norwalk, CT: Appleton & Lange, 1995.

Maitra A, Abbas AK. The endocrine system. In: Kumar V, Assas AK, Fausto N, eds. Robbins and Cotran Pathologic Basis of Disease, 7th ed. Philadelphia, PA: Elsevier Saunders, 2004:1164–83.

Maitra A. The endocrine system. In: Mitchell RN, Kumar V, Abbas AK, et al., eds. Pocket Companion to Robbins and Cotran Pathologic Basis of Disease, 7th ed. Philadelphia: Saunders, 2006:575–9.

Walsh RM, Watkinson JC, Franklyn J. The management of the solitary thyroid nodule: a review. Clin Otolaryngol 1999:24(5):388–97.

CASE 17

A 72-year-old man complains of the sudden onset of headache, blurred vision, and tenderness and severe throbbing pain over his left temple region. He also has experienced flu-like symptoms and joint stiffness over the last week. He previously had been in good health. The physical examination reveals tenderness and induration of the left temporal region.

- **What is the most likely diagnosis?**

- **What other studies may be helpful in confirming the diagnosis?**

ANSWERS TO CASE 17: TEMPORAL ARTERITIS

Summary: A 72-year-old man presents with acute-onset headache, blurred vision, and pain over the left temple. He also has joint pain and flu-like symptoms over 1 week.

- **Most likely diagnosis:** Temporal arteritis.
- **Other confirmatory studies:** The gold standard is a temporal artery biopsy of at least 2 to 3 cm in length. A markedly elevated erythrocyte sedimentation rate (ESR) would be highly suggestive.

CLINICAL CORRELATION

This 72-year-old man has a classic presentation of temporal arteritis (TA). Typically, the symptoms of temporal arteritis occur in a patient aged 50 years or older with **sudden-onset headache** over the **temporal region, disturbances in vision, and polymyalgia rheumatica; these findings warrant immediate treatment. Physical examination may note a cord-like thickening of the temporal artery. Polymyalgia rheumatica** includes the symptoms of joint pain, morning stiffness, and muscle ache. Inflammation of the temporal artery increases the likelihood of **thrombosis of the ophthalmic artery, causing irreversible blindness.** Consequently, if temporal arteritis is suspected clinically, **corticosteroids are administered immediately,** with a subsequent temporal biopsy to establish the diagnosis.

APPROACH TO ARTERITIS

Objectives

- Describe the different types of arteritis and their "classic" patient population.
- Describe the presentation of temporal arteritis.
- List the most common complications of temporal arteritis.

Definitions

Vasculitis: Inflammation of a vessel wall that increases the risk for thrombosis.

Antineutrophil cytoplasmic antibodies (ANCAs): Antibodies against the primary granules within neutrophils. p-ANCA refers to perinuclear staining, and c-ANCA indicates cytoplasmic staining after ethanol fixation and immunofluorescence.

DISCUSSION

Normal Vessel

Arteries can be subdivided into **elastic arteries,** which are the large arteries that carry blood away from the heart, such as the aorta; **muscular arteries** that distribute blood to the organs; and **arterioles** (less than 100 μm), which regulate blood pressure. **Veins** have valves in the tunica intima and a thinner tunica media.

A vessel consists of three layers: **tunica intima, tunica media, and tunica adventitia.** The innermost layer is the **tunica intima,** which consists of simple squamous endothelial cells lining the lumen. It has longitudinal smooth muscle cells to form the subendothelial connective tissue and then an internal elastic lamina. The internal elastic lamina is poorly defined in elastic arteries and well defined in muscular arteries. The next portion is the **tunica media,** which is generally the thickest layer, consisting of circular smooth muscle cells, reticular fibers, collagenous fibers, and elastic fibers. The **tunica adventitia** consists of collagenous connective tissue with **vasa vasorum,** or vessels that run in the larger vessels to provide blood to the tunica media and adventitia.

Temporal Arteritis (Giant Cell Arteritis)

Temporal arteritis affects arteries ranging from small to large, **typically affecting intracranial and superficial vessels of the head.** The etiology is unknown; however, it is suspected that there is a T-cell-mediated immune response to an antigen. It is the **most common** vasculitis. Temporal arteritis consists of inflammatory vessel wall thickening, which narrows the lumen and **increases thrombotic formation.** In the ophthalmic artery, occlusion of the vessel can lead to **irreversible blindness.** Microscopically, examination will show a **granulomatous inflammation** of the vessel wall with **giant cells,** histiocytes, plasma cells, and **lymphocytic infiltration with fragmentation of the internal elastic lamina.**

Takayasu Arteritis (Pulseless Disease)

Takayasu arteritis is a disease typically seen in **females younger than age 40 years** with symptoms of **visual disturbances, painful skin nodules, myalgia, fever, fatigue, and weak upper extremity pulses.** The disease involves the medium-size and large vessels, often including the aortic arch and its branches. Gross examination of an affected aortic arch shows intimal folds that cause a narrowed lumen and a diminishing vascular supply to the distal vessels. As a result of the lower blood flow, there is compensatory intimal thickening with decreased pulses. Histologically, the presence of granulomas with giant cells is seen in only a few cases; **therefore, if giant cell lesions are found in the aorta of a young patient, Takayasu arteritis is the diagnosis.** Usually there is neutrophilic and chronic inflammatory cell infiltration of the media and adventitia. The sequelae of vasculitis after fibrotic healing of intimal layer can include aortic valve insufficiency and myocardial infarct.

Polyarteritis Nodosa (PAN)

Polyarteritis nodosa is a disease affecting mainly **young adults,** but it also can affect children and the elderly. It is associated with **hepatitis B infection.** The clinical picture may include a variety of symptoms, such as rapid-onset hypertension, abdominal pain with weight loss, melena, muscle aches, peripheral neuritis, and, most important, **renal** involvement, which is the major cause of death. It usually spares the pulmonary circulation. It can be acute, subacute, or a chronic process that is **fatal unless treated** with **corticosteroids** or cyclophosphamide to induce remission or cure the disease. It typically affects the medium-sized muscular arteries, producing segmental nodular swellings. Microscopically, there is **also fibrinoid necrosis of the media, eosinophils, and acute inflammation of all layers.** After the acute inflammatory infiltration, the vessel is restored with a fibrous nodular thickening of the vessel wall that marks areas of previous lesions. **Multiple stages can exist within the same vessel; this is a notable feature of PAN.** The fibrotic segments are **areas of weakness and dilation** when there are thrombotic occlusions. As a result of the vessel occlusion, the affected segments will have decreased **perfusion with resultant ischemia or hemorrhaging,** which can be fatal if it occurs in a critical location.

Kawasaki Disease (Mucocutaneous Lymph Node Syndrome)

Kawasaki disease is the **leading cause of acquired heart disease** in **young children.** The symptoms include an acute **self-limited fever, oral and conjunctival erythema, a desquamating rash, and lymphadenitis.** The etiology is unknown but is suspected to be an infectious agent and is characterized by T-cell and macrophage activation. **Intravenous immunoglobulin therapy** is used to decrease the incidence of associated heart disease. Histologically, there is inflammation of the entire vessel wall and necrosis, which resolves. In severe cases, there can be coronary intimal thickening with resultant aneurysm formation, myocardial infarction, or death.

Microscopic Polyangiitis

The clinical features of **microscopic polyangiitis** include hemoptysis, hematuria, proteinuria, bowel pain, muscle pain and/or weakness, and palpable cutaneous purpura. It is suspected that this vasculitis is initiated by immunoglobulin and complement reaction to an introduced antigen such as a drug or a tumor-produced antigen. It affects the arterioles, capillaries, and venules, causing transmural necrotic lesions. Microscopic visualization of fragmented neutrophils infiltrating the vessel wall is called **leukocytoclastic angiitis.**

Wegener Granulomatosis

Wegener granulomatosis is a disease characterized by **acute necrotizing granulomas** of the **respiratory** tract, a **necrotizing granulomatous vasculitis,** and renal pathology. The small- and medium-size vessels are involved. Microscopic evaluation illustrates lymphocytes, plasma cells, macrophages, and giant cells with a localized necrotic center. It is responsive to **immunosuppressive therapy.**

Thromboangiitis Obliterans (Buerger Disease)

Thromboangiitis obliterans is associated with **smoking** and classically is seen before age 35 in males; now it is seen increasingly in females. Typical symptoms include **cyanosis** of the hands, **claudication** of the foot, and **ulceration** of the distal extremities leading to gangrene. The small- and medium-size arteries, particularly of the extremities, are affected. Microscopic examination shows **acute and chronic segmental inflammation with thrombotic microabscesses.** The abscesses consist of neutrophils enveloped by granulomatous inflammation. The best **treatment is cessation of cigarette smoking.** See Table 17-1 for a comparison of types of arteritis.

Table 17-1
TYPES OF ARTERITIS

	ARTERIES INVOLVED	SIGNS/SYMPTOMS	"CLASSIC" PATIENT POPULATION	ANTINEUTROPHIL CYTOPLASMIC ANTIBODIES (ANCA)
Temporal Arteritis	Small and large sized (typically intracranial and superficial vessels of the head)	Severe, unilateral headache; jaw claudication, sudden irreversible blindness, polymyalgia rheumatica	Elderly patient	
Takayasu Arteritis	Medium and large sized (typically the aortic arch and its branches)	Weak upper extremity pulses, myalgia, fever, fatigue, visual disturbances, painful skin nodules	Young Asian female (<40 years)	
Polyarteritis Nodosa	Medium sized	Rapid onset hypertension, abdominal pain, weight loss, melena, muscle aches, renal failure	Young adults; Patients with hepatitis B	
Kawasaki Disease	Small and medium sized	Fever, oral and conjunctival erythema, desquamating rash, lymphadenitis	Children	
Microscopic Polyangiitis	Arterioles, capillaries	Hemoptysis, hematuria, proteinuria, weakness, palpable cutaneous purpura		p- or c-ANCA
Wegener Granulomatosis	Small and medium sized	Hemoptysis, perforation of nasal septum, renal failure		c-ANCA
Thromboangiitis Obliterans	Small and medium sized	Cyanosis of the hands, claudication of the foot, ulceration of the distal extremities	Young male smokers	

COMPREHENSION QUESTIONS

[17.1] A 70-year-old woman presents with recurrent headaches, blurred vision, and a 1-week history of joint pain and flu-like symptoms. Physical examination finds focal tenderness in her right temporal area, and laboratory examination reveals a markedly elevated erythrocyte sedimentation rate. A biopsy from her right temporal artery reveals granulomatous inflammation with giant cells in the inner tunica media of the vessel wall. Without treatment, what is the worst complication associated with this individual's disease?

A. Aspiration pneumonia
B. Embolic stroke
C. Hearing loss
D. Irreversible blindness
E. Renal failure

[17.2] A 20-year-old woman presents with increasing fatigue, muscle pain, and visual disturbances. Physical examination finds weak pulses in her upper extremities, and further evaluation finds thickening of the aortic arch and narrowing of the blood vessels that originate from the aortic arch. Which of the following is the most likely diagnosis?

A. Goodpasture disease
B. Kawasaki disease
C. Polyarteritis nodosa
D. Takayasu disease
E. Wegener granulomatosis

[17.3] A 36-year-old woman presents with muscle pain, fever, and chronic sinusitis. Physical examination finds mucosal ulcerations of the nasopharynx and signs of renal disease. A biopsy from her nasopharynx reveals a necrotizing vasculitis with chronic inflammatory cells and giant cells surrounding localized necrotic areas. The presence of which of the types of autoantibodies listed below would be most consistent with a diagnosis of Wegener granulomatosis?

A. Antigliadin antibodies
B. Antimitochondrial antibodies
C. Antineutrophil cytoplasmic antibodies
D. Antinucleolar antibodies
E. Antismooth muscle antibodies

Answers

[17.1] **D.** Temporal arteritis is a common type of vasculitis that typically affects the superficial blood vessels in the head. Patients with temporal arteritis are usually older than 50 years of age and develop signs of headaches, jaw claudication, and visual abnormalities. About half of these patients develop systemic symptoms, including malaise, joint pains, and muscle aches (polymyalgia rheumatica). Microscopic examination of a temporal artery biopsy may reveal granulomatous inflammation with giant cells or breaks in the internal elastic lamina. Inflammation of the temporal artery is associated with an increased risk for thrombosis of the ophthalmic artery, which can cause irreversible blindness. Treatment with corticosteroids can reduce the risk of this complication.

[17.2] **D.** Takayasu disease, which also is called aortic arch syndrome, is a type of vasculitis that primarily involves the medium- and large-size vessels of the aortic arch and its branches. It also is called pulseless disease because of the decreased blood flow to the upper extremities. Signs and symptoms produced by this decreased blood flow include visual disturbances and weak upper extremity pulses.

[17.3] **C.** Wegener granulomatosis (WG) is a disease characterized by focal necrotizing vasculitis and acute necrotizing granulomas of the upper and lower respiratory tract. Renal involvement is common. The clinical signs associated with WG include perforation of the nasal septum, chronic sinusitis, hemoptysis, and hematuria. Patients with WG who have renal involvement may have a positive test for the presence of antineutrophil cytoplasmic antibodies, which are antibodies directed against the primary granules within neutrophils. There are two basic types of ANCA: p-ANCA and c-ANCA. p-ANCA refers to perinuclear staining, and c-ANCA indicates cytoplasmic staining after ethanol fixation and immunofluorescence. Patients with WG most commonly have c-ANCA.

PATHOLOGY PEARLS

- Temporal arteritis classically presents in patients older than 50 years with sudden-onset temporal headache, palpable cord-like nodules over the temporal region, vision changes, and polymyalgia rheumatica.
- The most common complication of temporal arteritis is irreversible blindness caused by thrombosis of the ophthalmic artery.
- The clinical presentation of temporal arteritis should be treated immediately with corticosteroids, with a biopsy performed afterward for a definitive diagnosis.

REFERENCES

Schoen FJ. Blood vessels. In: Kumar V, Assas AK, Fausto N, eds. Robbins and Cotran Pathologic Basis of Disease, 7th ed. Philadelphia, PA: Elsevier Saunders, 2004:836–9.

Schoen FJ. Blood vessels. In: Mitchell RN, Kumar V, Abbas AK, et al., eds. Pocket Companion to Robbins and Cotran Pathologic Basis of Disease, 7th ed. Philadelphia, PA: Saunders, 2006:276–80.

CASE 18

A 60-year-old woman seeks medical attention for soreness and oozing from the nipple of her left breast. She denies trauma to the breast. On physical examination, there is fissuring and ulceration of the areola and nipple. Biopsy of the breast is performed, and the skin of the nipple is shown in Figure 18-1.

- **What is the most likely diagnosis?**
- **What is the clinical significance of this finding?**

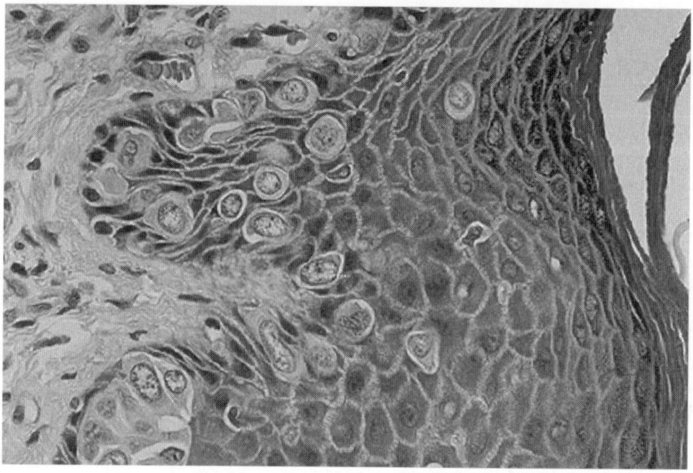

Figure 18-1. Breast biopsy.

ANSWERS TO CASE 18: PAGET DISEASE OF THE BREAST

Summary: A 60-year-old woman complains of soreness and oozing from the nipple of her left breast. On examination, there is fissuring and ulceration of the areola and nipple. Biopsy of the breast skin shows large periodic acid-Schiff (PAS)-positive cells with pale-staining cytoplasm within the epidermis.

- **Most likely diagnosis:** Paget disease of the breast.
- **Clinical significance of this finding:** Underlying adenocarcinoma of the breast is often present.

CLINICAL CORRELATION

This patient presents with many of the typical clinical symptoms of Paget disease. Paget disease is a rare form of breast cancer that occurs in approximately 1 percent of all breast cancer patients. Patients usually present with symptoms in the sixth decade of life, similar to other common forms of breast cancer. Initial symptoms include erythema and mild eczematous changes of the nipple skin. Scaling and flaking of the nipple may advance to crusting, skin erosion, and ulceration with exudation or frank discharge. A patient also may have pruritus, tingling, burning, pain, or hypersensitivity around the skin lesion. Approximately 40 to 50 percent of all Paget skin lesions have an underlying breast mass.

The differential diagnosis for patients with scaling skin and erythema of the nipple-areolar complex includes eczema, contact dermatitis, postradiation dermatitis, and Paget disease. The presence of bilateral eczematous changes on the nipple-areolar complex is seen more commonly with eczema and contact dermatitis but can occur with Paget disease. Eczema often involves the areola, sparing the nipple (rarely seen with Paget disease). Patients with a history of radiation treatment may have postradiation dermatitis. Because of the eczematous initial appearance of Paget disease, patients often are started on topical steroids or antibiotics, with transient improvement of symptoms, delaying the diagnosis by an average of 6 months.

Paget disease of the breast invariably has been associated with underlying ductal carcinoma in situ and less commonly with invasive ductal carcinoma. Reports have cited the incidence of underlying carcinoma being as high as >99 percent. Traditionally, Paget disease has been treated with mastectomy; however, recent reports have shown that more conservative treatment may be possible for select patients. A patient's prognosis is dependent on the extent of the underlying carcinoma and the stage of the disease, similar to that of females with other types of breast cancer.

APPROACH TO PAGET DISEASE AND DUCTAL CARCINOMA IN SITU

Objectives

- List the different types of breast cancer.
- Describe the most common causes of breast cancer.
- Describe the presentation of Paget disease.

Definitions

Ductal carcinoma in situ: Considered a malignant lesion with dysplastic cells of the breast ducts that do not invade beneath the basement membrane.

Paget disease of the nipple: A rare type of breast cancer that presents as a scaly red crusty lesion of the nipple or areola.

DISCUSSION

When one is evaluating a patient with a breast lesion, carcinoma must always be considered. The risk of breast cancer is dependent on many factors, such as **age,** family history, and the specific characteristics of the lesion in question. Many breast cancers can be localized with aid of mammogram screening before symptoms or lesions are clinically apparent. Several clinical features are common to all invasive cancers of the breast, including a **fixed position, retraction and dimpling of the skin or nipple, metastases** through lymphohematogenous routes with a pattern of nodal spread influenced by the location of the tumor, and distant metastases to any organ of the body.

The diagnosis of **Paget disease** often is delayed because of its **eczematous appearance,** and this delay can lead to a diagnosis at advanced stages (see Figure 18-2). When patients present with symptoms suggestive of Paget disease, a **diagnosis** should be attempted with **scrape cytology, superficial epidermal shave biopsy, a 2-mm punch biopsy, a wedge incisional biopsy, or rarely nipple excision.** An ideal specimen contains adequate epidermis to provide Paget cells and lactiferous ducts. The **histologic hallmark** finding for Paget disease is the presence of **Paget cells** in the epidermis of the nipple; these cells are **large with pale-staining cytoplasm and nuclei with prominent nucleoli.** Various stains for mucin, epithelial membrane antigens, and low-molecular-weight keratins further characterize these cells. Paget cells usually are located between the normal keratinocytes of the nipple epidermis and the basement membrane. The keratinocyte layer frequently is disrupted, allowing serous fluid to seep through, causing the characteristic crusting and scaling of the nipple skin. Paget cells do not invade through the dermal basement membrane and therefore are a form of ductal carcinoma in situ.

Noninvasive (in situ) intraductal carcinomas account for approximately 20 to 30 percent of carcinomas of the breast and today are detected more frequently with the use of mammography. This malignant population of cells lacks the ability to invade through the basement membrane and thus is incapable of distant metastasis. These cells can spread throughout the ductal system and

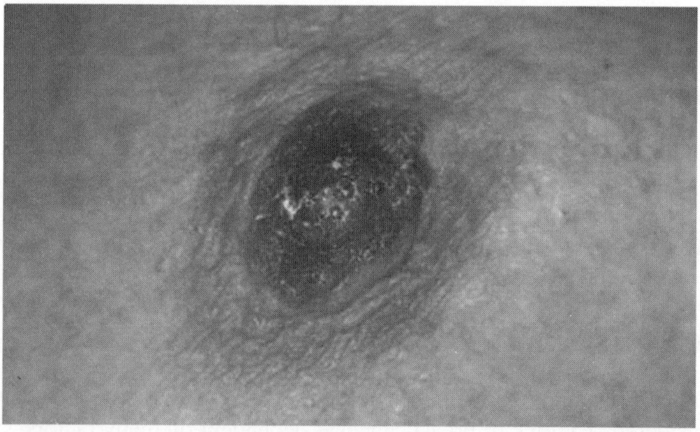

Figure 18-2. Mammary Paget disease: A sharply demarcated red plaque mimicking eczema or psoriasis on the nipple. The plaque is slightly indurated and there is slight scaling; any red, eczema-like lesion on the nipple and areola that does not respond to topical *corticosteroids* should be biopsied. *(Reused, with permission, from Wolff K, Johnson RA, Suurmond D.* Fitzpatrick's Color Atlas and Synopsis of Clinical Dermatology, 5th ed. *New York: McGraw-Hill, 2005:495.)*

may spread up the main duct and into the nipple skin, resulting in the clinical appearance of Paget disease.

Invasive ductal carcinoma is the **most common type of breast cancer,** accounting for 65 to 80 percent of all mammary cancers. There is usually a marked increase in dense, fibrous tissue stroma, giving the tumor a hard consistency. On gross examination, the tumor averages 1 to 2 cm in size and has a **stony-hard consistency.** The tumor consists of malignant duct lining cells deposed in cords, solid cell nests, tubules, and glands. The cells invade the connective tissue stroma and frequently invade perivascular and perineural spaces. See Table 18-1 for signs, symptoms, and characteristic features of each type of breast disease.

Table 18-1
BREAST DISEASE

TYPE	SIGNS/SYMPTOMS	CHARACTERISTIC FEATURES
BENIGN		
Fibrocystic disease	Diffuse breast pain, many bilateral lesions	Changes with menstrual cycle (worse right before menstruation)
Fibroadenoma	Mobile, firm mass with distinct edges	Does not change with menstrual cycle
Intraductal papilloma	Unilateral bloody nipple discharge	Does not increase cancer risk unless multiple lesions present
MALIGNANT		
Ductal carcinoma in situ (DCIS)	Usually nonpalpable; seen as irregularly shaped calcifications on mammography	No basement membrane invasion
Invasive ductal	Firm, fibrous mass, with indistinct margins	Most common breast cancer
Invasive lobular	Vague appearance on mammogram	Often bilateral
Inflammatory	Erythema, painful breast	Rapidly progressive; lymphatic involvement, so frequently metastatic upon presentation
Paget's disease of the breast	Eczematous patches on nipple	Normally seen with an underlying ductal carcinoma

COMPREHENSION QUESTIONS

[18.1] A 65-year-old woman complains of itching and scaliness of the right breast nipple area. A 1-cm palpable mass is felt underlying the skin. A biopsy confirms Paget disease. Which of the following is likely to be an association?

A. Infiltrating ductal carcinoma
B. Lobular carcinoma in situ
C. Invasive lobular carcinoma
D. Intraductal papilloma

[18.2] The microscopy of the biopsy of the patient in question 18.1 most likely demonstrates which of the following?

A. Fibrovascular cores of tall columnar cells extending into ducts
B. Large PAS-positive cells with pale-staining cytoplasm and nuclei with prominent nucleoli
C. Tissue with increased stromal cellularity and cytologic atypia and a leaflike architectural structure
D. Well-formed tubules lined by a single layer of well-differentiated cells

[18.3] Which of the following is thc most common location for extramammary Paget disease?

A. Liver
B. Lung
C. Kidney
D. Penis
E. Vulva

Answers

[18.1] **A.** Infiltrating and in situ ductal carcinomas are the most common underlying malignancies associated with Paget disease.

[18.2] **B.** Paget disease is characterized by large PAS-positive cells with pale cytoplasm and prominent nucleoli. When a mass is palpable, invasive carcinoma is common, whereas in the absence of a mass, ductal carcinoma in situ often is encountered.

[18.3] **E.** Paget disease may be found in the vulva in postmenopausal females, with symptoms similar to those of Paget disease of the breast. The same appearance of the Paget cells is noted; however, the risk of underlying adenocarcinoma is far less (about 3 to 5%) with vulvar disease.

PATHOLOGY PEARLS

- Paget disease consists of a scaly red oozing pruritic skin lesion of the nipple, which on biopsy reveals large PAS-positive cells with pale cytoplasm and prominent nucleoli.
- Females with Paget disease of the breast often have an underlying carcinoma.
- The most common type of invasive breast cancer is invasive (infiltrating) ductal carcinoma.

REFERENCES

Abeloff MD, Armitae JO, Lichter AS, et al. Clinical Oncology, 2nd ed. New York: Churchill Livingstone, 2000.

DeVita VT, Hellman S, Rosenberg SA. Cancer: Principles and Practice of Oncology, 6th ed. New York: Lippincott Williams & Wilkins, 2001.

Harris JR, Lippman ME, Morrow M, et al. Diseases of the Breast, 2nd ed. New York: Lippincott Williams & Wilkins, 2000.

Lester SC. The breast. In: Kumar V, Assas AK, Fausto N, eds. Robbins and Cotran Pathologic Basis of Disease, 7th ed. Philadelphia, PA: Elsevier Saunders, 2004:1129–49.

Lester SC. The breast. In: Mitchell RN, Kumar V, Abbas AK, et al., eds. Pocket Companion to Robbins and Cotran Pathologic Basis of Disease, 7th ed. Philadelphia, PA: Saunders, 2006:552–60.

Stenchever MA, Droegemueller W, Herbst AL, et al. Comprehensive Gynecology, 4th ed. St. Louis, MO: Mosby, 2002.

❖ CASE 19

During a routine monthly self-examination of her breasts, a 25-year-old woman discovers an ill-defined firm area in the right breast. The patient states that both of her breasts become somewhat tender during menses. Her physician is able to palpate similar areas in both breasts. There is no nipple discharge, skin induration or redness, or axillary lymph node enlargement.

◆ **What is the most likely diagnosis?**

◆ **What is the clinical significance of these findings?**

ANSWERS TO CASE 19: FIBROCYSTIC CHANGES OF THE BREAST

Summary: During a routine monthly self-examination of her breasts, a 25-year-old woman discovers an ill-defined firm area in her right breast. Her physician is able to palpate similar areas in her left breast. There is no nipple discharge, skin induration or redness, or axillary lymph node enlargement.

- ◆ **Most likely diagnosis:** Fibrocystic changes of the breast.
- ◆ **Clinical significance of these findings:** May obscure the examination of other underlying breast pathology.

CLINICAL CORRELATION

A 25-year-old woman notes breast lumps in both breasts. They are ill defined, bilateral, and slightly tender with menses. No dominant mass is palpated, and there is no adenopathy. This is a classic description of fibrocystic changes of the breast, a condition of benign nonproliferative breast changes without an increased risk of cancer. Fibrosis with chronic inflammation and stromal reaction often is seen on biopsy specimens. Cysts of various sizes are also typical, sometimes leading to a serous yellowish or greenish nipple discharge. Mammography appears as dense breasts with cystic changes. These changes are responsive to hormonal alterations; hence, the symptoms seem to worsen just before or during menses.

APPROACH TO FIBROCYSTIC BREAST CHANGES

Objectives

- Describe the clinical features of fibrocystic changes of the breast.
- Describe the clinical features of fibroadenoma.
- Describe the presentation of intraductal papilloma.

Definitions

Duct ectasia: A condition characterized by the dilation of major ducts, usually in the subareolar region, and various degrees of inflammation and fibrosis around the ducts. It is seen at autopsy in approximately 25 percent of women.

Fat necrosis: Focal necrosis of fat tissue in the breast, followed by an inflammatory reaction. It is an uncommon lesion that tends to occur as an isolated, sharply localized area. Many patients have a history of trauma. It is possible to confuse it with tumor.

Blue-domed cysts: Benign cysts found in breast tissue, filled with fluid that appears blue when seen through the cyst wall.

Fibrosis: The process of fibrosis includes the formation of new blood vessels, migration and proliferation of fibroblasts, deposition of extracellular matrix, and remodeling. Fibrosis replaces tissue damage. Newly formed connective tissue is laid down to replace nonfunctioning parenchymal cells.

Intracanalicular fibroadenoma: Fibroadenoma that is characterized by proliferative stroma that compresses and distorts glands into slit-like spaces.

Pericanalicular fibroadenoma: Fibroadenoma in which the glands retain their round shape.

Sclerosing adenosis: Increased numbers of distorted and compressed acini.

DISCUSSION

Fibrocystic Changes

Fibrocystic changes are the most common disorder of the breast. They are found in females between adolescence and menopause. Fibrocystic changes are characterized clinically as lumpy breasts, usually bilateral, with midcycle tenderness. The cyclic symptoms are hypothesized to be due to increased activity of or sensitivity to estrogen or decreased progesterone activity. **There are three principal patterns of morphologic change: cyst formation, fibrosis, and adenosis.**

Fibrocystic changes are usually multifocal, but some single large cysts are found. As a result of cystic dilation of ducts and lobules, the involved areas, on palpation, have an ill-defined diffuse increase in consistency and discrete nodularity. Larger, single cysts create the greatest concern for possible tumors. Secretory products within the cysts calcify, resulting in microcalcifications. Unopened, these cysts appear brown to blue **(blue-dome cysts)** because of the contained semitranslucent turbid fluid. **Frequently, cysts are lined by large polygonal cells with an eosinophilic cytoplasm, with small, round dark nuclei resembling apocrine epithelium of sweat glands. This lining is called apocrine metaplasia.** These cysts often are found in normal breast tissue and are almost always benign. Epithelial overgrowth and papillary projections are also common in cysts lined by apocrine epithelium. In larger cysts, lining cells may be flattened or totally atrophic. Cysts frequently rupture and release secretory material into the surrounding breast tissue; this can create chronic inflammation and fibrosis, which can increase the palpable firmness of the breast.

Adenosis is an increase in the number of acinar units per lobule. A physiologic adenosis occurs during pregnancy, but this change also can be seen in nonpregnant women. **The gland lumens become enlarged but do not become distorted** as in another proliferative lesion, described below, called sclerosing adenosis. Calcifications are occasionally present in the lumens of patients with adenosis.

Fibrocystic changes do not increase the risk of developing cancer. However, these changes may come to clinical attention when they mimic carcinoma by producing palpable lumps, mammographic densities or calcifications, or nipple discharge. Cysts and fibrosis produce "lumpy bumpy" findings on physical examination that may make detection of other breast masses more difficult. Single, enlarged cysts may form densities or palpable masses but usually can be diagnosed by disappearance of the mass after fine needle aspiration of cyst contents. Cysts containing solid debris or clusters of small cysts are more difficult to diagnose and may require surgical excision. Calcifications are found commonly in cysts and adenosis and often form mammographically suspicious clusters. Cystic changes rarely are associated with spontaneous unilateral nipple discharge. Table 19-1 describes interventions that help or exacerbate the symptoms.

Fibroadenoma

Fibroadenoma is the **most common benign breast tumor in females younger than age 25.** It is composed of both fibrous and glandular tissue. The tumors are frequently multiple and bilateral. Young females usually present with a palpable mass, and older females with mammographic density. Fibroadenomas are associated with a mild increase in the risk of subsequent breast cancer, especially when they are associated with fibrocystic changes, proliferative breast disease, or a family history of breast cancer.

Fibroadenomas grow as nodules that usually are sharply demarcated and freely movable from the surrounding breast tissue. These tumors frequently occur in the upper outer quadrant of the breast. They vary in size from less than 1 cm in diameter to 10 to 15 cm in diameter. Most are removed surgically when they are over 2 to 4 cm in diameter.

Table 19-1

CLINICAL FEATURES OF FIBROCYSTIC CHANGE

TREATMENTS THAT HELP SYMPTOMS	FOODS THAT WORSEN SYMPTOMS
Vitamin E	Caffeine
Nonsteroidal anti-inflammatory drugs	Chocolate
Evening primrose oil	Cola
Oral contraceptives	Tea

The importance of performing monthly breast self-exams cannot be overemphasized.

Grossly, fibroadenomas are grayish-white and often contain slit-like spaces. Microscopically, there is **delicate cellular fibroblastic stroma that resembles intralobular stroma.** This stroma encloses glandular and cystic spaces lined by epithelium. The epithelium may be surrounded by stroma or compressed and distorted by it. Fibroadenomas are subclassified into two types, intracanalicular and pericanalicular, depending on how the stroma affects the epithelial component of the glandlike structures. The glandular epithelium of fibroadenomas is hormonally responsive, and a slight increase in size may occur during the late phases of each menstrual cycle. An increase in size resulting from lactational changes or even from infarction and inflammation may lead to a fibroadenoma mimicking carcinoma during pregnancy. Regression usually occurs postmenopause.

Intraductal Papilloma

An **intraductal papilloma** is the **most common** cause of **bloody,** usually **unilateral, nipple discharge.** Intraductal papillomas are **benign tumors of major lactiferous ducts.** They are manifested clinically by a **serous or bloody discharge.** The discharge is most often spontaneous and easily reproducible on palpation from a single duct orifice. Most intraductal papillomas are located within 1 to 2 cm of the areolar edge in the major ducts. **Intraductal papillomas must be distinguished from carcinoma because breast cancer also can present with bloody nipple discharge.**

Inflammatory Reactions

Inflammatory reactions include fat necrosis, duct ectasia, and acute mastitis. Acute mastitis most commonly occurs during breast-feeding. The breast is vulnerable to bacterial infection because of the development of cracks and fissures in the nipples. From this portal of entry, bacteria invade the breast. Mastitis is rare outside the postpartum period. The disease is usually unilateral.

Grossly, *Staphylococcus aureus* tends to produce a localized area of acute inflammation that progresses to the formation of single or multiple abscesses. *Streptococcus* tends to cause a more diffusely spreading infection. When extensive necrosis occurs, the destroyed breast substance is replaced by fibrous scar as a permanent residual of the inflammatory process. Such scarring may create a localized area of increased density that sometimes is accompanied by retraction of the skin.

Fat Necrosis

Fat necrosis usually results from **trauma to the breast.** Grossly, the lesion may consist of hemorrhage in the early stages and, later, central liquefactive necrosis of fat. It may become an **ill-defined nodule of gray-white firm tissue** containing small foci of chalky white or hemorrhagic debris. Microscopically, the central focus of necrotic fat is surrounded by lipid-filled macrophages and neutrophils. Then progressive fibroblastic proliferation, increased vascularization, and histiocytic infiltration wall off the focus. By that time, the central necrotic fat cells have disappeared and may be represented only by foamy, lipid-laden macrophages and crystalline lipids. Eventually the focus is replaced by scar tissue or is encysted and walled off by fibrosis. On **mammography,** fat necrosis often has the **characteristic appearance of a calcified cyst** and sometimes is characterized by a cluster of calcifications that can be confused with the appearance of breast cancer.

Sclerosing Adenosis

Sclerosing adenosis is defined as **proliferation of stromal tissue in the breast with an increased number of acini.** Small lesions commonly present as **calcifications** on **mammography,** and larger lesions may form densities or palpable masses. Grossly, sclerosing adenosis sometimes has a hard cartilaginous consistency that can be mistaken for breast cancer. When sectioned into pieces, the area is usually not as well localized as breast carcinoma is.

Microscopically, the number of acini per terminal duct is increased to at least twice the number found in normal breast tissue. The acini are compressed and distorted in the center but dilated at the periphery. Myoepithelial cells also can be prominent. There is also a presence of stromal fibrosis, which can compress the lumens to create the appearance of solid cords or double strands of cells lying within dense breast tissue.

COMPREHENSION QUESTIONS

[19.1] A 33-year-old woman presents because during her routine monthly breast self-examination she thought her breasts felt more "lumpy" than usual. Physical examination finds an ill-defined firm area in her right breast. Because of a family history of breast cancer, she is very concerned about this area, and a biopsy is performed. Histologic examination reveals typical fibrocystic changes. Some of the smaller cysts are lined by large polygonal cells with abundant eosinophilic cytoplasm and small, round dark nuclei. Which of the terms listed below best describes this abnormality?

A. Apocrine metaplasia
B. Atypical hyperplasia
C. Intraductal papillomatosis
D. Radial scar
E. Sclerosing adenosis

[19.2] A 22-year-old woman presents with a rubbery 1.5-cm mass in the upper outer quadrant of her right breast. A biopsy from this mass reveals a well-circumscribed lesion consisting of a mixture of delicate stromal fibrous tissue and glandular and cystic spaces. The stromal cells are not increased in number. No mitoses or cellular atypia is seen. What is the correct name for this lesion?

A. Cystadenoma
B. Fibroadenoma
C. Fibroangioma
D. Leiomyoma
E. Papilloma

[19.3] A 30-year-old woman with a subareolar intraductal papilloma of the breast most likely would present with which of the following clinical signs?

A. A bloody nipple discharge
B. A cystic lesion of the nipple
C. A milky nipple discharge
D. A scaly lesion of the nipple
E. A thick cheesy nipple discharge

Answers

[19.1] **A.** Fibrocystic change of the breast is a common finding in the adult female breast. It is typically bilateral and may vary with the menstrual cycle or regress with pregnancy. The three basic histologic patterns seen with fibrocystic change are fibrosis, cyst formation, and adenosis. Grossly, these cysts may have a blue color (blue-domed cysts); histologically, they may be lined by large polygonal cells with abundant eosinophilic cytoplasms and small, round dark nuclei. Because these cells resemble the apocrine epithelium of sweat glands, this histologic change is referred to as apocrine metaplasia.

[19.2] **B.** Fibroadenoma is the most common benign breast tumor in women. They typically occur in the upper outer quadrant of the breast in females between the ages of 20 and 35. Grossly, they are firm rubbery nodules that are well circumscribed and have a uniform tan color. They are estrogen-sensitive and may enlarge during pregnancy. Histologically, they are composed of both fibrous and glandular tissue. The stroma is loose (delicate), and there is no increase in the number of stromal cells. Mitoses and atypia are not present in fibroadenomas.

[19.3] **A.** Intraductal papillomas of the breast are the most common cause of a bloody nipple discharge in a female. These benign tumors are found within the major lactiferous ducts, usually near the nipple. Thus, they also are called subareolar papillomas. Histologic sections of intraductal papillomas, which must be distinguished from carcinomas, show papillary structures that are lined by a layer of epithelial and myoepithelial cells.

PATHOLOGY PEARLS

- ❖ Fibrocystic changes diagnosed clinically as irregular lumpiness of bilateral breasts consist histologically of cyst formation, fibrosis, and adenosis.
- ❖ Fibrocystic changes do not increase the risk of breast cancer.
- ❖ Fibroadenomas are benign smooth muscle tumors of the breast and are the most common benign breast tumor in a female less than 25 years old.
- ❖ Sclerosing adenosis, which is identified as proliferation of stromal tissue in the breast with an increased number of acini, commonly present as calcifications on mammography.
- ❖ Fat necrosis, usually caused by trauma, is characterized by ill-defined nodules of gray-white, firm tissue with small areas of calcification.
- ❖ Intraductal papilloma is the most common cause of bloody nipple discharge and typically involves one duct and without a mass. Breast cancer needs to be ruled out.

REFERENCES

Dupont WD, Page DL, Parl FF, et al. Long-term risk of breast cancer in women with fibroadenoma. N Engl J Med 1994;331:10.

Falkenberry SS. Nipple discharge. Obstet Gynecol Clin North Am 2002;29(1):21–29.

Lester SC. The breast. In: Kumar V, Assas AK, Fausto N, eds. Robbins and Cotran Pathologic Basis of Disease, 7th ed. Philadelphia, PA: Elsevier Saunders, 2004:1120–40.

Lester SC. The breast. In: Mitchell RN, Kumar V, Abbas AK, et al., eds. Pocket Companion to Robbins and Cotran Pathologic Basis of Disease, 7th ed. Philadelphia, PA: Saunders, 2006:551–60.

Schneider AS, Szanto PA. Board Review Series: Pathology. Philadelphia, PA: Lippincott Williams & Wilkins, 1993.

Townsend CM, Beauchamp RD, Evers BM, et al. Sabiston Textbook of Surgery, 16th ed. Philadelphia, PA: Saunders, 2001.

CASE 20

A 35-year-old woman notices a milky discharge from both nipples. She underwent a bilateral tubal ligation after the birth of her last child, and a pregnancy test is negative. She has not had a menstrual period for the last 8 months. She complains of intermittent headaches and some difficulty with her peripheral vision.

- **What is the most likely diagnosis?**
- **What is the best diagnostic test?**

ANSWERS TO CASE 20: PROLACTIN ADENOMA

Summary: A 35-year-old woman has bilateral nipple discharge, headache, and visual abnormalities.

- **Most likely diagnosis:** Prolactin adenoma.
- **Diagnostic tests:** Basal prolactin levels and magnetic resonance imaging (MRI) of the pituitary with gadolinium or computed tomography (CT) imaging.

CLINICAL CORRELATION

This 35-year-old woman complains of headache, difficulty with her peripheral vision, amenorrhea, and galactorrhea. This symptom complex is consistent with hyperprolactinemia caused by a prolactin-secreting adenoma. The pituitary tumor impinges on the optic chiasm, leading to headache and bitemporal hemianopia. The elevated prolactin level causes milk production in the breast and also inhibits gonadotropin-releasing hormone at the level of the hypothalamus. Thus, gonadotropin levels fall, and the ovaries become quiescent. The patient is in a hypoestrogenic state. Prolactin levels in this patient probably would demonstrate a marked elevation. Imaging of the sella turcica with MRI probably would show an adenoma. Medical therapy is generally the first option with these tumors.

APPROACH TO ANTERIOR PITUITARY PATHOLOGY

Objectives

- Know the most common pituitary adenoma.
- Describe the visual defect associated with a pituitary adenoma.
- Describe the common causes of hyperprolactinemia.

Definitions

Pituitary tumors: Neoplastic growths that are classified by the type of hormone they produce and by their size: Microadenomas are less than 1 cm in diameter, and macroadenomas are more than 1 cm in diameter.

Hyperprolactinemia: Increased levels of prolactin (higher than 20 μg/L) caused by a prolactin adenoma, physiologic hyperprolactinemia in pregnancy, nipple stimulation, damage to the dopaminergic neurons of the hypothalamus, and trauma or drugs blocking dopamine receptors.

Hypopituitarism: Decreased secretion of pituitary hormones ensuing from diseases of the hypothalamus or the pituitary; it can be a congenital or acquired abnormality. Most cases are due to destructive processes such as tumors, ischemic necrosis of the pituitary, and the empty sella syndrome.

DISCUSSION

The **pituitary gland** is located in the **sella turcica** at the base of the brain. It is a small gland that measures approximately 1 cm in diameter and weighs approximately 0.5 g. The pituitary has two lobes: the anterior lobe, which is derived from the Rathke pouch, and the posterior lobe. Its proximity to the optic chiasm causes the typical visual symptoms (bitemporal hemianopia) (see Figure 20-1). Histologically, the anterior pituitary contains eosinophilic cells (growth hormone and prolactin), basophilic cells (gonadotropins, adrenocorticotropic hormone, melanocyte-stimulating hormone, and thyroid-stimulating hormone) and chromophobic cells. The anterior pituitary hormones, except prolactin, are controlled by releasing hormones from the hypothalamus that pass through the hypophyseal portal system. The posterior pituitary or neurohypophysis stores oxytocin and vasopressin, hormones that are made by the hypothalamus. These hormones then are released by exocytosis into the systemic circulation.

Prolactinomas

Prolactinomas are the **most common pituitary adenoma,** accounting for approximately 30 to 40 percent. They are composed of lactotrophic cells (eosinophilic and chromophobic cells). Even the smallest tumor can secrete enough prolactin for hyperprolactinemia to occur. Prolactinoma causes galactorrhea and amenorrhea in women, and men may experience decreased libido, impotence, and, rarely, gynecomastia and galactorrhea.

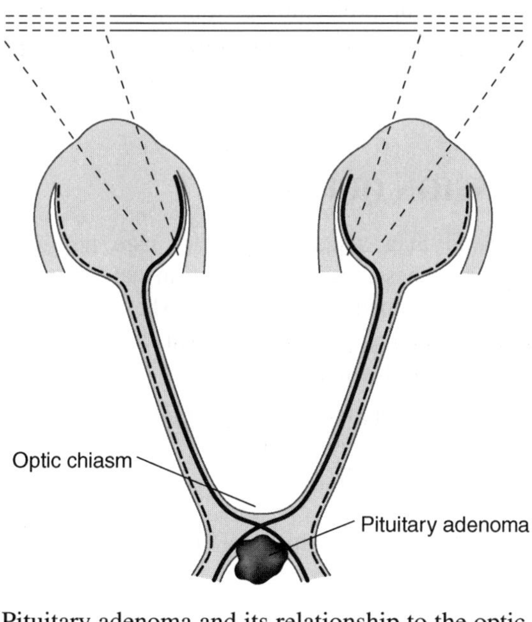

Figure 20-1. Pituitary adenoma and its relationship to the optic chiasm.

Hyperprolactinemia

Numerous conditions can cause elevation of the prolactin level. **Hypothyroidism, pregnancy, medications, and pituitary adenomas are the most common causes.** Thyrotropin-releasing hormone (TRH) acts as a prolactin-releasing hormone; its elevation in hypothyroidism is thought to be the mechanism of hyperprolactinemia. Correction of the hypothyroidism usually leads to normalization of the prolactin level. **Drugs** that may produce a hyperprolactinemic state include **neuroleptic drugs** (dopamine receptor antagonists) and reserpine (inhibits dopamine storage). Other causes include **estrogens, renal failure, stress, and herpes zoster of the chest wall.**

Hypopituitarism

Ischemic necrosis of the pituitary gland is a significant cause of hypopituitarism, causing damage to more than 75 percent of the gland. Infarction of the anterior lobe may be seen in **Sheehan syndrome** as a result of hemorrhage or shock occurring postpartum. The presenting sign may be inability to lactate, amenorrhea, and symptoms of adrenal insufficiency.

Another cause of hypopituitarism may be pituitary adenomas, by direct destruction or compression of the pituitary or by impaired blood supply resulting from pituitary stalk compression.

Treatment

As first-line treatment for prolactin-secreting adenomas, bromocriptine or cabergoline (dopamine agonists) should be used, even if the patient exhibits visual disturbances, because it decreases the size of the adenoma 25 to 50 percent. Transsphenoidal resection of the adenoma is an alternative treatment.

COMPREHENSION QUESTIONS

[20.1] A 67-year-old man visits his primary care physician because of headaches, weakness, and an increase in hat and glove size. Blood pressure is determined to be elevated. The workup reveals a tumor originating within the pituitary gland. This tumor is most likely secreting which of the following substances?

A. Adrenocorticotropic hormone (ACTH)
B. Antidiuretic hormone (ADH)
C. Growth hormone (GH)
D. Prolactin
E. Thyroid-stimulating hormone (TSH)

[20.2] The inability to lactate after delivery and prolonged amenorrhea due to gonadotrophin deficiency are classic signs of which of the following abnormalities?

A. Acromegaly
B. Diabetes insipidus
C. Hyperprolactinemia
D. Kallmann syndrome
E. Sheehan syndrome

[20.3] A 29-year-old woman complains of cold intolerance, fatigue, and dry coarse skin. Her prolactin is noted to be twice the normal level. Which of the following is the most likely explanation?

A. Herpes simplex virus infection
B. Craniopharyngioma
C. Prolactin-secreting adenoma
D. Increased thyrotropin-releasing hormone

Answers

[20.1] **C.** Growth hormone-secreting adenomas are the second most common form of pituitary adenomas. In children, excessive GH secretion may result in gigantism (extreme height and prognathism) if it occurs before closure of epiphyses. In adults, it results in acromegaly, causing facial changes, hyperhidrosis and oily skin, headaches, paresthesias/carpal tunnel syndrome, diastolic hypertension, goiter, diabetes mellitus, visual field defects, deepening of the voice, and weakness. These patients are at increased risk of gastrointestinal cancers. To make a diagnosis, basal insulinlike growth factor-1 (IGF-1) levels are measured. Treatment consists of surgery or radiation.

[20.2] **E.** Sheehan syndrome refers to postpartum necrosis of the pituitary necrosis (although the term now also extends to the nonobstetric population). Hypotension during pregnancy or at the time of delivery may cause sudden infarction of the anterior lobe of the pituitary because it is supplied by a low pressure portal network of blood vessels. In addition, physiologic hyperplasia of the pituitary normally occurs during pregnancy and this increases the interstitial pressure in the fixed space of the sella. The postpartum necrosis spares the posterior pituitary because it has a separate arterial blood supply, which is under high pressure. The classic first sign of Sheehan syndrome is decreased or complete failure of lactation after delivery due to prolactin deficiency. The next sign is secondary (persistent) amenorrhea due to decreased release of gonadotropins.

[20.3] **D.** Hypothyroidism leads to increased hypothalamic secretion of thyrotropin-releasing hormone, which acts as a prolactin-releasing factor. This patient has symptoms of hypothyroidism: cold intolerance, fatigue, and coarse skin. Correction of the hypothyroidism would lead to resolution of the hyperprolactinemia.

PATHOLOGY PEARLS

- Prolactinoma is the most common type of pituitary adenoma.
- Prolactin is inhibited through the action of dopamine and is released by thyroid-releasing hormone associated with hypothyroidism.
- Bilateral hemianopia is a classic visual field defect associated with pituitary adenomas.
- The symptoms most often seen are galactorrhea and amenorrhea in females and decreased libido and weakness in men.

REFERENCES

Maitra A, Abbas AK. The endocrine system. In: Kumar V, Assas AK, Fausto N, eds. Robbins and Cotran Pathologic Basis of Disease, 7th ed. Philadelphia, PA: Elsevier Saunders, 2004:1150–60.

Maitra A. The endocrine system. In: Mitchell RN, Kumar V, Abbas AK, et al., eds. Pocket Companion to Robbins and Cotran Pathologic Basis of Disease, 7th ed. Philadelphia, PA: Saunders, 2006:561–7.

❖ CASE 21

A 35-year-old man develops severe headaches and is found to have a blood pressure of 200/120 mm Hg. He also notes anxiety, palpitations, and sweating. He has been in good health and has had normal blood pressure readings on several occasions. The urine drug screen is negative. Further evaluation reveals a left suprarenal mass that subsequently is removed. Grossly, it appeared gray and tan centrally and yellowish on the cortex. On microscopy, there are large pink cells arranged in nests with capillaries between them.

- **What is the most likely diagnosis?**
- **What other tests can confirm the diagnosis?**
- **What are some of the acute complications that are associated with this condition?**

ANSWERS TO CASE 21: PHEOCHROMOCYTOMA

Summary: A 35-year-old man with severe headaches and marked hypertension undergoes surgical resection of a left suprarenal mass that appeared gray and tan centrally and yellowish on the cortex. On microscopy, large pink cells are arranged in nests with capillaries between them.

- **Most likely diagnosis:** Pheochromocytoma
- **Other helpful diagnostic tests:** Urinary or serum catecholamines such as vanillylmandelic acid (VMA)
- **Acute complications:** Acute left ventricular failure, pulmonary edema, myocardial infarction, ventricular fibrillation and cerebrovascular accidents, congestive heart failure, and death

CLINICAL CORRELATION

This 35-year-old man has a very rapid elevation of blood pressure, palpitations, sweating, and anxiety. This is a very characteristic presentation for pheochromocytoma. Cocaine intoxication closely resembles this condition and is far more common. The urine drug screen in this individual was negative. Other clinical manifestations include tremor, headache, and nausea and vomiting. Excess catecholamine production from this suprarenal (adrenal) tumor also can induce cardiomyopathy, myocardial infarction, and death. The diagnosis is established by **increased urinary catecholamines** such as **vanillylmandelic acid and metanephrine.** Adrenergic blocking agents are used to prevent an adrenergic crisis.

APPROACH TO PHEOCHROMOCYTOMA

Objectives

- Describe the "rule of 10s ."
- Describe the presentation of pheochromocytoma.
- Describe the association with pheochromocytoma and MEN 2A and 2B.

Definitions

Chromaffin cells: Cells derived from neural crest cells that synthesize catecholamines for secretion as a response to preganglionic sympathetic nervous system stimulation.

Pheochromocytoma: Catecholamine-secreting paraganglioma of the adrenal medulla.

Multiple endocrine neoplasia 2A: An autosomal dominant familial syndrome with medullary thyroid carcinoma, parathyroid hyperplasia, and pheochromocytoma.

Multiple endocrine neoplasia 2B: An autosomal dominant familial syndrome with medullary thyroid carcinoma, neuromas, marfanoid features, and pheochromocytoma.

DISCUSSION

The adrenal gland consists of two neuroendocrine organs that develop separately embryologically and have distinct functions. The adrenal cortex is mesodermal in origin, and the adrenal medulla is neuroectodermal in origin and is composed of chromaffin and supporting sustentacular cells. The chromaffin cells are part of the sympathetic nervous system and are responsible for the production and secretion of the majority of the catecholamines in the body. The release of epinephrine and norepinephrine in the normal adrenal medulla is modulated by preganglionic nerves that innervate the chromaffin cells.

Pheochromocytoma is a **rare catecholamine-producing neoplasm** of **chromaffin cells** in the **adrenal medulla** (see Figure 21-1). It is classified as a paraganglioma because it is a neoplasm of the paraganglionic system. Extra-adrenal paragangliomas occur in the other sites of the paraganglionic system, such as the wall of urinary bladder, the paraaortic sympathetic chain, and the sympathetic chain of the neck or mediastinum. Approximately 85 to 90 percent of pheochromocytomas arise from the adrenal medulla, and the rest arise from extra-adrenal paraganglia, usually below the diaphragm. The following is a learning device called the **rule of 10s** that is helpful for remembering some of the characteristics of pheochromocytomas (see Table 21-1).

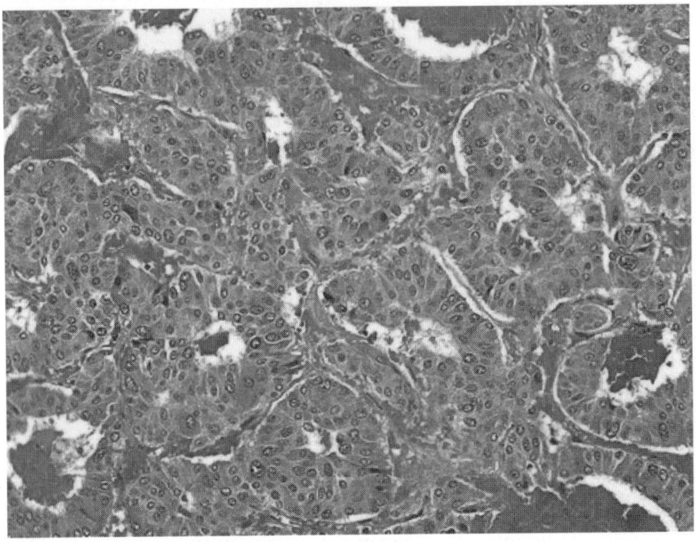

Figure 21-1. Pheochromocytoma demonstrating nests of cells with abundant cytoplasm.

Table 21-1
RULE OF 10s IN PHEOCHROMOCYTOMA

10% are extra-adrenal
10% are multiple or bilateral
10% are malignant
10% recur after surgical removal
10% occur in children
10% occur as part of a familial syndrome
10% present as adrenal incidentalomas

Pheochromocytomas are not innervated by preganglionic nerves, and so the release of catecholamines is not stimulated by neural input. The trigger for the secretion of catecholamines in pheochromocytoma is unclear, but factors such as tumor blood flow, direct pressure, and medications are believed to play a role. This explains the dysequilibrium and lability seen in these patients. Catecholamines act on α- and β-adrenergic receptors. Stimulation of **α-adrenergic receptors results in elevated blood pressure, increased cardiac contractility, glycogenolysis, gluconeogenesis, and intestinal relaxation.** Stimulation of **β-adrenergic receptors** results in an increase in **heart rate and contractility.** The clinical presentation reflects these effects. The most common presentation is chronic sustained hypertension with an additional component of lability and orthostatic hypotension. **Orthostatic hypotension** is a result of down regulation of catecholamine receptors. The classic description is paroxysmal spells of elevated blood pressure, tachycardia, palpitations, headache, sweating, tremor, and anxiety precipitated by stress, exercise, change in posture, or palpation of the tumor. The five Ps is a memory device for the paroxysmal presentation of pheochromocytomas:

1. Pain (headache, chest, and abdominal pain)
2. Pressure, elevated blood
3. Perspiration
4. Palpitation
5. Pallor

The acute side effects of a paroxysmal spell include acute left ventricular failure, pulmonary edema, myocardial infarction, ventricular fibrillation, and cerebrovascular accidents. The chronic complications are due to long-term exposure to elevated catecholamine levels that lead to cardiomyopathy and congestive heart failure and may manifest symptomatically as anginal chest pain or pulmonary edema. The cardiomyopathy classically is called catecholamine cardiomyopathy.

The diagnosis is established by **elevated 24-hour urinary excretion of free catecholamines** (norepinephrine and epinephrine) or metabolites (VMA or total metanephrine). Radiologic imaging of the abdomen also should be performed (MRI is preferred over CT scan to detect extra-adrenal tumors and metastases).

The **primary treatment is surgical resection of the tumor.** The surgical procedure is considered high risk, and so precautions should be taken before and during the operation. A high-salt diet should be followed before surgery, along with an α- and β-blockade immediately before surgery. The α-blockade should be established before the β-blockade to avoid more severe hypertension resulting from unopposed α-adrenergic stimulation. Intraoperative hemodynamic monitoring should be done and followed closely.

Various syndromes are associated with pheochromocytoma: multiple endocrine neoplasia 2A and 2B (MEN 2A and 2B), **neurofibromatosis** (von Recklinghausen disease; NF-1), von Hippel-Lindau disease, and Sturge-Weber syndrome. Neuroblastomas are malignant hemorrhagic tumors of the adrenal medulla that are composed of neuroblasts and mainly present in infants and children. Neurofibromatosis is a sporadic or autosomal dominant familial syndrome that affects cell growth of neural tissue. NF-1 (von Recklinghausen disease) is characterized by neurofibromas and hyperpigmented skin macules. Pheochromocytomas, meningiomas, gliomas, bone cysts, scoliosis, and noncommunicating hydrocephalus also may occur. NF-2 is accompanied by eighth cranial nerve tumors and an increased incidence of intracranial and spinal tumors.

Sturge-Weber syndrome is a congenital syndrome with cavernous hemangiomas (port-wine stains) along the distribution of the trigeminal nerve (cranial nerve V), angiomas of the leptomeninges, mental retardation, epileptic seizures and pheochromocytomas. **von Hippel-Lindau disease is a** rare genetic **multisystem disorder** characterized by the **abnormal growth of tumors (angiomatosis)** in various parts of the body that manifest as **cysts of kidney, liver, and epididymis; renal cell carcinomas** (clear cell type); **pheochromocytomas; angiomas; and cerebellar hemangioblastomas.**

COMPREHENSION QUESTIONS

[21.1] A 34-year-old woman presents with recurrent episodes of severe headaches, palpitations, tachycardia, and sweating. Her blood pressure is found to be elevated during one of those episodes. Which of the following is the most common primary site for the origin of a tumor that could produce this constellation of clinical signs and symptoms?

A. Anterior portion of the pituitary gland
B. Interstitium of the thyroid gland
C. Medulla of the adrenal gland
D. Superior portion of the hypothalamus
E. White pulp of the spleen

[21.2] An individual with a pheochromocytoma who has recurrent symptoms most likely would have elevated 24-hour urinary levels of which of the following substances?

A. Aminolevulinic acid
B. Homogentisic acid
C. Methylmalonic acid
D. Orotic acid
E. Vanillylmandelic acid

[21.3] A 13-month-old female infant who presented with an enlarging abdominal mass is found to have elevated urinary levels of metanephrine. The mass is resected surgically, and histologic sections reveal that mass is composed of numerous proliferating small "blue" cells. Occasional Homer-Wright rosettes are identified. Which of the following is the most likely diagnosis?

A. Hepatoblastoma
B. Medulloblastoma
C. Nephroblastoma
D. Neuroblastoma
E. Pheoblastoma

Answers

[21.1] **C.** The classic clinical signs produced by the secretion of catecholamines from a pheochromocytoma include recurrent episodes (paroxysms) of elevated blood pressure, headaches, palpitations, tachycardia, and sweating. Pheochromocytomas are classified as a type of paraganglioma because they arise from the paraganglionic system. The most common site of origin is the adrenal medulla, where they originate from the chromaffin cells there. These tumors, however, also can originate outside the adrenal gland. Extra-adrenal paragangliomas can occur in other sites of the paraganglionic system, such as the wall of urinary bladder, the paraaortic sympathetic chain, and the sympathetic chain of the neck or mediastinum.

[21.2] **E.** Pheochromocytomas are catecholamine-producing neoplasms that most commonly originate in the adrenal medulla. As a result, individuals with pheochromocytomas have increased serum and urine levels of free catecholamines (norepinephrine and epinephrine) or their metabolites, such as metanephrine, normetanephrine, and VMA. In fact, the best screening test for a pheochromocytoma is to look for elevated urinary VMA levels.

[21.3] **D.** Neuroblastomas are the most common tumors of the adrenal medulla in children. These highly malignant tumors may secrete catecholamines or their metabolites. Thus, the best screening test for a young child who presents with an abdominal mass is to look for increased urinary levels of metanephrine or vanillymandelic acid. Histologically these tumors are composed of small round cells. The formation of Homer-Wright rosettes, which are groups of cells arranged in a ring around a central mass of pink neural filaments, is a characteristic microscopic finding.

PATHOLOGY PEARLS

- Pheochromocytomas are catecholamine-secreting paragangliomas of the adrenal medulla and characteristically present as the abrupt onset of severe hypertension, headache, tachycardia, palpitations, and sweating.
- The diagnosis of pheochromocytoma rests of elevations of urinary free catecholamines. **The rule of 10s applies in pheochromocytoma.**
- **Multiple endocrine neoplasia 2A** is an autosomal dominant familial syndrome with medullary thyroid carcinoma, parathyroid hyperplasia, and pheochromocytoma.
- **Multiple endocrine neoplasia 2B** is an autosomal dominant familial syndrome with medullary thyroid carcinoma, neuromas, marfanoid features, and pheochromocytoma.

REFERENCES

Maitra A, Abbas AK. The endocrine system. In: Kumar V, Assas AK, Fausto N, eds. Robbins and Cotran Pathologic Basis of Disease, 7th ed. Philadelphia, PA: Elsevier Saunders, 2004:1210–8.

Maitra A. The endocrine system. In: Mitchell RN, Kumar V, Abbas AK, et al., eds. Pocket Companion to Robbins and Cotran Pathologic Basis of Disease, 7th ed. Philadelphia, PA: Saunders, 2006:593–603.

CASE 22

A 62-year-old man who has had a worsening cough for several months now complains of dyspnea. He also has fatigue and has experienced a 15-lb weight loss. A chest radiograph shows hilar lymphadenopathy and a right lung mass.

- **What other studies might be helpful in arriving at a definitive diagnosis?**

- **What are the risk factors for tumors of the lung?**

ANSWERS TO CASE 22: LUNG MASS

Summary: A 62-year-old male who has had a worsening cough for several months now has dyspnea. He also has fatigue and has had a 15-lb weight loss. A chest radiograph shows hilar lymphadenopathy and a right lung mass.

- **Confirmatory diagnostic studies:** Bronchoscopic biopsies or washings for microscopic analysis.
- **Risk factors for tumors of the lung:** Tobacco use is the most important, although asbestos exposure also has been noted.

CLINICAL CORRELATION

This 62-year-old man complains of worsening cough and dyspnea. He also has had an unintentional 15-lb weight loss. Possible causes include primary lung cancer, metastatic cancer from sources such as the colon or prostate, and infection such as tuberculosis or a fungal infection. The chest radiograph findings of hilar adenopathy and a right lung mass make lung cancer the most likely possibility. Lung cancer is the leading cancer diagnosed worldwide and the number one cancer killer. It most often is diagnosed between the ages of 40 and 70 years. We are not given a history of this patient's smoking history, but almost certainly he is a smoker. The next step in the evaluation of this individual would be biopsy of the lung tumor, for example, with bronchoscopy. A metastatic workup would be the next step, with studies such as a computed tomography (CT) scan of the abdomen and pelvis, a bone scan, and chemistry tests. Treatment may include surgical resection if feasible and, depending on the tumor type, radiation and/or chemotherapy.

APPROACH TO LUNG PATHOLOGY

Objectives

- Describe the key characteristics of lung neoplasms.
- Describe the hormones associated with lung neoplasms.
- Know the most common cause of lung cancer.

Definitions

Bronchogenic carcinoma: The leading cause of cancer death in the United States. It includes squamous cell carcinoma, adenocarcinoma, small cell carcinoma, and large cell carcinoma.

Squamous cell carcinoma: A centrally occurring tumor of the lung with a clear association with smoking. Initially appears as a hilar mass and frequently results in cavitation.

Adenocarcinoma: A peripherally occurring tumor of the lung with gland formation present. Bronchial-derived and bronchioloalveolar forms exist. The bronchial-derived form also is known as scar carcinoma, occurring at previous sites of inflammation or injury, usually in smokers, whereas the bronchioloalveolar form has tumor cells lining alveolar walls and has **no apparent connection to smoking.**

Small cell carcinoma: Also known as **oat cell carcinoma,** this centrally located undifferentiated tumor type represents the most aggressive bronchogenic carcinoma and is strongly associated with tobacco use.

Large cell carcinoma: This peripherally located undifferentiated tumor often shows features of both squamous cell carcinoma and adenocarcinoma.

Bronchial carcinoid: A low-malignancy lung tumor that occurs in the major bronchi; it is not related to smoking tobacco.

Fibrochondrolipoma: Also known as **benign mesenchymoma,** it is the most benign tumor of the lung. It is composed of benign cartilage, fibrous tissue, and adipose tissue and is usually asymptomatic.

Superior vena cava syndrome: Compression or invasion of the superior vena cava (SVC), resulting in facial swelling, cyanosis, and swelling of neck and head veins.

Pancoast tumor: Tumor involvement at the apex of the lung-cervical sympathetic plexus that results in **Horner syndrome:** ptosis, miosis, and anhidrosis.

Syndrome of inappropriate antidiuretic hormone (SIADH): A paraneoplastic syndrome caused by the secretion of ADH from a small cell carcinoma. Symptoms are related to the plasma hypotonicity that is secondary to water retention. Symptoms include weakness, lethargy, abnormal mentation, coma, and seizures. Laboratory evaluation shows inappropriately high urine osmolality.

Carcinoid syndrome: A paraneoplastic syndrome caused by the release of serotonin in association with carcinoid cancers or occasionally small cell cancers, resulting in intermittent diarrhea, flushing, cyanosis, tachycardia, hypotension, and wheezing.

Ectopic Cushing syndrome: A paraneoplastic syndrome associated with the ACTH-like activity of a small cell carcinoma, causing any of the features of Cushing syndrome associated with long-term exposure to excess glucocorticoids.

Lambert-Eaton myasthenic syndrome: Muscle weakness caused by autoantibodies that are reactive with the neuronal calcium channel.

Hypercalcemia: Often one of the most common life-threatening disorders associated with cancer, this paraneoplastic syndrome is related to the parathyroid activity associated with squamous cell carcinoma.

Hypertrophic pulmonary osteoarthropathy: A paraneoplastic syndrome first described by Hippocrates over 2400 years ago that includes clubbing and hypertrophic osteoarthropathy (HPO) as changes in the hands and long bones; commonly associated with thoracic malignancy.

Hypercoagulability: Venous thrombosis and embolism are associated with neoplastic states, especially adenocarcinomas, because of their nature as hypercoagulable states.

Hoarseness: May be caused by recurrent laryngeal nerve palsy in association with lung carcinoma.

Pleural effusion: A bloody pleural effusion is suggestive of malignancy, tuberculosis, or trauma.

Carcinoma metastatic to the lung: Occurs more frequently than do tumors that originate in the lung.

DISCUSSION

Normal Lung

The respiratory system is composed of a **conducting portion** with two components—an **extrapulmonary region** and an **intrapulmonary region**—and a **respiratory portion.** The lung encompasses the intrapulmonary region of the conducting portion as well as the respiratory portion. The intrapulmonary region is composed of **intrapulmonary bronchi** that further give rise to **bronchioles.** Whcrcas thc intrapulmonary bronchus has cartilaginous support, the bronchioles are tubes of decreasing diameter that do not have this type of supporting skeleton. The larger bronchioles have a **ciliated** epithelial lining with a few **goblet cells;** however, smaller branches have a **simple columnar epithelium** with the goblet cells replaced by **Clara cells.** The wall thickness and luminal diameter of the bronchioles decrease until they reach the last region in the conduction portion, the **terminal bronchioles.** The respiratory portion then begins with branches of the terminal bronchioles known as the **respiratory bronchioles,** which lead to **alveolar ducts** and then into expanded regions known as **alveolar sacs,** which are composed of a number of **alveoli** whose thin walls readily permit gas exchange.

Two types of cells compose the epithelium of the alveolar sacs and the alveoli: **type I pneumonocytes,** which are highly attenuated and act as lining cells, and **type II pneumonocytes,** which manufacture **surfactant,** the phospholipids that reduce surface tension. The **blood-air barrier** of the lung is composed of the attenuated epithelial cells of the capillaries that invest each alveolus, the attenuated type I pneumonocytes, the surfactant and fluid coating the alveolus, and a single fused basal lamina. The lung has numerous alveoli, which are crowded against one another and separated by walls known as **interalveolar septa.** The septa have varying thicknesses, with the thinnest walls possessing communicating alveolar pores by which air can pass between alveoli. Macrophages, which are very efficient, and numerous scavenger cells known as **dust cells,** which are derived from monocytes, often are noticed in these interalveolar septa.

Bronchogenic Carcinoma

Bronchogenic carcinoma is the **leading cause of death** from **cancer** in both males and females. It is **increasing in incidence** in women more than in men in parallel with the smoking of cigarettes. This incidence has been found to be in direct proportion to a **pack-year tobacco history.** The histologic changes caused by cigarette smoking that occur before the development of bronchogenic carcinoma include **squamous metaplasia** of the respiratory epithelium, often accompanied by atypical changes that range from dysplasia to carcinoma in situ. Other substances that have been implicated in the etiology of bronchogenic carcinoma include **air pollution, industrial exposure to nickel or chromate, industrial radiation exposure, and asbestos.** Clinically, bronchogenic carcinoma manifests as a **cough often with hemoptysis, weight loss, chest pain, and dyspnea.** There may be bronchial obstruction with atelectasis or pneumonitis. Other signs and symptoms of clinical presentation may include **SVC syndrome, Horner syndrome, Lambert-Eaton myasthenic syndrome, hoarseness, a pleural effusion, hypertrophic pulmonary osteoarthropathy, hypercoagulability, and various paraneoplastic syndromes.**

This carcinoma is subclassified into **squamous cell carcinoma, adenocarcinoma, and small or large cell carcinoma** (see Table 22-1). **Squamous cell carcinoma** is **most common** in **males** and has the **highest association with smoking.** It arises **centrally** near the **hilum,** and **thickening and irregularity of the bronchial mucosa** can be seen with a bronchoscope. The very well differentiated forms may be seen to have prominent **keratin** production and **necrosis** with associated **cavitation.** This form often spreads locally before metastasis and is associated with **parathyroidlike activity** that can lead to life-threatening **hypercalcemia.** The **adenocarcinoma** consists of a **bronchial-derived type** and a **bronchioloalveolar type.** The bronchial-derived type affects males and females equally but is the **most common cancer in females and nonsmokers.** This form is usually **peripheral** in location, developing on the site of a **prior lung inflammation or injury.** This **scar carcinoma** has prominent **gland formation** and usually contains **mucin.** The bronchioloalveolar type usually is also peripherally located, but its **well-differentiated** tumor cells **line the alveolar septa,** forming **solitary or multiple nodules** that may resemble **pneumonia on chest x-ray.**

Small cell carcinoma, also known as oat cell carcinoma, which is more common in males and is strongly associated with smoking, usually starts **centrally** near the **hilum and** is the **most aggressive** type of bronchogenic carcinoma, with early and widespread metastases. Histologically, oat cell carcinoma has a very characteristic appearance, demonstrating **small cells with very high N/C ratio** (nuclear to cytoplasmic ratio) with **fine chromatin** and small or absent nucleoli. Small cell carcinoma is highly associated with paraneoplastic endocrine syndromes including adrenocorticotropic **(ACTH)-like activity** or antidiuretic hormone **(ADH)-like activity.** Conversely, **large cell carcinoma,** an **undifferentiated** tumor that may show the features of

Table 22-1
BRONCHOGENIC CARCINOMA

TYPE	LOCATED	"KEY" FEATURE	HISTOLOGY	ASSOCIATED HORMONES
Squamous cell carcinoma	Centrally	Highest association with smoking	Prominent keratin production and necrosis with associated cavitation	Parathyroid-like activity → hypercalcemia
Small cell carcinoma	Centrally	Most aggressive type of bronchogenic carcinoma	Small cells with very high N/C ratio with fine chromatin	ADH/ACTH
Adenocarcinoma	Peripherally	Most common cancer in females and nonsmokers	Prominent gland formation; usually contains mucin	
Bronchioalveolar carcinoma	Peripherally	Unrelated to smoking	Solitary or multiple nodules that may resemble pneumonia on chest x-ray	
Large cell carcinoma	Peripherally	Very poor prognosis	Undifferentiated; highly anaplastic	

either squamous cell carcinoma or adenocarcinoma, usually is found **peripherally.** The **prognosis is very poor** for small cell carcinoma and better for the other types of bronchogenic carcinoma.

Bronchial Carcinoid

This **low-malignancy** type of lung tumor usually occurs in patients **less than 40 years** of age, has **no relationship to tobacco** use or any other recognized etiologic factors. Usually found **intraluminally** within the **major bronchi,** it accounts for **1 to 5 percent of lung tumors,** with most **less than 4 cm in diameter.** Clinically, there is an association with **pneumonia, bronchiectasis, emphysema, and atelectasis.** Histologically, the cells are seen as having uniform round nuclei and infrequent mitosis and **neuroendocrine differentiation.**

Some atypical carcinoids have increased pleomorphism, mitosis, and necrosis and a more aggressive course. However, in general the **prognosis is good.** Metastasis to regional lymph nodes occurs at a rate between 5 and 10 percent, and the 5-year survival rate is 90 to 95 percent.

Fibrochondrolipomas

Fibrochondrolipomas, also known as benign mesenchymomas, are the **most benign tumors** of the lung. These lung nodules, which may be located **centrally or peripherally, rarely cause clinical symptoms** unless a large central mass causes symptoms of airway obstruction. The mass may be seen on **chest x-ray or CT as a low-density area** composed of fat with some calcifications. Histologically, the nodule is seen to be composed of **benign cartilage, fibrous tissue, and adipose tissue.**

Metastatic Tumors

Metastatic tumors have **a much higher incidence** than does primary lung cancer. These tumors, which often present with **multiple nodules in multiple lobes,** may be spread by **lymphatics or blood vessels or contiguously** from the structures of the mediastinum or esophagus.

COMPREHENSION QUESTIONS

[22.1] A 63-year-old man who has a long history of smoking several packs of cigarettes a day presents with a worsening cough and weight loss. A chest x-ray finds a solitary 3-cm mass in the lower lobe of his right lung. This mass is resected surgically, and the pathologist diagnoses the lesion as a moderately differentiated squamous cell carcinoma. Which of the histologic findings listed below is most consistent with this diagnosis?

A. Abundant mucin secretion
B. Dense collagen deposition
C. Neurosecretory granule formation
D. Extensive glandular differentiation
E. Prominent keratin production

[22.2] Which of the following types of carcinomas is most likely to be found at the periphery of the lung in areas of prior lung inflammation or injury?

A. Adenocarcinoma
B. Clear cell carcinoma
C. Large cell carcinoma
D. Small cell carcinoma
E. Squamous cell carcinoma

[22.3] Which of the following is the classic triad of signs and symptoms associated with Horner syndrome?

A. Cogwheel rigidity, flat facies, and akinesia
B. Fever, vomiting, and nuchal rigidity
C. Orthostatic hypotension, impotence, and excess salivation
D. Ptosis, miosis, and anhidrosis
E. Scanning speech, intention tremor, and nystagmus

Answers

[22.1] **E.** Lung carcinomas, which usually originate from the bronchi (bronchogenic carcinomas), are classified histologically into four major categories: squamous cell carcinomas, adenocarcinomas, small cell carcinomas, and large cell carcinomas. Squamous cell carcinomas, which have a strong association with smoking, usually arise centrally near the hilum of the lung. Histologically well-differentiated squamous cell carcinomas have prominent keratin production, and intercellular bridges may be seen.

[22.2] **A.** A peripherally occurring tumor of the lung is most likely to be an adenocarcinoma. These tumors may develop within previous sites of inflammation or injury where fibrous tissue has been deposited. Therefore, these tumors are sometimes called scar carcinomas. Histologic sections of the bronchial-derived type of adenocarcinoma reveal prominent gland formation, the lumen of which may contain abundant mucin. Histologic sections of the bronchioloalveolar type, which also may be found peripherally, show well-differentiated mucus-secreting columnar epithelial cells that infiltrate along the alveolar walls.

[22.3] **D.** The usual clinical signs and symptoms produced by lung cancer include cough, hemoptysis, weight loss, chest pain, and dyspnea. Bronchial obstruction by a tumor may produce atelectasis or pneumonia. Other signs and symptoms of lung cancer include Horner syndrome, Lambert-Eaton myasthenic syndrome, superior vena cava syndrome, and hypertrophic pulmonary osteoarthropathy. The classic triad of signs and symptoms associated with Horner syndrome are ptosis (eyelid drop), miosis (pupil constriction), and anhidrosis (lack of sweating). These signs result from a tumor located at the apex of the lung (Pancoast tumor) invading the cervical sympathetic plexus.

PATHOLOGY PEARLS

- Lung cancer is the cancer diagnosed most frequently worldwide and the number one cancer killer.
- Squamous cell carcinoma of the lung is most common in men and has the highest association with smoking. It arises centrally near the hilum.
- Small cell carcinoma, also known as oat cell carcinoma, is more common in males and is strongly associated with smoking. It usually starts centrally near the hilum, is very aggressive, and is associated with paraneoplastic syndromes.
- Metastatic tumors have a much higher incidence than does primary lung cancer and generally present with multiple nodules in multiple lobes.

REFERENCES

Hussain AN, Kumar V. The lung. In: Kumar V, Assas AK, Fausto N, eds. Robbins and Cotran Pathologic Basis of Disease, 7th ed. Philadelphia, PA: Elsevier Saunders, 2004:763–6.

Hussain AN. The lung. In: Mitchell RN, Kumar V, Abbas AK, et al., eds. Pocket Companion to Robbins and Cotran Pathologic Basis of Disease, 7th ed. Philadelphia, PA: Saunders, 2006:396–8.

Rubin E. Essential Pathology, 3rd ed. Philadelphia, PA: Lippincott Williams & Wilkins, 2001.

CASE 23

A 35-year-old African American woman complains of shortness of breath and cough for the last 2 months. She also has had fatigue and mild subjective fever. Physical examination reveals several discrete subcutaneous nodules. No masses or organomegaly is found. A chest radiograph shows bilateral hilar lymphadenopathy but no lung or mediastinal masses. A biopsy of one of the skin nodules shows noncaseating granuloma.

- **What are the diagnostic considerations?**

- **What serum blood test can help confirm the diagnosis?**

ANSWERS TO CASE 23: RESTRICTIVE PULMONARY DISEASE (SARCOIDOSIS)

Summary: A 35-year-old African American woman complains of dyspnea, cough, fatigue, and mild subjective fever. She has several discrete subcutaneous nodules but no organomegaly. A chest radiograph shows bilateral hilar lymphadenopathy but no lung or mediastinal masses. A biopsy of one of the skin nodules shows noncaseating granuloma.

- **Diagnostic considerations:** Granulomatous diseases of the lung such as tuberculosis and sarcoidosis.
- **Confirmatory test:** There is no single test for the definitive diagnosis of sarcoidosis; it is often a diagnosis of exclusion. Relevant investigations include elevated serum calcium and angiotensin-converting enzyme levels.

CLINICAL CORRELATION

This 35-year-old woman complains of a 2-month history of progressive dyspnea, fatigue, and cough. She has subcutaneous nodules that on microscopy reveal noncaseating granulomas. She is African American, which is a risk factor for sarcoidosis. Sarcoidosis is a multisystemic granulomatous disorder of unknown etiology that typically affects young adults, especially females. The chest radiographic finding of bilateral hilar adenopathy is also very characteristic of sarcoidosis. The liver and spleen often are enlarged in these patients. About one-third of affected patients have subcutaneous skin nodules or eye findings (iritis). The diagnosis of sarcoidosis is one of exclusion, and other causes of granulomas, such as tuberculosis and fungal infections, must be excluded.

APPROACH TO RESTRICTIVE PULMONARY DISEASE

Objectives

- Describe the key features of sarcoidosis.
- Describe the causes of restrictive airway disease.
- Describe the key manifestations of interstitial fibrosis.

Definitions

Obstructive airway disease: These are diseases in which there is obstruction to air flow. Other obstructive diseases are chronic obstructive pulmonary disease (COPD) (irreversible obstructive airway disease) and bronchial asthma (reversible obstructive airway disease).

Restrictive airway disease: These are diseases in which there is diffuse and chronic involvement of pulmonary connective tissue. There is reduction in oxygen diffusion capacity, lung volumes, and lung compliance.

DISCUSSION

Sarcoidosis

The **most common presentation** is **respiratory symptoms** or abnormalities discovered on **chest x-ray. Bilateral hilar lymphadenopathy** with lung mottling is a typical chest x-ray feature (see Table 23-1). Chest x-ray and computed tomography (CT) of the chest are likely to show involvement by the disease process. Lung function tests show a restrictive pattern of defect. Biopsy of the affected organs is likely to show **noncaseating granulomas.** These granulomas are composed of tightly clustered epithelioid cells, often with Langhans cells or foreign body giant cells. With chronic disease there is fibrosis. Other microscopic features that may be present are the presence of **Schaumann bodies** (laminated concretions of calcium and protein) and that of asteroid bodies (stellate inclusions in giant cells). As the histology of granulomas caused by infectious diseases may be similar, special stains should be used to exclude them. These stains are typically acid-fast bacillus (AFB) to rule out *Mycobacteria* and Gomori methenamine silver (GMS) to rule out fungi. Serum angiotensin-converting enzyme (ACE) levels usually are elevated with this condition.

Skin sarcoidosis and ocular sarcoidosis are the most common extrapulmonary manifestations. These manifestations include **erythema nodosum (see Figure 23-1) and anterior uveitis.** Sarcoid macrophages are responsible for 1-α-hydroxylation of vitamin D, with resultant 1,25-$(OH)_2$ vitamin D_3. This results in hypercalcemia and hypercalciuria. Levels of ACE are elevated in sarcoidosis. High levels also are seen in lymphoma, pulmonary tuberculosis, asbestosis, and silicosis. Although ACE levels are not of diagnostic value, they may be useful for monitoring the progression of disease.

Table 23-1

DIFFERENTIAL DIAGNOSIS OF BILATERAL HILAR LYMPHADENOPATHY

Sarcoidosis
Lymphoma
Pulmonary tuberculosis
Carcinoma of the bronchus with spread to the contralateral node

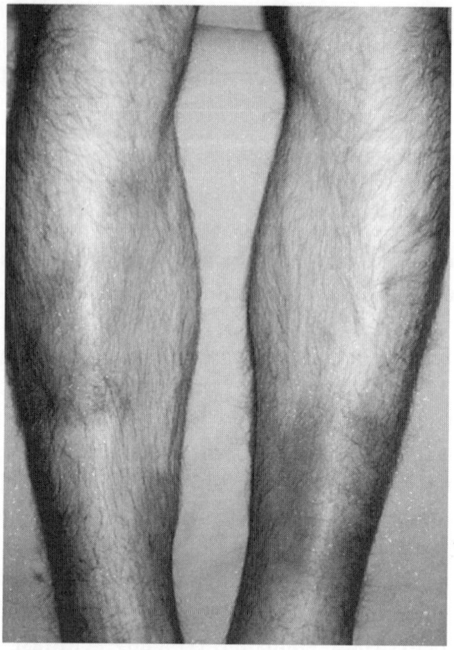

Figure 23-1. Erythema nodosum. *(Reproduced, with permission, from Kasper DL, Braunwald E, Fauci AS, et al., eds.* Harrison's Principles of Internal Medicine, 16th ed. *New York: McGraw-Hill, 2004:2019.)*

Regardless of the specific type of restrictive lung disease (see Table 23-2), it is thought that the earliest manifestation of most of these conditions is alveolitis. In alveolitis, there is increased accumulation of inflammatory cells that distorts the normal alveolar structure and also results in the liberation of harmful chemical mediators that injure parenchymal cells and stimulate fibrosis. Eventually, the alveoli are replaced by cystic air spaces separated by thick bands of connective tissue. This represents the end-stage lung, which also is referred to as "honeycomb lung."

A **progressive diffuse interstitial fibrosis** occurs classically in progressive systemic sclerosis. Interstitial pneumonitis and fibrosis also may be seen in systemic lupus erythematosus (SLE) and rheumatoid arthritis. Desquamative interstitial pneumonitis (DIP) typically affects males between ages 30 and 50 years. It is usually a progressive disease that results in end-stage **honeycomb lung** that is unresponsive to medications such as steroids. Patients present with dyspnea, hypoxia, and clubbing. Crepitations are heard over the lung fields. Lung biopsy classically shows "temporal heterogeneity." This means there will be areas of unaffected lung, early lesions, and end-stage lung in the biopsy at

Table 23-2
SELECTED CAUSES OF RESTRICTIVE AIRWAY DISEASES

Sarcoidosis
Collagen-vascular diseases
Usual interstitial pneumonitis
Desquamative interstitial pneumonitis
Hypersensitivity pneumonitis
Dust lung diseases (pneumoconiosis)
Drugs

any point in time. DIP is characterized by the accumulation of intraalveolar macrophages with periodic acid-Schiff (PAS)-positive granules. Temporal heterogeneity is absent, and patients do respond to steroids.

Hypersensitivity pneumonitis is thought to be due to immunologic mechanisms related to inhalation of organic dusts and occupational antigens. The most well-known example of this type of pneumonitis is **"farmer's lung."** This condition is due to the inhalation of spores of thermophilic actinomycete (*Micropolyspora faeni*). The spores are found on humid, warm hay. Typically, the patient will complain of dyspnea and wheezing several hours after exposure. Hypersensitivity pneumonitis is characterized histologically by granuloma formation, which is useful in differentiating it from other types of pneumonitis.

Pneumoconiosis is dust lung disease (see Table 23-3). Progressive massive fibrosis, silicosis, and asbestos-related lung diseases are usually progressive

Table 23-3
EXAMPLES OF PNEUMOCONIOSIS

Coal dust exposure from coal mining: coal workers' pneumoconiosis, simple and complicated (progressive massive fibrosis)
Silica exposure from foundry work, sandblasting, stone cutting: silicosis
Asbestos exposure from mining, insulation-related work: asbestosis, mesothelioma, lung cancer, pleural plaque
Beryllium exposure from mining: berylliosis

even after exposure to the offending agent stops. The development of pneumoconiosis is dependent on the following:

1. The amount of dust retained in the lung and airways
2. The size and shape of the particles (particles between 1 and 5 μm are the most dangerous)
3. Solubility and physicochemical properties of the particles
4. Concomitant effects of other irritants, such as smoking

COMPREHENSION QUESTIONS

[23.1] A 28-year-old African American woman presents with nonspecific symptoms, including malaise and mild subjective fever. A chest x-ray reveals bilateral enlarged hilar lymph nodes ("potato nodes") with mottling of the lungs. Laboratory evaluation finds elevated serum levels of calcium and ACE. No organisms are found with any cultured material. A biopsy from her enlarged lymph nodes most likely would reveal the presence of which of the following abnormalities?

A. Caseating granulomas
B. Infiltrating malignant cells
C. Noncascating granulomas
D. Stellate abscesses
E. Sterile microabscesses

[23.2] A chest x-ray of a 62-year-old man who presented with increasing shortness of breath is found to have a diffuse pulmonary infiltrate. A transbronchial biopsy reveals fibrosis of the walls of the alveoli along with the accumulation of macrophages in the lumen of the alveoli. These macrophages have PAS-positive cytoplasmic granules. Which of the following is the most likely diagnosis?

A. Chemical pneumonitis
B. Desquamative interstitial pneumonitis
C. Hypersensitivity pneumonitis
D. Radiation pneumonitis
E. Usual interstitial pneumonitis

[23.3] A 34-year-old man presents with the sudden development of malaise and fever along with dyspnea, coughing, and wheezing that developed a couple of hours after he worked with moldy hay. His symptoms are most likely an immunologic reaction to which of the following organisms?

A. *Aspergillus clavatus*
B. *Candida* species
C. *Mycoplasma pneumoniae*
D. *Nocardia* species
E. Thermophilic actinomycetes

Answers

[23.1] **C.** Bilateral hilar lymphadenopathy with lung mottling is a typical chest x-ray feature of sarcoidosis. Patients most commonly are young adult African American females. Sarcoidosis is characterized by the formation of noncaseating granulomas in multiple organs. These granulomas are composed primarily of activated macrophages (epithelioid cells). These cells may activate vitamin D and produce hypercalcemia and hypercalciuria. Levels of ACE also are elevated with sarcoidosis. Other microscopic features of sarcoidosis include the presence of Langhans-type giant cells; Schaumann bodies, which are small, laminated calcified structures; and asteroid bodies, which are stellate-shaped inclusions found in giant cells.

[23.2] **B.** The term *pneumonitis* refers to inflammation of the lungs, whereas the term *interstitial pneumonitis* refers to inflammation of the walls of the alveoli. The usual type of interstitial pneumonitis is called usual interstitial pneumonitis (UIP). UIP is an idiopathic disorder that most commonly affects males aged 30 to 50 years. It is a progressive lung disease that results in an end-stage honeycomb lung. The disease does not respond to medications such as steroids. In contrast to UIP, DIP is a type of pneumonitis that does respond to treatment with steroids. The diagnosis of DIP is made by finding an accumulation of macrophages with PAS-positive granules in the lumen of the alveoli.

[23.3] **E.** Hypersensitivity pneumonitis is characterized by immunologically mediated damage to the interstitium of the lungs. Characteristic histologic features include poorly formed noncaseating granulomas in the interstitium. The best-known example of hypersensitivity pneumonitis is farmer's lung. This condition results from the inhalation of spores of thermophilic actinomycetes (*Micropolyspora faeni*), the spores of which are found in humid, warm hay. Patient usually develops dyspnea and wheezing with a cough several hours after exposure to the moldy hay.

PATHOLOGY PEARLS

- Sarcoidosis is a multisystemic granulomatous (noncaseating) disorder that typically affects young adults.
- There is no single test for the definitive diagnosis of sarcoidosis.
- Bilateral hilar lymphadenopathy with lung mottling is a typical chest x-ray feature of sarcoidosis.
- Serum calcium and angiotensin-converting enzyme (ACE) levels typically are elevated in sarcoidosis.
- In restrictive airway disease, there is reduction in oxygen diffusion capacity, lung volumes, and lung compliance.
- The earliest manifestation of most cases of interstitial fibrosis is alveolitis, and eventually the alveoli are replaced by cystic air spaces separated by thick bands of connective tissue. This end-stage lung is referred to as honeycomb lung.

REFERENCES

Husain AN, Kumar V. The lung. In: Kumar V, Assas AK, Fausto N, eds. Robbins and Cotran Pathologic Basis of Disease, 7th ed. Philadelphia, PA: Elsevier Saunders, 2004:737–40.

Husain AN. The lung. In: Mitchell RN, Kumar V, Abbas AK, et al., eds. Pocket Companion to Robbins and Cotran Pathologic Basis of Disease, 7th ed. Philadelphia, PA: Saunders, 2006:583–9.

CASE 24

A 65-year-old man with a 40-year history of tobacco use and a chronic productive cough for several years develops more severe dyspnea and fever. He has an enlarged chest diameter and some mild blueness to the lips. A chest radiograph shows an enlarged heart and hyperlucent lung fields but no evidence of a pulmonary infiltrate.

- **What is the most likely diagnosis?**
- **What is the most likely underlying mechanism associated with this disorder?**

ANSWERS TO CASE 24: CHRONIC BRONCHITIS WITH ACUTE EXACERBATION

Summary: A 65-year-old man with a long history of tobacco use and a chronic productive cough for several years develops more severe dyspnea and fever. He has a barrel chest and cyanosis. A chest radiograph shows cardiomegaly and hyperinflated lung fields.

- **Most likely diagnosis:** Chronic obstructive pulmonary disease.
- **Underlying mechanisms associated with this disorder:** Inhalation injury from cigarette smoke.

CLINICAL CORRELATION

This 65-year-old man has a long history of tobacco use, which is the most common risk factor for chronic obstructive pulmonary disease (COPD). He complains of a several-year history of worsening dyspnea and a productive cough. He is in respiratory distress with labored respirations, cyanosis, a "barrel chest," wheezing, and distant heart sounds, all of which suggest lung disease. The main issue is his respiratory status. Rapid clinical assessment is critical in case this patient is headed toward respiratory failure, necessitating intubation and mechanical ventilation. An arterial blood gas will give quick information regarding the oxygenation status as well as the ventilatory efficiency via the P_{CO_2} level. Bronchitis or pneumonia possibly has exacerbated his pulmonary disease.

APPROACH TO CHRONIC OBSTRUCTIVE PULMONARY DISEASE

Objectives

- Describe the differences between obstructive and restrictive pulmonary disease.
- Describe the common etiologies of COPD.
- Describe the treatment of COPD.

Definitions

Chronic bronchitis: A clinical diagnosis characterized by excessive secretion of bronchial mucus and a productive cough for 3 months or more in at least two consecutive years in the absence of any other disease that might account for this symptom.

Emphysema: A pathologic diagnosis that denotes abnormal, permanent enlargement of air spaces distal to the terminal bronchiole with destruction of their walls and without obvious fibrosis.

Chronic obstructive pulmonary disease: A disease state characterized by the presence of airflow obstruction caused by chronic bronchitis or emphysema. The airflow obstruction is usually progressive and may be accompanied by airway hyperreactivity; it may be partially reversible.

DISCUSSION

COPD is a common disease that has been cited as the fourth leading cause of morbidity and mortality in the United States. The most common etiology for COPD is inhalation injury, specifically cigarette smoking. Another important cause is **α_1-antitrypsin deficiency,** which is hereditary. The disease may become evident by the age of 40 years and often occurs without cough or a history of smoking. Therapy with replacement of α_1-antitrypsin enzyme is available. Characteristically, patients with COPD present with progressively worsening dyspnea (first on exertion, then with activity, and then at rest). A patient may vary in appearance from a "blue bloater" (chronic bronchitis, overweight, edematous, cyanotic) to a "pink puffer" (emphysema, thin, ruddy cheeks).

The **obstructive lung diseases (emphysema,** chronic **bronchitis, bronchiectasis,** and **asthma)** have similar effects on the pulmonary function through **decreased pulmonary expiratory flow. Emphysema** typically is characterized by **large air spaces distal to the terminal bronchioles,** leading to an appearance of "overinflation" of the air spaces. There is usually no fibrosis present. The anatomic location of the emphysematous changes is a helpful method for classification: panacinar, paraseptal, centriacinar, and irregular. The centriacinar variety is the most common, affecting the central or proximal aspects of the acini; the distal alveoli usually are not involved.

Chronic bronchitis typically involves **hypersecretion of mucus** and enlarged submucous glands of the large airways, leading to a **chronic productive cough.** Chronic inhalant irritation such as from cigarette smoke, silica dust, or cotton is found in the vast majority of cases. The **increased mucus secretion of the airways and inflammation** leads to **chronic small airway obstruction.** Histologic studies reveal **mucus plugging** of the **bronchioles, pigmented alveolar macrophages,** and **fibrosis** of the bronchiolar wall. Continued insult by cigarette smoke leads to alveolar damage and cyanosis.

Arterial blood gases are often normal in the early phase of the disease; however, in advanced cases, there is evidence of hypoxemia and hypercapnia. Usually, these patients are in a state of chronic respiratory acidosis resulting from CO_2 retention. **Spirometry is the most basic, inexpensive, and widely valuable pulmonary function test.** It helps identify the type of lung disease, obstructive versus restrictive (see Table 24-1), along with potential reversibility and the gas-exchanging capability of the lungs (DL_{CO}). **Flow volume loops** help

TABLE 24-1
PULMONARY FUNCTION TESTS

Obstructive	Increased TLC	Decreased FEV1/FVC
Restrictive	Decreased TLC	Normal to increased FEV1/FVC

identify the type of lung disease; restrictive lung diseases tend to have lower lung volumes, whereas obstructive diseases have larger lung volumes.

Management of severe COPD exacerbations focuses simultaneously on relieving airway obstruction and correcting life-threatening abnormalities of gas exchange. **Bronchodilators** (β-agonist and anticholinergic agents) are administered by hand-held nebulizers, high-dose **systemic glucocorticoids** accelerate the rate of improvement in lung function among these patients, and **antibiotics** should be given if there is suspicion of a respiratory infection. **Controlled oxygen administration** with nasal oxygen at low flows or oxygen with Venturi masks will correct hypoxemia without causing severe hypercapnia. Caution must be exercised in patients with chronic respiratory insufficiency whose respiratory drive is dependent on "relative hypoxemia"; these individuals may become apneic if excessive oxygen is administered.

Positive-pressure mask ventilation offers an alternative to intubation and mechanical ventilation in the treatment of cooperative patients with an acute exacerbation of COPD and severe hypercapnia. Signs of **acute respiratory failure** include **tachypnea** (respiratory rate >40/min), **inability to speak** because of dyspnea, **accessory muscle use with fatigue** despite maximal therapy, **confusion, restlessness, agitation, lethargy, a rising PCO_2 level,** and extreme **hypoxemia.** Acute respiratory failure generally is treated with mechanical intubation. Endotracheal or nasotracheal intubation with ventilatory support helps correct the disorders of gas exchange. Complications of mechanical intubation include difficulty in extubation, ventilator-associated pneumonia, pneumothorax, and acute respiratory distress syndrome. **Long-term complications** of COPD from **hypoxemia** can cause **pulmonary hypertension,** secondary **erythrocytosis, exercise limitation,** and **impaired mental functioning.** These patients must be encouraged to quit smoking and undergo evaluation for oxygen therapy. They are susceptible to lung infections and should receive **pneumococcal immunization** and **annual influenza vaccination.**

COMPREHENSION QUESTIONS

[24.1] A 54-year-old male smoker is diagnosed with chronic bronchitis. A biopsy of the bronchus is performed. Which of the following is the most likely finding on histology?

A. Abundant mucus with plugging of the bronchioles
B. Alveolar destruction and enlargement
C. Interstitial fibrosis
D. Noncaseating granuloma

[24.2] A 46-year-old man complains of progressive dyspnea and cough. He has been hospitalized multiple times over the last 2 years for respiratory distress. Bronchoscopy is performed with biopsy of the lung. Histologic analysis reveals large airspaces distal to the terminal bronchioles. Which of the following is the most likely diagnosis?

A. Asthma
B. Bronchiectasis
C. Bronchitis
D. Emphysema
E. Sarcoidosis

[24.3] A 29-year-old woman is noted to have chronic dyspnea and easy fatigue with exertion. A chest radiograph reveals hyperinflated lung fields without infiltrates. She denies a history of cigarette smoking. Which of the following is the most likely etiology for her condition?

A. α_1-Antitrypsin deficiency
B. Second hand smoke
C. Subclinical asthma
D. Amyloidosis

Answers

[24.1] **A.** Abundant mucus with plugging of the bronchioles is the hallmark of bronchitis. Pigmented alveolar macrophages and fibrosis of the bronchiolar walls also may be seen.

[24.2] **D.** Emphysema typically is associated with large airspaces distal to the terminal bronchioles, leading to an appearance of "overinflation" of the air spaces. There is usually no fibrosis present.

[24.3] **A.** α_1-Antitrypsin deficiency may present as COPD, but usually without the cough. This is a hereditary enzyme deficiency; thus, a family history is often present. Affected individuals are nonsmokers, with onset in the forties.

PATHOLOGY PEARLS

- Patients with obstructive lung disease have trouble blowing air out; patients with restrictive lung disease have trouble getting air in.
- For simple acid-base disorders, one should think the following: If pH and P_{CO_2} move in the same direction, think metabolic acidosis/alkalosis. If pH and P_{CO_2} move in opposite directions, think respiratory acidosis/alkalosis.
- Mainstay treatment of COPD exacerbations includes bronchodilators, oxygen, and glucocorticoids.
- Controlled supplemental oxygen alone or with positive-pressure ventilation may avoid the need for intubation.
- Home oxygen therapy to treat chronic hypoxemia is the only way to improve survival among persons with COPD.

REFERENCES

Husain AN, Kumar V. The lung. In: Kumar V, Assas AK, Fausto N, eds. Robbins and Cotran Pathologic Basis of Disease, 7th ed. Philadelphia, PA: Elsevier Saunders, 2004:714–30.

Husain AN. The lung. In: Mitchell RN, Kumar V, Abbas AK, et al., eds. Pocket Companion to Robbins and Cotran Pathologic Basis of Disease, 7th ed. Philadelphia, PA: Saunders, 2006:378–83.

❖ CASE 25

After traveling by air from Romania to New York, a 35-year-old woman develops a sudden onset of chest pain and shortness of breath. She has not experienced anything like this before, but her sister had a similar episode after the delivery of her first child. On examination, the patient appears anxious and tachypneic. Her lungs reveal good air movement bilaterally.

- **What is the most likely diagnosis?**
- **What are the possible underlying mechanisms?**
- **What are the risk factors?**

ANSWERS TO CASE 25: PULMONARY EMBOLUS

Summary: After an international air flight, a 35-year-old woman develops acute chest pain and dyspnea. Her sister had a similar episode during her postpartum period. The patient appears anxious and tachypneic but has good air movement bilaterally.

- **Most likely diagnosis:** Pulmonary embolism.
- **Possible underlying mechanisms:** Deep venous thrombosis with embolization to the pulmonary arteries versus intracardiac thrombosis.
- **Risk factors:** Venous stasis, vascular damage, and hypercoagulable state.

CLINICAL CORRELATION

Pulmonary embolus causes 50,000 deaths per year and is the sole cause or a major contributing cause in 10 percent of adult acute deaths in hospitals. Ninety to ninety-five percent of pulmonary emboli are embolic in origin, most commonly from deep veins of the legs or the pelvis. The development of in situ thromboses is rare and can be seen in the presence of pulmonary hypertension, pulmonary atherosclerosis, and heart failure. Risk factors include immobilization (after surgery or prolonged sitting during car trips or long airplane rides), pregnancy and the postpartum period, malignancy, cardiovascular diseases such as myocardial infarction (MI) and congestive heart failure (CHF), oral contraceptives, hypercoagulable state (such as antithrombin III, protein C deficiency, factor V Leiden, and lupus anticoagulant), and the presence of central venous lines, which can serve as a nidus for thrombus formation.

APPROACH TO SUSPECTED THROMBOSIS AND PULMONARY EMBOLISM

Objectives

- Describe the risk factors for developing a deep venous thrombosis/pulmonary embolus.
- Describe the most common location of a deep venous thrombosis.
- Describe the presentation of a pulmonary embolus.

Definitions

Tachypneic: Rapid, shallow breathing
Dyspnea: Labored or difficult breathing
Hemoptysis: Coughing and spitting of blood or blood stained sputum
Thrombophilia: A tendency to form thrombosis. A disorder of the hemopoietic system in which there is an increased tendency for thrombosis (Antithrombin III difeciency, factor V leiden mutation, protein C or S deficiency, Prothrombin G20210A mutation, hyperhomocysteinemia, homozygous MTHFR).
D-dimer: A specific fibrin degradation product that is a result of thrombus breakdown. Fibrin formation can also be due to inflammation.

DISCUSSION

Deep Venous Thrombosis

Deep venous thromboses (DVTs) are **clot formations** in the **deep venous system,** most commonly the deep veins below the knee and iliofemoral veins and less commonly the pelvic veins. They occur with damage to the intimal wall of the vein, stasis, or when a hypercoagulable state is present. Damage to the intimal wall causes the release of factors that attract platelets to the site. The platelets in turn release thromboxane A_2 and serotonin, which serve to attract more platelets. There is eventual formation of fibrin, which incorporates the platelets into a clot. This is balanced by blood flow, which prevents accumulation of these elements and natural anticoagulants such as protein C and protein S and antithrombin III. Antithrombin III interferes with the action of serine proteases such as thrombin and is a general inhibitor of the intrinsic pathway. Protein C, with its cofactor protein S, inhibits factor V and factor VIII, the principal components of the common coagulation. In the absence of flow or natural anticoagulants, the risk of clot formation increases. There is also clot breakdown by plasmin, which, paradoxically, also is produced by damaged endothelial cells and helps keep clot formation localized.

DVT classically presents with a **painful, swollen tender extremity.** However, these signs are not always present. Attention to the history for risk factors also may raise suspicion for the diagnosis of DVT. Diagnosis is confirmed with Doppler ultrasound studies on the lower **extremities** that reveal **decreased flow or lack of compressibility of the vein;** this study is not as good for pelvic venous thrombosis, which can be detected by magnetic resonance imaging (MRI) or computed tomography (CT) with contrast of the veins. A **D-dimer blood test** may be elevated in the presence of DVT, but an elevated level would need to be confirmed by imaging modalities. Currently there are no other blood tests available for the diagnosis of DVT. Treatment is focused on stabilizing the clot by anticoagulation to reduce the risk of developing a pulmonary embolus (PE) and evaluating the underlying causes (thrombophilia, malignancy, immobility) and addressing the risk factors.

Pulmonary Embolus

Embolization to the pulmonary vasculature occurs most commonly when a clot from a DVT breaks off and travels proximally, becoming lodged in the pulmonary arteries. Other causes include amniotic fluid emboli that occurs at or after delivery; trophoblast fragments, which can be found in the lungs of pregnant women; fat emboli after trauma involving crush injury to the bone; tumor; and talc or starch particles in injection drug users. Similar underlying risk factors for DVT (immobility, malignancy, pregnancy, thrombophilia) also place one at risk for PE.

The presentation is variable, depending on the size and location of pulmonary emboli. A large embolus that is blocking the pulmonary artery or the major branches (saddle embolus) can cause sudden death. Smaller emboli affecting distal branches of the pulmonary arteries can present with chest pain, dyspnea, tachycardia, tachypnea, fever, and/or cough. These symptoms can be transient with smaller emboli. An elevated D-dimer in the presence of symptoms is suggestive of a PE, but false-positive D-dimers can occur in pregnancy and in the presence of pulmonary infection. Ventilation-perfusion scans look for an area of the lung where ventilation is good but perfusion is poor ($\dot{V}/\dot{Q}$ mismatch). CT angiography of the lungs also can detect pulmonary emboli by showing defects in the filling of the pulmonary arteries. As with DVT, treatment is focused on stabilizing the clot with anticoagulation and attempting to reduce extension of the clot as well as looking for potential underlying causes.

Another potential complication is pulmonary infarction, which can occur when a midsize artery is obstructed in a patient who has baseline impaired pulmonary circulation (left heart failure, pulmonary hypertension). This can present with cough, fever, pleuritic chest pain, and hemoptysis. On chest x-ray there is a wedge-shaped infiltrate that appears 12 to 36 hours after infarction has occurred. Pulmonary hypertension, pulmonary vascular sclerosis, and chronic cor pulmonale (enlargement of the right side of the heart) can occur with recurrent pulmonary emboli.

COMPREHENSION QUESTIONS

[25.1] A 43-year-old woman, while recovering in bed several days after having an abdominal hysterectomy, develops an acute onset of chest pain and shortness of breath. Physical examination finds the patient to be afebrile with moderate respiratory distress. She is anxious, is breathing quickly, and calf tenderness is present. Which of the following laboratory findings would be most suggestive of the diagnosis of pulmonary embolus in this individual?

A. Decreased serum levels of protein C
B. Elevated serum fibrin degradation products
C. Increased erythrocyte sedimentation rate
D. Increased serum angiotensin-converting enzyme activity
E. Presence of a mutated form of coagulation factor V

[25.2] What is the most common cause and site of origin for pulmonary emboli?

A. Deep venous thrombosis
B. Long bone trauma
C. Mesenteric vein obstruction
D. Right ventricle stasis
E. Superficial leg hemorrhage

[25.3] A 35-year-old woman is noted to have a 2-day history of a swollen and tender right leg. Doppler ultrasound studies confirm a deep venous thrombosis. She has had two previous episodes of venous thrombosis and also has a history of losing three pregnancies in the past 6 years. Which of the listed substances is a vitamin-K dependent substance that is associated with an increased risk of thrombosis when it is deficient?

A. Coagulation factor VII
B. Lecithin
C. Lipoprotein(a)
D. Protein C
E. Sphingomyelin

Answers

[25.1] **B.** Most pulmonary emboli are small thromboemboli that do no harm and produce no clinical signs or symptoms. Large emboli, however, can produce acute cor pulmonale or sudden death (saddle embolus), whereas smaller emboli can produce chest pain, dyspnea, tachypnea, fever, and cough. Elevated serum fibrin degradation products (e.g., D-dimers) in the presence of these classic symptoms in the appropriate clinical setting are suggestive of a pulmonary embolus. An elevated D-dimer blood test should be confirmed, using imaging modalities.

[25.2] **A.** Pulmonary emboli most commonly originate from clots that form in the deep venous system, most commonly the deep veins below the knee and the iliofemoral veins. A thrombus that develops in a deep vein can break off and eventually become lodged in the pulmonary arteries. Although most pulmonary emboli are thromboemboli, which develop when conditions that damage veins, stasis, or hypercoagulable states are present, other causes of pulmonary emboli are possible and include amniotic fluid emboli, fat emboli, bone marrow emboli, and gas emboli.

[25.3] **D.** Recurrent thromboemboli and spontaneous abortions are clinical signs that may result from a deficiency of either antithrombin III, protein C, or protein S. All of these substances are normal inhibitors of the intrinsic coagulation pathway. Antithrombin III is a nonvitamin K-dependent protease that inhibits the action of thrombin and other coagulation factors, such as activated factor X. Protein C and protein S both inhibit activate coagulation factors V and VIII.

PATHOLOGY PEARLS

- Pulmonary emboli can be a cause of sudden death.
- Risk factors for PE are similar to those for DVT and relate to a disturbance in the balance of clot formation and breakdown.
- Signs and symptoms for DVT and PE are nonspecific; a high level of suspicion is necessary to make the diagnosis.

REFERENCES

Chandrasoma P, Taylor C. Concise Pathology, 3rd ed. Stamford, CT: Appleton & Lange, 1998.

Freied C. Deep venous thrombosis. eMedicine 2004:1–25. http://www.emedicine.com/med/topic2785.htm

Haselton PS, ed. Spencer's Pathology of the Lung, 5th ed. New York: McGraw-Hill, 1996.

Husain AN, Kumar V. The lung. In: Kumar V, Assas AK, Fausto N, eds. Robbins and Cotran Pathologic Basis of Disease, 7th ed. Philadelphia, PA: Elsevier Saunders, 2004:742–50.

Husain AN. The lung. In: Mitchell RN, Kumar V, Abbas AK, et al., eds. Pocket Companion to Robbins and Cotran Pathologic Basis of Disease, 7th ed. Philadelphia, PA: Saunders, 2006:389–91.

Rubin E, Farber J, eds. Pathology. Philadelphia, PA: Lippincott, 1988.

❖ CASE 26

A 78-year-old man is brought to the emergency department. For the last several days he has had fatigue, malaise, fever, and a productive cough. A chest radiograph shows consolidation in the right lower lobe. A Gram stain of the sputum shows a predominance of gram-positive cocci in pairs and chains (see Figure 26-1).

◆ **What is the most likely diagnosis?**

◆ **What is the likely prognosis for this patient?**

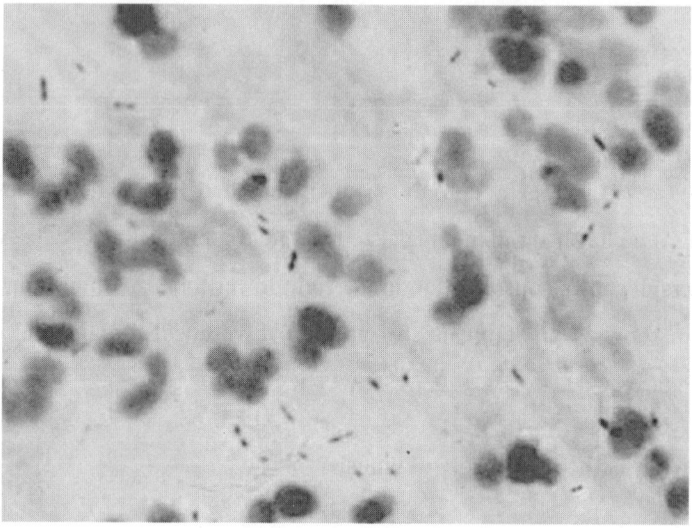

Figure 26-1. Gram stain. *(Reproduced, with permission, from Kasper DL, Braunwald E, Fauci AS, et al., eds.* Harrison's Principles of Internal Medicine, 16 ed. *New York: McGraw-Hill, 2004:810.)*

ANSWERS TO CASE 26: PNEUMOCOCCAL PNEUMONIA

Summary: A 78-year-old man is brought to the emergency department. For the last several days he has had fatigue, malaise, fever, and a productive cough. A chest radiograph shows right lower lobe consolidation. A Gram stain of the sputum shows a predominance of gram-positive cocci in pairs and chains.

- **Most likely diagnosis:** Pneumococcal pneumonia.
- **Likely prognosis:** This patient probably has a poor prognosis with high odds of mortality given his age of over 65 years.

CLINICAL CORRELATION

This 78-year-old man presents with pneumococcal pneumonia, which is the single most common cause of pneumonia, particularly community-acquired pneumonia. Pneumonia is infection of the lung parenchyma. It typically is caused by bacteria but may be caused by a variety of types of organisms. With pneumococcal pneumonia, the patient develops fever, cough, and chest pain. The sputum is typically **rust-colored,** and there may be frank hemoptysis. Purulent sputum is not uncommon. The respiratory rate is generally high.

Physical examination reveals reduced chest movement on the affected side as well as features of consolidation (bronchial breath sounds). Inflammation of the overlying pleura results in pleuritic chest pain and pleural rub (heard on auscultation). By virtue of the patient's age greater than 65 years, the mortality rate is increased. Other poor prognostic factors include respiratory rate >30/min and diastolic blood pressure (BP) <60 mm Hg, a chest x-ray revealing more than one lobe involved, hypoxemia, and renal insufficiency. The treatment is antibiotic therapy and support for possible septicemia.

APPROACH TO PNEUMOCOCCAL PNEUMONIA

Objectives

- Know the natural history of pneumonia.
- Describe the varying etiologies of pneumonia and their respective "key" features.
- List the risk factors for a lung abscess.

Definitions

Malaise: A vague feeling of bodily discomfort.

Gram stain: A staining procedure in which microorganisms are stained with crystal violet, treated with strong iodine solution, decolorized with ethanol or ethanol-acetone, and counterstained with a contrasting dye; those retaining the stain are gram-positive and those losing the stain but staining with the counterstain are gram-negative.

Pleuritic chest pain: Sharp chest pain with breathing.

Pleural rub: An auscultatory sound caused by friction between the visceral and parietal pleura.

Cold agglutinins: IgM antibody directed against I antigen, i antigen, or Pr antigen on the surface of a red blood cell that can lead to hemolytic anemia when titers are high and temperature is 28 to 31°C (winter months).

DISCUSSION

Pathologically, the natural history of **pneumonia** is divided into **four stages: (1) congestion, (2) red hepatization, (3) gray hepatization,** and **(4) resolution.** The stage of **congestion** represents the developing bacterial infection and is characterized by vascular congestion with some intra-alveolar accumulation of fluid. In the stage or red hepatization, there are significant numbers of neutrophils and fibrin within the alveolar spaces. Extravasated red cells are present. The affected lung parenchyma is now solid with a consistency similar to that of liver. The **red discoloration** caused by the extravasated red cells, coupled with the change in the consistency, is the reason for the term ***red hepatization.*** In the next stage, the red cells and white cells are disintegrating. The previous gross appearance of red changes to **gray.** The consistency is still the same. All the inflammatory exudates will be engulfed by macrophages and normal lung parenchyma is restored. Air can reach the affected alveoli. This is the stage of **resolution.**

APPROACH TO PULMONARY INFECTIONS

Infectious pneumonia can be classified either anatomically or on the basis of etiology.

Anatomic classification includes lobar, lobular (bronchopneumonia), and interstitial.

As the name implies, **lobar pneumonia** occurs when one or more lobes are affected. The **vast majority of lobar pneumonias** are due to **pneumococci.** Occasionally, *Staphylococcus, Streptococcus, Klebsiella pneumoniae, Hemophilus influenzae,* and gram-negative rods may be implicated. This condition may occur at any age but is typically uncommon in infancy and late life. **Lobular pneumonia** is characterized by **patchy involvement** and consolidation of the lung. In contrast to lobar pneumonia, it tends to affect **infants** and the **elderly.** Any of the agents that produce lobar pneumonia can produce lobular pneumonia.

In **interstitial pneumonia** the inflammatory exudates are confined mostly to the alveolar interstitium. Alveolar exudate is not prominent. Thus, consolidation is not a feature of this type of pneumonia. This type of pneumonia is seen with viral infections and certain bacterial infections, but not the ones associated with lobar or lobular pneumonia.

Etiologic Classification

An etiologic agent can be found in approximately 75 percent of all pneumonias (see Table 26-1). Most often these agents are bacteria. Pneumonias caused by certain bacteria, such as *Mycoplasma, Legionella, Chlamydia,* and *Coxiella,* usually result in interstitial inflammation and traditionally have been termed **atypical pneumonia.** Viral pneumonia is uncommon in adults. Influenza, adenovirus, and respiratory syncytial virus are examples of viral pneumonias. In an immunocompromised individual, the variety of agents infecting the lungs is much broader. In the case of patients with AIDS, the most common opportunistic infection of the lung is *Pneumocystis jiroveci.*

Mycoplasma pneumoniae Pneumonia

This is the **most common type of atypical pneumonia** encountered, occurring mostly in children and young adults, often in schools, camps, military barracks, or prisons. Symptoms related to pneumonia are present, but signs (features of consolidation) are usually disproportionately less. The white blood cell count may not be raised, as is in typical pneumonia. **Cold agglutinins**

Table 26-1
ETIOLOGY OF PNEUMONIA

Streptococcus pneumoniae	Most common cause of lobar pneumonia "rust colored" sputum
Staphylococcus aureus	IV drug abusers, may follow influenza
Haemophilus influenzae	May be seen in people with preexisting lung disease such as COPD
Gram-negative organisms	Especially seen in hospital-acquired infections
Klebsiella	Alcoholics; "currant jelly" sputum
Pseudomonas aeruginosa	Cystic fibrosis; nosocomial
Mycoplasma pneumoniae	Atypical pneumonia
Chlamydia	*Chlamydia psittaci* is seen with contact with birds (bird fancier's disease) atypical pneumonia
Legionella pneumophila	Institutional outbreaks, atypical pneumonia, elderly
Coxiella burnetii	Abattoir workers, atypical pneumonia
Anaerobic organisms	Aspiration pneumonia
Pneumocystis jiroveci	AIDS
Viral pneumonias	Can vary from mild symptoms to life-threatening disease

occur in up to half the cases. Extrapulmonary features may be present and may dominate the clinical picture, including myocarditis, pericarditis, meningoencephalitis, hemolytic anemia, thrombocytopenia, and erythema multiforme.

Legionnaires' Disease

Infection with *Legionella pneumophila* results in Legionnaires' disease. *Legionella* grows well in water, and infection is spread by the aerosol route. Extrapulmonary features also may be seen with this condition. Half the patients have gastrointestinal symptoms with nausea, vomiting, and diarrhea. Other possible features include neurologic and renal abnormalities.

Pneumocystis jiroveci Pneumonia

Immunocompromised patients may develop pneumonia with the usual organisms along with a number of organisms that normally do not cause illness in healthy hosts. Aside from pneumococcus, *P. jiroveci* is the most common cause of pneumonia in AIDS patients. It is seen particularly when the peripheral serum CD4 count is less than 200/mm^3. It also is seen in individuals on immunosuppressive therapy.

Lung Abscess

Lung abscess is a local suppurative process within the lung characterized by necrosis of lung tissue. Lung abscesses may be seen in many different circumstances (see Table 26-2 for risk factors). When a bronchus is obstructed by a tumor mass, the distal airways are prone to stasis, atelectasis, and persistent infection, resulting in abscess formation.

The commonly isolated organisms include aerobic and anaerobic streptococci, *Staphylococcus,* and gram-negative organisms.

Pleuritis

Inflammation of the pleura (pleuritis) may be primary or secondary. Primary pleuritis usually is due to bacterial seeding of the pleura as part of bacteremia. Secondary pleuritis is due to underlying infection and inflammation of the lung. Depending on the nature of the inflammatory exudates, pleuritis may be serofibrinous, suppurative (empyema), or hemorrhagic. Serofibrinous pleuritis may resolve completely with resorption of the inflammatory exudates. Empyema may resolve, but more often there occurs fibrosis with adhesions that obliterate the pleural space.

Table 26-2
RISK FACTORS FOR LUNG ABSCESS

Aspiration of infective material (involving multiple organisms)
Preceding pneumonia Lung abscesses following pneumonia are more often seen in pneumonia due to *Staphylococcus, Klebsiella,* and fungal infections
Septic emboli
Lung cancer

COMPREHENSION QUESTIONS

[26.1] A 31-year-old woman presents to the emergency room with the acute onset of malaise, fever, and a productive cough. A chest x-ray reveals consolidation of the right lower lobe along with air bronchograms, and a Gram stain of her sputum shows a predominance of gram-positive lancet-shaped cocci in pairs and chains. Which of the following is the most likely causative agent of this individual's infectious disease?

A. *Hemophilus influenzae*
B. *Klebsiella pneumoniae*
C. *Pseudomonas aeruginosa*
D. *Streptococcus pneumoniae*

[26.2] A 26-year-old woman presents with the acute onset of fever, malaise, headaches, muscle pain, and a dry, hacking nonproductive cough. Laboratory evaluation finds the presence of cold agglutinins in her serum, mainly immunoglobulin M (IgM) anti-I cold agglutinins. Which histologic changes would most likely be present in the lung parenchyma of this individual?

A. Eosinophils within the walls of the capillaries
B. Lymphocytes within the walls of the alveoli
C. Microthrombi within the lumen of the capillaries
D. Neutrophils within the lumen of the alveoli
E. Noncaseating granulomas in the walls of the alveoli

[26.3] A 25-year-old HIV-positive man presents with a low-grade fever, a nonproductive cough, and increasing shortness of breath. Routine histologic sections from a transbronchial biopsy reveal foamy frothy eosinophilic material within the alveoli. Silver stains reveal the presence of numerous cup-shaped organisms with central dark dots. Which of the following is the most likely diagnosis?

A. Aspiration pneumonia
B. Atypical pneumonia
C. Organizing pneumonia
D. *Paragonimus* pneumonia
E. *Pneumocystis* pneumonia

Answers

[26.1] **D.** Although infection of the lung parenchyma (pneumonia) can be caused by a number of different types of organisms, most commonly pneumonia results from bacterial infection (bacterial pneumonia) of the lung. There are two basic patterns of bacterial pneumonia: lobar pneumonia, which is characterized by involvement of an entire lobe by a virulent organism, and lobular pneumonia (bronchopneumonia), which is characterized by patchy inflammation involving one or more lobes. The vast majority of cases of lobar pneumonia, which is the more common type of bacterial pneumonia, are caused by infection with *Streptococcus pneumoniae.* With pneumococcal pneumonia, patients usually present with fever, a productive cough with rust-colored sputum, and pleuritic chest pain.

[26.2] **B.** With bacterial pneumonia, the acute inflammatory exudate, which consists mainly of neutrophils, is found primarily within the lumen of the alveoli. In contrast, with interstitial pneumonia, the chronic inflammatory exudate, which consists mainly of lymphocytes, is mainly within the walls (interstitium) of the alveoli. This type of inflammatory reaction, which traditionally is called atypical pneumonia, characteristically is seen with viral infections and certain bacterial infections, such as infection with *Mycoplasma pneumoniae;* this is the most common cause of atypical pneumonia. Symptoms are similar to those of bacterial pneumonia (headache, malaise, and a dry hacking nonproductive cough) but are less severe ("walking pneumonia"). Many cases are associated with the presence in the serum of IgM anti-I cold agglutinins.

[26.3] **E.** *Pneumocystis* pneumonia is caused by *Pneumocystis jiroveci,* a fungus that behaves like a protozoon. *Pneumocystis jiroveci* is the most common cause of pneumonia in patients with AIDS. Routine stains of infected lung tissue will show foamy material within the alveoli, but the organisms may not be visible. Special stains, such as silver stains, will reveal organisms that have cup shapes with central dots.

PATHOLOGY PEARLS

- Pathologically the natural history of pneumonia is divided into four stages: congestion, red hepatization, gray hepatization, and resolution.
- Pneumonia can be classified either anatomically or on the basis of etiology.
- The vast majority of lobar infectious pneumonias are due to pneumococci.
- Lobular pneumonia tends to affect infants and the elderly.
- In interstitial pneumonia, the inflammatory exudate is confined mostly to the alveolar interstitium and is seen with viral infections and certain bacterial infections, not the ones associated with lobar or lobular pneumonia.
- *Mycoplasma* pneumonia is the most common type of atypical pneumonia encountered.
- In the case of patients with AIDS, the most common opportunistic infection of the lung is *Pneumocystis jiroveci;* however, HIV-infected individuals also develop pulmonary infections with common bacteria.
- Empyema may resolve, but more often there occurs fibrosis with adhesions that obliterate the pleural space.

REFERENCES

Husain AN, Kumar V. The lung. In: Kumar V, Assas AK, Fausto N, eds. Robbins and Cotran Pathologic Basis of Disease, 7th ed. Philadelphia, PA: Elsevier Saunders, 2004:741–52.

Husain AN. The lung. In: Mitchell RN, Kumar V, Abbas AK, et al., eds. Pocket Companion to Robbins and Cotran Pathologic Basis of Disease, 7th ed. Philadelphia, PA: Saunders, 2006:391–5.

❖ CASE 27

A 10-year-old boy complains of pain and swelling around his right knee for a 3-week duration that has not improved with rest. His mother denies a history of trauma to the knee. A radiograph shows a destructive mixed lytic and blastic mass arising from the metaphysis of the distal tumor.

◆ **What is the most likely diagnosis?**

◆ **What are the risk factors for developing this disease?**

ANSWERS TO CASE 27: OSTEOSARCOMA

Summary: A 10-year-old boy complains of pain and swelling around his right knee. A radiograph shows a destructive mixed lytic and blastic mass arising from the metaphysis of the distal tumor.

- **Most likely diagnosis:** Osteosarcoma.
- **Risk factors for developing this disease:** Prior irradiation, genetic predisposition (parents with retinoblastoma), Paget disease of the bone, and bone infarcts.

CLINICAL CORRELATION

This 10-year-old boy complains of progressive pain and swelling of his right knee, which may be a benign musculoskeletal problem such as a sprain or Osgood-Schlatter disease. This patient does not have a history of trauma. Although rare, osteosarcoma is the most common type of primary bony cancer. The x-ray reveals destruction and a lytic mass near the metaphysis of the bone, which is the most common location for osteosarcoma. This child's age is in the range for this cancer, with three-quarters of cases occurring in those younger than 20 years. Whereas previously extensive and disfiguring surgery would have been the only therapeutic option, today chemotherapy with limb-saving surgery is usually possible.

APPROACH TO BONE PATHOLOGY

Objectives

- List the risk factors for osteosarcoma.
- Describe the various types of bone tumors and their "key" features.
- Know the primary age groups of various bone tumors.

Definitions

Osteochondroma: A benign tumor composed of a hyaline cartilage-capped bony outgrowth, developmentally arising from an epiphyseal plate defect. The most common primary lesion of bone, it occurs twice as often in males. It occurs in the appendicular skeleton in the first through third decades of life.

Enchondroma: A benign hyaline cartilage tumor arising from the medullary cavity of the bones, usually those of the hands and feet. Equally found in males and females of all age ranges.

Giant cell tumor: A benign tumor formed of multinucleated giant cells and fibrous stroma, usually at the epiphyses of long bones. It most often is found in the distal femur or proximal tibia of women between 20 and 40 years of age.

Osteoma: A benign tumor formed of very dense mature bone, usually found in the skull or the bones of the face. This tumor most often is found in males of all ages and often protrudes into the paranasal sinuses.

Osteoid osteoma: A primary benign osteogenic lesion of **bone** that classically is described in the femur and is stated to be worse at night and relieved by aspirin. Most often found in males in the second decade of life.

Chondrosarcoma: A primary neoplasm of the bone that consists of malignant **cartilage.** Usually found in fourth to seventh decades of life and occurs twice as often in males.

Osteosarcoma: A primary malignant tumor of **bone** with neoplastic cells that form predominantly in immature osteoid; usually located at the metaphyses. It occurs slightly more frequently in males, usually during the second and third decades of life.

Parosteal osteosarcoma: A low-grade osteosarcoma that arises from the cortical surface of the **bone.** Is found most often in long bones, and the most common site is the posterior distal femur. It occurs twice as often in females, usually during the third through fifth decades of life.

Ewing sarcoma: A small, round cell malignant **bone** tumor of neural origin that occurs in the first and second decades of life. Usually found in the lower extremities, with a slight predominance in males. It is related to primitive neuroectoderm tumor (PNET), sharing the same chromosomal abnormality: t(11;22) (q24;q12).

DISCUSSION

Normal Bone

Bone is a vascular connective tissue that consists of cells and calcified intercellular materials. Bone may be dense, also known as **compact bone,** or may be sponge like, known as **cancellous** bone. Cancellous bone, like that which is found inside the epiphysis of the long bones, is always surrounded by compact bone. It has large open marrow spaces surrounded by thin anastomosing plates of bone known as **trabeculae,** which are composed of several layers of **lamellae.** Compact bone is much denser with spaces and thicker lamellae. The calcified matrix of the bone is composed of half minerals and half organic matter and bound water. The minerals are mostly **calcium hydroxyapatite,** and the organic matter consists of collagen and **protein-associated glycosaminoglycans.**

The marrow cavity of bone is lined by **endosteum,** which is composed of **osteogenic cells, osteoblasts,** and some **osteoclasts.** The **periosteum** covering the bone is a fibrous layer that consists mostly of collagen fibers. This periosteum is fixed to the bone by **Sharpey fibers,** which are collagenous bundles trapped in the calcified bone matrix during ossification. The bone matrix is produced by osteoblasts derived from the less differentiated osteogenic cells. As the osteoblasts lay down the matrix of the bone, they become trapped. As this matrix calcifies, they become known as **osteocytes.** The osteocytes occupy lenticular spaces called lacunae and have long processes that are found in the canals or tunnels known as **canaliculi.** The canaliculi eventually open into channels known as **haversian canals** that house the blood vessels. This functional unit of each haversian canal with its surrounding lamellae of bone containing canaliculi radiating to it from the osteocytes trapped in the lacunae is known as an **osteon** or a **haversian canal system.** The canaliculi of the osteon extend to the haversian canals to facilitate the exchange of waste products for nutrients and oxygen. The haversian canals, which run approximately parallel to the longitudinal axis of the long bones, are connected to one another by **Volkmann canals.**

Osteogenesis

The histogenesis of bone occurs by one of two routes: **intramembranous ossification** or **endochondral ossification.** Intramembranous ossification occurs in richly vascularized mesenchymal membrane in which the mesenchymal cells differentiate into osteoblasts and begin to elaborate bone matrix and form the trabeculae of bone. With the increasing formation of trabeculae in approximation to one another, they begin to become interconnected. With this fusion to one another they form cancellous bone, which will be remodeled to form compact bone. The surfaces of these trabeculae are populated with osteoblasts and the occasional osteoclast.

The **osteoclast** is a **large multinucleated cell** that is **derived from the monocytes.** These cells, which function to resorb bone, are found in shallow depressions in the trabecular surface of the bone known as **Howship lacunae.** The region of the mesenchymal membrane that does not participate in this ossification process remains the soft tissue component of the bone: the periosteum and endosteum. As the bone is newly formed, it is called **woven** or **primary bone** because the arrangement of the collagen fibers does not possess the precise organization found in older bone. The integrated interaction between the osteoblasts and the osteoclasts coordinates the replacement of the woven bone with **secondary** or **mature bone.** Endochondral ossification, in contrast, relies on the presence of a hyaline cartilage model. This hyaline cartilage model is a template on which the long and short bones are made.

A **bony subperiosteal collar** is formed around the middle of the cartilage template, and then this collar increases in width and length. The chondrocytes in the middle of the template enlarge and resorb some of their matrix, thereby enlarging their lacunae and making some of the lacunae confluent. These hypertrophied **chondrocytes** assist in the calcification of the cartilage and then degenerate. The newly formed spaces they leave behind are invaded by a **periosteal bud** that is composed of blood vessels, mesenchymal cells, and osteogenic cells. The osteogenic cells then differentiate into osteoblasts and elaborate a bony matrix lining on the calcified cartilage. As the periosteal bone collar continues to increase in width and length, the osteoblasts resorb the calcified cartilage, leaving behind an enlarged space that will be the future marrow cavity occupied by marrow cells. The entire ossification process spreads bidirectionally away from this primary ossification center, eventually replacing most of the cartilage template with bone and forming the **diaphysis** of the long bone. The **epiphysis** of the bone is the **secondary ossification center,** which is formed in a modified fashion to allow the cartilaginous covering to be maintained at the articular surface. The longitudinal growth of the long bones is attributable to the presence of epiphyseal plates of cartilage between the epiphysis and the diaphysis.

Osteosarcoma

Osteosarcoma (OS) is the **most common primary malignant tumor of bone,** with a peak incidence in males between ages 10 and 20 years. This tumor always should be considered in the differential of any young person with an apparent osseous neoplasm involving the metaphysis or diaphysis of any long bone. This tumor occurs most frequently at the **metaphysis** of the long bones, with greatest preference for the sites about the **knee,** specifically the proximal portion of the tibia and the distal portion of the femur. Histologically, it is a malignant bone tumor with the neoplastic cells producing **osteoid or bone.**

The clinical presentation of the tumor includes **pain and swelling** and may be associated with a **pathologic fracture** of the bone. Blood serum chemistries will reveal a serum **alkaline phosphatase** level of 2 to 3 times the normal level. Radiographically, this tumor creates a very characteristic appearance known as the **Codman triangle,** which is a lifting of the periosteum by the expanding tumor, creating a triangle visible on x-ray (see Figure 27-1). **Predisposing factors** for this type of tumor include **Paget disease of the bone, previous ionizing radiation, previous bone infarcts,** and **familial retinoblastoma.** OS necessitates treatment as a systemic disease because there is **very early hematogenous spread to the lungs, liver, and brain,** with 45 to 90 percent of patients having systemic metastases at the time of presentation. In these patients, treatment with surgery alone results in a 100 percent mortality rate of this population within 3 years. Therefore, **neoadjuvant chemotherapy and surgery with postoperative chemotherapy follow-up** is the treatment of choice, resulting in a 10-year survival rate of 65 to 70 percent of these patients.

Chondrosarcoma

Chondrosarcoma is a **malignant cartilaginous tumor** with a peak incidence in males between the ages of 30 and 60 years. Its characteristic sites of origin include the pelvis, spine, scapula, proximal humerus or femur, and the femur or tibia near the knee. Histologically, it is noted to be hypercellular with decreased organization and the presence of binuclear cells. Radiographically, it usually can be seen at the **metaphysis or diaphysis** and is noted to have **endosteal scalloping.** There is no effective adjuvant therapy, and therefore treatment is solely **surgical.** The prognosis is related to grade, tumor site and size, and surgical accessibility.

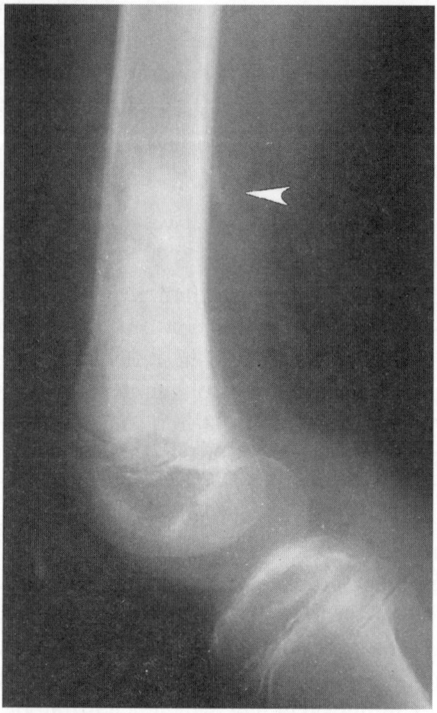

Figure 27-1. Radiograph of osteosarcoma. *(Reproduced, with permission, from Rudolph CD, Rudolph AM, Hostetter MK, et al., eds.* Rudolph's Pediatrics, 21st ed. *New York: McGraw-Hill, 2003:1610.)*

Ewing Sarcoma

Ewing sarcoma is an **extremely anaplastic small round cell malignant tumor** that occurs most frequently in the **long bones,** ribs, pelvis, and scapula, with a peak incidence in **males under 15 years** of age. This tumor follows an **extremely malignant course** with very early metastasis. In its early stages, the clinical presentation of this disease may **resemble that of osteomyelitis.** Histologically, there is a proliferation of uniform, monotonous small cells with very scant cytoplasm. The nuclei have uniform finely distributed chromatin, and the cytoplasm contains glycogen, making it periodic acid-Schiff **(PAS)-positive.** Radiographically, it is described as having a **moth-eaten permeative pattern,** and the **periosteal reaction bone** is described as **onion skin.** This tumor is responsive to **chemotherapy,** which is a mainstay of therapy in combination with surgery or radiation. Long-term survival appears to be site-dependent but approximates 60 percent overall. This tumor is characterized by an **11;22 chromosomal translocation** identical to that found in primitive neuroectodermal tumors.

Osteochondroma

Osteochondroma is the **most common benign tumor of bone,** found most commonly in **males under the age of 25 years.** It is a bony growth that is found to be covered by a **cap of cartilage** projecting from the surface of a bone. It often originates from the **metaphysis of the long bones,** with the lower end of the femur and the upper end of the tibia being the most common locations. A stalk consisting of cortex and the medullary cavity are in continuity with their counterparts within the parent bone. A sessile form also exists that forms a transmural cortical defect. It has been postulated that this may be a hamartoma rather than a true neoplasm. Occasionally this tumor will undergo a **malignant transformation to chondrosarcoma,** but this occurs most often in **multiple familial osteochondromatosis,** a hereditary variant characterized by multiple lesions. Histologically, the cartilaginous cap **mimics the epiphyseal plate.** The prognosis for this type of tumor is excellent, with the growth either involuting or remaining static as the skeleton matures. Therefore, treatment is not necessary unless the patient is symptomatic, or the cap continues to grow with the skeleton, resulting in a cap >2 cm.

Giant Cell Tumor

A giant cell tumor is a **benign** but very locally aggressive tumor characterized by **oval or spindle-shaped cells** interspersed with many **multinuclear giant cells.** It occurs most frequently in **females between the ages of 20 and 40 years.** It usually is found on the epiphyseal end of long bones, with more than half of them occurring around the knee. Treatment is not necessary unless the patient is symptomatic; curettage and packing are mandated; however, **recurrence** is very common.

Enchondroma

An enchondroma is a **benign intramedullary cartilaginous neoplasm** that occurs most often in the short tubular bones of the **hands and feet.** It occurs equally in males and females and over a wide distribution of ages. Histologically, it is noted to be **hypercellular and to have disorganized hyaline cartilage without significant atypia.** Radiographically, it is seen to be located at the **metaphysis** and is fairly **radiolucent. Ring and fleck calcification** may be noted within the lesion. Treatment is not mandated unless the patient is symptomatic, which would necessitate curettage and packing. Prognostically, although this is a self-limited disease, it carries with it a very small increased incidence of **secondary chondrosarcoma:** less than 1 percent.

Osteoid Osteoma

Osteoid osteoma is a **primary benign osteogenic lesion of the bone.** This lesion may grow to only 1 to 2 cm and has very distinct clinical features, including **pain that worsens at night and is relieved by aspirin.** It occurs most often in males in the second decade, most often in the femur. The tumor is composed of **interweaving trabeculae** of osteoid and bone lined by osteoblasts and a few osteoclasts with a **capillary background.** Radiographically, a **radiolucent nidus <2 cm** is seen in the metaphysis or diaphysis. The lesion may calcify, resulting in a **target-shaped appearance.** The prognosis is very good, with nearly a 100 percent cure rate when the nidus is completely removed. Treatment therefore consists of **surgical** resection. Recurrences occur up to 25 percent of the time, secondary to incomplete nidus removal. The rate of complete removal is increased with **radionucleotide labeling and preoperative tetracycline loading/ultraviolet fluorescence of the specimen.**

Table 27-1 summarizes the location, key features, and primarily affected age groups for each type of bone tumor discussed above.

Table 27-1
BONE TUMORS

	LOCATION	"KEY FEATURE"	PRIMARY AGE GROUP
MALIGNANT			
Osteosarcoma	Metaphysis	Most common primary malignant tumor; Codman triangle	Males 10–20 years
Chondrosarcoma	Diaphysis	Endosteal scalloping	Males 30–60 years
Ewing Sarcoma	Diaphysis	"Onion skin" appearance; 11:22 translocation	Males <15 years
BENIGN			
Osteochondroma	Metaphysis	Most common benign tumor of bone; cartilaginous cap that mimics the epiphyseal plate	Males <25 years
Enchondroma	Intramedullary	Most often in hands and feet; may progress to Chondrosarcoma	Males = females
Giant cell tumor	Epiphysis	"Soap bubble" appearance	Females 20–40 years
Osteoid osteoma	Metaphysis/ diaphysis	Pain that worsens at night and is relieved by aspirin; radiolucent nidus	Males 20–30 years

COMPREHENSION QUESTIONS

[27.1] A 23-year-old man presents with a "lump" in the distal portion of his left femur. Workup finds a cartilage-capped outgrowth of bone that is connected to the underlying skeleton by a bony stalk. No destruction of the underlying bone is seen. Which of the following is the most likely diagnosis?

A. Chondroblastoma
B. Chondrosarcoma
C. Osteoblastoma
D. Osteochondroma
E. Osteosarcoma

[27.2] Which of the following clinical signs or symptoms is most characteristically associated with a benign osteoid osteoma?

A. Nontender swelling in the popliteal space
B. Numbness and tingling in the fourth and fifth fingers
C. Pain in the first toe that occurs after binge drinking
D. Severe pain in the femur that occurs at night
E. Stiffness in the knee that is worse in the morning

[27.3] An 11-year-old boy presents with an enlarging painful lesion in the medullary cavity of his left femur. X-rays reveal a destructive lesion that produces an "onion-skin" periosteal reaction. The lesion is surgically resected, and histologic sections reveal sheets of small round cells with cytoplasmic glycogen. This tumor most often is associated with which of the following chromosomal abnormalities?

A. t(8;14)
B. t(9;22)
C. t(11;22)
D. t(14;18)
E. t(15;17)

Answers

[27.1] **D.** An osteochondroma is a benign tumor of bone that is composed of a bony outgrowth that has a hyaline cartilage cap. It is the most common benign bone tumor and is found most commonly in males under the age of 25 years. Osteochondromas usually originate from the metaphysis of long bones, with the lower end of the femur and the upper end of the tibia being common sites. Some consider osteochondromas to be a form of exostosis or hamartoma rather than a true neoplasm. Malignant transformation can occur but is quite rare.

[27.2] **D.** An osteoid osteoma is a benign tumor of bone that characteristically produces severe pain at night as a result the excess production of prostaglandin E_2. Also characteristic is the fact that this nocturnal pain is relieved by aspirin. This benign bone tumor occurs most frequently in males in the second decade and most often occurs in the femur. Histologic sections of the tumor reveal a central nidus of uncalcified osteoid with a rim of sclerotic bone.

[27.3] **C.** Ewing sarcoma is a malignancy of bones that is found most commonly in males under the age of 15 years. It usually is located in the diaphysis or metaphysis of long bones. Histologically, this tumor is composed of sheets of small round cells with cytoplasmic glycogen that is PAS-positive. Reactive new bone formation produces a concentric onionskin layering appearance on x-ray examination. This malignancy is similar, and probably identical, to primitive neuroendocrine tumor or neuroblastoma cells located elsewhere in the body. It shares the same chromosomal abnormality t(11;22) with these other primitive neuroectodermal tumors.

PATHOLOGY PEARLS

❖ Risk factors for osteosarcoma include prior irradiation, genetic predisposition (parents with reintoblastoma), Paget disease of the bone, and bone infarcts.

❖ A radiograph revealing lytic lesions of the bone with a periosteum reaction near the metaphysis raises suspicion for osteosarcoma.

❖ Osteochondroma is the **most common benign tumor of bone,** found most commonly in men under the age of 25 years. It is a bony growth that is found to be covered by a **cap of cartilage** projecting from the surface of a bone.

REFERENCES

Rosenberg AE. Bones, joints, and soft tissue tumors. In: Kumar V, Assas AK, Fausto N, eds. Robbins and Cotran Pathologic Basis of Disease, 7th ed. Philadelphia, PA: Elsevier Saunders, 2004:1294–300.

Rosenberg AE. Bones, joints, and soft tissue tumors. In: Mitchell RN, Kumar V, Abbas AK, et al., eds. Pocket Companion to Robbins and Cotran Pathologic Basis of Disease, 7th ed. Philadelphia, PA: Saunders, 2006:640–7.

Rubin E. Essential Pathology, 3rd ed. Philadelphia, PA: Lippincott Williams & Wilkins, 2001.

❖ CASE 28

A 60-year-old woman has pain in her lower back upon bending over in her kitchen. A radiograph of the spine shows a compression fracture of the lumbar vertebrae at L2–L3. Further evaluation reveals normocytic anemia, hypercalcemia, and a high globulin fraction. A bone marrow biopsy is shown in Figure 28-1.

◆ **What is the diagnosis?**

◆ **What other tests might be contributory to her diagnosis and follow-up?**

◆ **What is the most likely mechanism?**

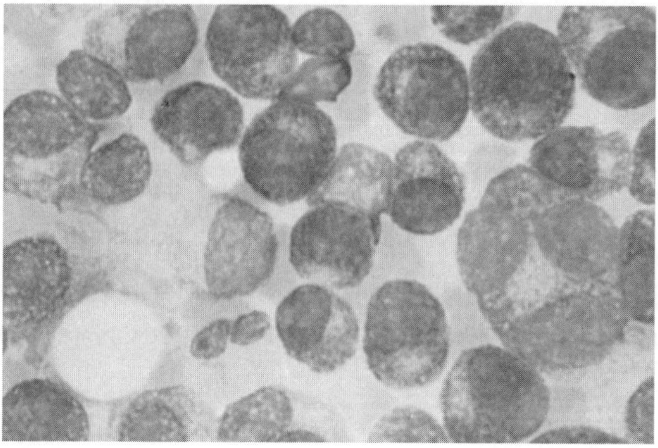

Figure 28-1. Bone marrow biopsy. *(Reproduced, with permission, from Kasper DL, Braunwald E, Fauci AS, et al., eds.* Harrison's Principles of Internal Medicine, 16th ed. *New York: McGraw-Hill, 2004:657.)*

ANSWERS TO CASE 28: MULTIPLE MYELOMA

Summary: A 60-year-old woman with back pain has a compression fracture of her lumbar vertebrae at L2–L3. She has normocytic anemia, hypercalcemia, and a high globulin fraction. A bone marrow biopsy is done.

- **Most likely diagnosis:** Multiple myeloma (MM).
- **Contributory tests:** Serum and urine protein electrophoresis with immunofixation to demonstrate a monoclonal gammopathy.
- **Most likely mechanism:** Etiology unknown but possibly caused by exposure to chemicals, high-dose radiation, viruses such as human herpesvirus 8 (HHV-8) and human immunodeficiency virus (HIV), or longstanding chronic infections.

CLINICAL CORRELATION

Multiple myeloma is a plasma cell neoplasm that has its peak incidence in the ages of 50 to 60 years. This patient, a 60-year-old female, fits that profile. The increased immunoglobulins produced and the infiltration of the plasma cells in various organs, particularly bones, leads to hypercalcemia and bone resorption. This patient developed a pathologic fracture as a result of the bony changes from MM. Skull radiographs often demonstrate lytic lesions. The serum globulins are increased because of the elevated immunoglobulins, and if electrophoresis is performed, a single spike consistent with monoclonal immunoglobulin elevation would be seen. Although the clinical and laboratory criteria are strongly suggestive of MM, a bone marrow biopsy, as performed in this case, gives the definitive diagnosis. The microscopic examination of the bone marrow usually shows an increased number of plasma cells. The prognosis for MM is variable but generally poor. Chemotherapy can be helpful, using medications such as bisphosphonates for the hypercalcemia and bone involvement.

APPROACH TO MULTIPLE MYELOMA

Objectives

- Describe the presentation of multiple myeloma.
- List the diagnostic criteria used for multiple myeloma.
- Describe the findings seen on urine protein electrophoresis in multiple myeloma.

Definitions

Pancytopenia: Anemia, neutropenia and thrombocytopenia in the peripheral blood.

Monoclonal protein: An immunoglobulin of one subtype produced by a clone of plasma cells or B lymphocytes.

UPEP/SPEP: Urine or serum protein electrophoresis, a laboratory technique used to separate proteins by size, is used as a screening technique for identifying monoclonal proteins.

Immunofixation: Laboratory technique using immunologic means to identify the subtype of a monoclonal protein, e.g., IgG kappa.

DISCUSSION

Plasma cells are derived from **B lymphocytes** that have been sensitized to a specific foreign antigen and produce antibodies against that antigen. In MM, a **clone of plasma cells proliferates** independently of normal immune stimulation. **Multiple myeloma is the most common primary malignancy of bone.** The incidence is **increased in the elderly, males, and African Americans.**

Multiple myeloma is a neoplasm of monoclonal plasma cells that proliferate in the bone marrow and cause a space-occupying lesion (myelophthisis) that manifests as **pancytopenia** and **destruction of bone.** The bone marrow replacement results in suppression of myelopoiesis, leading to anemia followed by bone marrow failure. The destruction of bone manifests as **osteolytic lesions, bone pain, pathologic fractures,** and **hypercalcemia.** It is believed that cytokines that are osteoclast-activating factors produced by the neoplastic plasma cells activate osteoclasts, leading to bone destruction and elevated serum calcium. **Hypercalcemia can cause fatigue, depression, mental confusion, nausea, and cardiac arrhythmias.** The neoplastic cells secrete abundant amounts of immunoglobulins (Ig) and their components, which are detected with serum and urine protein electrophoresis as M proteins (monoclonal immunoglobulins). In large quantities, they may cause renal failure, tissue amyloid deposition, and hyperviscosity syndrome. **The most important factor in the pathogenesis of renal failure secondary to MM is Bence Jones proteinuria, which consists of light chains excreted by the neoplastic plasma cells.** These chains are seen as an M spike in urine protein electrophoresis (UPEP). The most common serum monoclonal Ig (M protein) is IgG (50 percent), followed by IgA (20 percent) and light chains (15 percent). These antibodies secreted by the neoplastic plasma cells are defective, leading to an impaired humoral immunity, making the patients susceptible to infections by encapsulated bacteria such as pneumococci. The accompanying neutropenia and impaired humoral immunity lead to increased and recurrent infections.

The bone marrow has an increased number of plasma cells, usually more than 30 percent of all cells, with large foci, nodules, or sheets of plasma cells. In the peripheral blood, mature and immature forms of plasma cells are seen with rouleaux formation, red blood cells that are stuck together like stacked coins. Diagnosis is made in symptomatic patients with progressive disease that fulfills one major and one minor criterion or three minor criteria, which should include 1 and 2. The criteria are summarized in Table 28-1.

Monoclonal gammopathy of undetermined significance (MGUS) is defined as the presence of monoclonal protein in peripheral blood, but with no apparent associated cellular proliferation and no Bence Jones proteinuria. MGUS may be seen in patients with a variety of other diseases, such as chronic lung disease, heart disease, and neurologic disease, or in patients who are otherwise in good health. The incidence of MGUS increases with age. In 5 to 10 percent of patients, MGUS progresses to myeloma, Waldenström macroglobulinemia, lymphoma, or amyloidosis.

Table 28-1

DIAGNOSTIC CRITERIA FOR MULTIPLE MYELOMA

Major Criteria
I. Plasmacytoma by biopsy
II. >30% marrow plasmacytosis
III. Monoclonal gammopathy Serum: IgG >3.5 g/dL, IgA >2 g/DL Urine: >1 g/d of Bence Jones proteins
Minor Criteria
A. 10–30% marrow plasmacytosis
B. Monoclonal gammopathies with lower values than above
C. Lytic bone lesions
D. Suppressed normal immunoglobulins

COMPREHENSION QUESTIONS

[28.1] A 61-year-old woman presents with increasing fatigue and pain in her lower back and hip. X-rays reveal multiple punched-out lytic bone lesions, especially in the pelvis. Laboratory examination finds increased serum calcium and protein but normal serum levels of albumin. Serum protein electrophoresis reveals a single large spike in the gamma region. Which of the following changes is most likely to be seen in a bone marrow biopsy from this individual?

A. Diffuse infiltration of myeloblasts
B. Few cells with increased reticulin
C. Multiple sheets of plasma cells
D. Paratrabecular lymphoid aggregates
E. Scattered atypical and immature megakaryocytes

[28.2] A 61-year-old woman presents with increasing bone pain and is found to have multiple lytic bone lesions along with hypercalcemia. A bone marrow biopsy finds more than 80 percent plasma cells infiltrating the marrow, but no increased monoclonal protein (M spike) is found in the peripheral blood. Which of the following is the most likely diagnosis?

A. Bence Jones proteinuria
B. Heavy chain disease
C. IgA multiple myeloma
D. Plasma cell leukemia
E. Waldenstrom macroglobulinemia

[28.3] During a routine physical examination, a 65-year-old asymptomatic man is found to have elevated serum proteins as a result of the presence of an abnormal M spike. His serum calcium level is normal, and no lytic bone lesions are found. A bone marrow aspiration and a biopsy reveal approximately 5 percent plasma cells within the marrow. Which of the following is the most likely diagnosis?

A. Gamma heavy chain disease
B. Immunoproliferative small intestinal disease
C. Langerhans cell histiocytosis
D. Monoclonal gammopathy of undetermined significance
E. Waldenström macroglobulinemia

Answers

[28.1] **C.** Multiple myeloma is the most common primary malignancy arising in the bone of adults. It is a malignant neoplasm that results from the monoclonal proliferation of plasma cells in the bone marrow, usually more than 30 percent of all cells present. This proliferation of plasma cells causes destruction of the bone and produces multiple osteolytic lesions, bone pain, and increased calcium levels in the serum. These changes result in the classic clinical triad seen with multiple myeloma: hypercalcemia, multiple lytic bone lesions, and increased plasma cells in the bone marrow.

[28.2] **A.** The classic clinical triad of symptoms in individuals with MM is the combination of: hypercalcemia, multiple lytic bone lesions, and increased plasma cells in the bone marrow. These neoplastic plasma cells secrete large amounts of immunoglobulin, the components of which can be detected with serum and urine protein electrophoresis as M proteins (monoclonal immunoglobulins). However, this M spike may not be seen if Bence Jones proteins are present. These Bence Jones proteins are fee immunoglobulin light chains. They are small proteins and can be filtered into urine. Bence Jones proteins are important because if the neoplastic plasma cells secrete only Bence Jones proteins, they will be filtered into the urine from the blood, and no M spike will be seen with serum protein electrophoresis.

[28.3] **D.** Monoclonal gammopathy of undetermined significance is a disorder characterized by the presence of monoclonal protein (M spike) in peripheral blood in an individual with no apparent abnormal cellular proliferation. The incidence of MGUS increases with age; M protein is found in approximately 1 to 3 percent of asymptomatic individuals aged over 50. Approximately 20 percent of individuals with MGUS will develop a plasma cell dyscrasia, such as MM, within 10 to 15 years.

PATHOLOGY PEARLS

- Multiple myeloma is a plasma cell neoplasm characterized by bone pain, pathologic fractures, bone marrow infiltration, and hypercalcemia.
- An elevated serum globulin is seen with a monoclonal immunoglobulin spike.
- A bone marrow biopsy is the gold standard for diagnosing MM, showing increased plasma cells.
- The most important factor in the pathogenesis of renal failure secondary to MM is Bence Jones proteinuria, which consists of light chains excreted by the neoplastic plasma cells.

REFERENCES

Aster JC. Diseases of the white blood cells, lymph nodes, spleen and thymus. In: Kumar V, Assas AK, Fausto N, eds. Robbins and Cotran Pathologic Basis of Disease, 7th ed. Philadelphia, PA: Elsevier Saunders, 2004:679–91.

Aster JC. Diseases of the white blood cells, lymph nodes, spleen and thymus. In: Mitchell RN, Kumar V, Abbas AK, et al., eds. Pocket Companion to Robbins and Cotran Pathologic Basis of Disease, 7th ed. Philadelphia, PA: Saunders, 2006:352–4.

CASE 29

During a routine athletic physical, a 15-year-old boy is found to have a systolic thrill that is palpable at the lower left sternal border accompanied by a harsh, pansystolic murmur that is heard best at the site of the thrill. He is asymptomatic and has no evidence of hypertension, cyanosis, or edema. An electrocardiogram and a chest radiograph are normal.

- **What is the most likely diagnosis?**

- **What is the natural history of this condition?**

- **What are potential sequelae if this condition remains untreated?**

ANSWERS TO CASE 29: VENTRICULAR SEPTAL DEFECT

Summary: During a routine physical, a 15-year-old boy is found to have a systolic thrill at the lower left sternal border with a harsh, pansystolic murmur heard best at the site of the thrill. An electrocardiogram and a chest radiograph are normal.

- **Most likely diagnosis:** Ventricular septal defect (VSD).
- **Natural history:** Some VSDs, if small, may close spontaneously. Larger ones require surgical repair.
- **Unrepaired VSDs:** Heart failure with pulmonary hypertension may result. Poor growth and, in young children, poor brain development may ensue. Patients are also susceptible to infected clots and pulmonary infections.

CLINICAL CORRELATION

Ventricular septal defects are the most common congenital heart defects; they affect approximately 5 per 1000 live births and represent approximately 30 percent of all congenital heart defects. In approximately 25 percent of patients, there are coexisting extracardiac anomalies. Congenital heart defects can be detected in stillbirths up to 10 times more frequently than in live births. Girls more frequently present with atrial septal defects and patent ductus arteriosus. In contrast, most left-sided obstructions, such as complete transposition of great arteries, aortic coarctation, aortic stenosis, and atresia, are present in boys.

VSD results from abnormal growth and fusion of the ventricular septal system. The majority of VSDs involve defects of the membranous septum, with fewer involving outlet and inlet defects. The defects are dynamic, and 50 percent close within 2 years. Usually smaller defects close spontaneously. VSDs allow shunting of blood from the high-pressure left ventricle to the low-pressure right ventricle (see Figure 29-1). This is not evident until after delivery, after which there is a rise in the left ventricular pressure compared with the right. The resultant shunting of blood from left to right can lead to increased blood flow to the lungs and pulmonary vascular changes, pulmonary hypertension, and heart failure.

APPROACH TO CONGENITAL HEART DISEASE

Objectives

- Describe the causes of right to left cardiac shunts.
- Know the causes of left to right cardiac shunts.
- Describe the most common congenital heart defect.

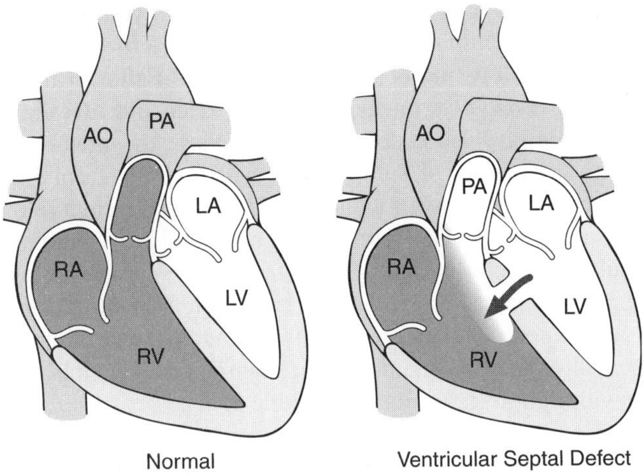

Figure 29-1. Schematic representation of a normal heart and a heart with ventricular septal defect.

Definitions

Congenital heart disease: A disease affecting the heart that is present from birth.

Tetralogy of Fallot: Obstruction with pulmonary stenosis and VSD, overriding aorta and right ventricular (RV) hypertrophy, with maldevelopment of the infundibular septum.

Shunt: Path of blood flow that results from abnormal communication from chamber to chamber, chamber to vessel, or vessel to vessel.

Paradoxical embolism: Result of right-left shunt in which thromboemboli bypass the lung and may access the general circulation directly.

DISCUSSION

Classification of Congenital Heart Defects

Congenital heart diseases can be divided into shunts and obstructive processes. Shunts may be from left to right or from right to left, depending on the affected heart chamber or vessels. Left-to-right shunts usually lead to late cyanosis and in addition to VSDs include atrial septal defects (ASDs) and patent ductus arteriosus (PDA). In fetal life, because the right-sided pressure is equal to that of the left side, the effects of the shunting are not evident until birth, when the right-sided pressure decreases. The result is that blood flows along the path of least resistance through the lungs. With time, **pulmonary hypertension can develop.** In severe forms, patients can develop pulmonary vascular disease with plexogenic pulmonary arteriopathy, or **Eisenmenger syndrome,** which consists of **heart failure, pulmonary hypertension, and a bleeding tendency.**

Types of **right-to-left shunts** include **tetralogy of Fallot, transposition of great arteries, persistent truncus arteriosus, tricuspid atresia, and total anomalous pulmonary venous connection.** Of these, the **most common** type of abnormality is **tetralogy of Fallot,** which usually results from displacement anterosuperior and left of the infundibular septum during embryologic development. This leads to a VSD from malalignment of the septum, overriding aorta, subpulmonic stenosis, and right ventricular hypertrophy. Classic tetralogy has severe pulmonary stenosis with right-to-left shunt, and patients are **cyanotic.** In pink tetralogy, the stenosis is mild and patients clinically present as do those with a VSD and a left-to-right shunt. Paradoxic emboli may occur in patients with right-to-left shunts (see Table 29-1).

Obstructive types of congenital heart disease include **coarctation of the aorta, aortic stenosis, and pulmonary stenosis.** The **most common** is **coarctation of the aorta.** Embryologically, this is thought to occur because of decreased blood flow into the ascending aorta, increased flow to the pulmonary artery or ductus arteriosus, or extension of contractile tissue into the aorta. Approximately one-third of these patients have coarctation as an isolated anomaly. Syndromes that may be associated with coarctation include DiGeorge and Turner syndromes. Coarctation leads to hypertension within the ascending aorta with left ventricular hypertrophy. Medial degeneration with necrosis of the aorta can be seen.

Hypoplastic left heart syndrome occurs in patients with aortic valve atresia and an intact ventricular septum. This probably results from a decrease in left-sided blood flow during embryogenesis. Postnatal survival depends on the patency of shunts and ductus arteriosus. The mortality from this condition is extremely high, often occurring within the first 6 weeks of life. The condition

Table 29-1
CONGENTIAL HEART DISEASES

RIGHT-TO-LEFT SHUNTS "EARLY CYANOSIS"	LEFT-TO-RIGHT SHUNTS "LATE CYANOSIS"
Persistent truncus arteriosus	VSD
Transposition of the great vessels	ASD
Tricuspid atresia	PDA
Tetralogy of Fallot	
Total anomalous pulmonary venous connection	

early cyanosis = immediately at birth; late cyanosis = later in life is not correctable, but some patients are treated with a series of surgeries during which the ductus is kept open medically. The goal of the operations is to allow the right ventricle to pump oxygenated blood.

Causative Factors and Treatment

There are multiple causative factors in the development of congenital heart disease, including genetic factors and congenital infections such as rubella. Drugs, including alcohol, amphetamines, anticonvulsants, chemotherapeutics, lithium, thalidomide, and retinoic acid, have been associated with fetal heart disease. In addition, females with system disease such as diabetes and lupus are at higher risk of having babies with heart abnormalities.

Treatment of congenital heart disease can be surgical in most cases. Medical treatment often is required to reduce the symptoms of heart failure. In patients with uncorrectable conditions, heart transplantation may be an option.

COMPREHENSION QUESTIONS

[29.1] An 11-month-old girl is noted to have blue lips and some fatigue after running around the room for 4 minutes. She was the product of a normal delivery. The family recently immigrated from Mexico, and she has not been evaluated by a doctor. Which of the following is the most likely diagnosis?

A. VSD
B. Tetralogy of Fallot
C. Atrial septal defect
D. Hypoplastic left heart

[29.2] A 1-month-old male neonate is brought into the emergency department because of difficulty feeding and lethargy. A loud murmur is heard. Which of the following is the most likely congenital heart disease in this patient?

A. Tetralogy
B. VSD
C. ASD
D. Aortic atresia

[29.3] Pulmonary hypertension that results from the reversal of the direction of blood flow through a congenital heart defect that initially had produced a left-to-right shunt is a characteristic feature of which of the following disorders?

A. Chagas disease
B. Eisenmenger syndrome
C. Libman-Sach disease
D. Lutembacher syndrome
E. Roger disease

Answers

[29.1] **B.** Cyanosis requires mixing of deoxygenated blood into the systemic circulation, which may be seen in tetralogy of Fallot. VSD and ASD usually result in left-to-right shunting of blood because of the higher pressure in the left ventricle or atrium, respectively.

[29.2] **B.** Ventricular septal defect is the most common congenital heart disease and usually presents in neonates at approximately 4 weeks of age with congestive heart failure. In an infant, this means poor feeding, sweating, and tachypnea.

[29.3] **B.** The clinical features of the Eisenmenger syndrome include heart failure, pulmonary hypertension, and bleeding tendency. It results from a congenital heart defect that initially had produced a left-to-right shunt but was severe enough to cause pulmonary hypertension because of the increased blood flow to the lungs. The pulmonary hypertension will eventually cause right ventricular hypertrophy and subsequently the blood flow will reverse (right to left). This will result in cyanosis late (tardive), which is the characteristic feature of Eisenmenger syndrome.

PATHOLOGY PEARLS

- ❖ VSDs are the most common congenital heart defects; some may close spontaneously without surgical intervention.
- ❖ Classification of congenital heart defects generally includes right-to-left shunts, left-to-right shunts, and obstructive defects.
- ❖ Tetralogy of Fallot results from misalignment of the infundibular septum that leads to VSD, overriding aorta, pulmonary stenosis, and right ventricular hypertrophy.
- ❖ Hypoplastic left heart syndrome generally is incompatible with life. Surgical repair requires that the ductus arteriosus remain patent.

REFERENCES

Damjanov I, Linder J. Anderson's Pathology, 10th ed. St. Louis, MO: Mosby, 1996.

Schoen FJ. The heart. In: Kumar V, Assas AK, Fausto N, eds. Robbins and Cotran Pathologic Basis of Disease, 7th ed. Philadelphia, PA: Elsevier Saunders, 2004:564–70.

Schoen FJ. The heart. In: Mitchell RN, Kumar V, Abbas AK, et al., eds. Pocket Companion to Robbins and Cotran Pathologic Basis of Disease, 7th ed. Philadelphia, PA: Saunders, 2006:290–4.

❖ CASE 30

A 58-year-old male teacher notices the sudden onset of "chest tightness" when he walks across the parking lot to and from the school. The pain, which is localized over the sternum, goes away when he sits down. He does not experience any pain or discomfort at other times. He has mild hypertension, for which he is on dietary therapy. His cholesterol level is elevated. He does not smoke.

- **What is the most likely diagnosis?**
- **What is the most likely mechanism for these symptoms?**
- **What are the complications and prognosis?**

ANSWERS TO CASE 30: CORONARY ATHEROSCLEROTIC HEART DISEASE

Summary: A 58-year-old man with mild hypertension and hyperlipidemia has "chest tightness" with mild exertion. He does not experience any pain or discomfort at rest.

- **Most likely diagnosis:** Coronary atherosclerotic heart disease.
- **Most likely mechanism for these symptoms:** Occlusive coronary vascular disease leading to ischemia of the myocardium.
- **Complications and prognosis:** Myocardial ischemia or infarction, depending on the extent of arterial blockage and underlying cardiac function. The prognosis is worse with underlying poor myocardial contractility.

CLINICAL CORRELATION

This 58-year-old man has chest pain with exertion but not at rest. He has four risk factors for coronary heart disease: hypertension, hyperlipidemia, age, and male sex. The first priority is for this patient to be evaluated in an emergency center for airway, breathing, and circulation (ABC) and for possible myocardial infarction. A dictum in emergency centers is that "time is myocardium." It is vital that aspirin be chewed as soon as possible. Continued chest pain may be treated with oxygen and nitrates. An ECG and serum cardiac enzymes may help with the diagnosis and ideally should be drawn within 15 minutes of entry into the emergency department. A classic ECG finding consistent with a myocardial infarction (MI) would be ST elevation in the leads of myocardial injury, but sometimes these changes are absent. Cardiac enzyme elevation is the hallmark of myocardial injury, but occasionally it may be misleading. Thus, the history is the single most important determinant in the attempt to establish the emergent diagnosis of possible MI. Indications of an acute MI may necessitate the need for thrombolytic therapy. Myocardial ischemia may result in angina pectoris, MI, cardiac arrhythmias, or congestive heart failure. For these reasons, patients who are suspected of having an MI are observed in an intensive care setting with continuous electrocardiography. β-Blockers are often used to decrease myocardial contractility and heart rate, thereby reducing work demands on the heart. Urgent reperfusion techniques with angioplasty or tissue plasminogen activator may be initiated in appropriate candidates.

APPROACH TO CARDIOVASCULAR DISEASE

Objectives

- Describe the pathology of cardiovascular disease.
- List the risk factors for cardiovascular disease.
- Describe the difference between left and right heart failure.

Definitions

Angina pectoris: Paroxysmal episodes of chest pain resulting from myocardial ischemia that fall precariously short of myocardial necrosis.

Classical or exertional angina (Heberden angina): Angina provoked by exertion, either physical or emotional. This type of angina usually is due to underlying coronary artery atherosclerosis.

Variant, or prinzmetal, angina: Angina unrelated to exertion. This type of angina is due to vasospasm of atherosclerotic coronary arteries.

Unstable angina: Angina at rest or angina of recent onset or worsening angina. One in seven patients with unstable angina may develop MI if left untreated.

Myocardial infarction: Myocardial ischemia to an extent that causes myocardial necrosis; the area of necrosis may be full myocardial thickness (transmural MI) or subendocardial (subendocardial MI).

Congestive heart failure: Inability of the heart to pump enough blood to meet the demand of the tissue despite adequate venous return.

DISCUSSION

Coronary atherosclerosis is characterized by the accumulation of lipids, macrophages, and smooth muscle cells in the **intima of the coronary arteries.** The resultant lesions are termed **plaques.** These lesions cause obstruction to coronary blood flow by protruding into the lumen, weaken the underlying media, and may undergo various complications. When 75 percent of the cross-sectional area of the major epicardial artery is obstructed and there is a moderate increase in myocardial oxygen demand, compensatory vasodilation is inadequate to meet this increase in demand. Symptoms of typical angina thus are explained by this imbalance between myocardial oxygen demand and supply. Superimposed **vasospasm** on atherosclerotic arteries is the reason for episodes of angina without any direct relation to exercise **(variant angina).** See Table 30-1 for risk factors for coronary heart disease.

Sometimes acute changes affect the plaques, including **hemorrhage into the atheroma,** rupture or fissuring of the atheroma, and erosion or ulceration. These events result in subsequent **thrombosis** of the vessel at the site of the atheroma. Hemorrhagic expansion of the atheroma or superadded thrombosis

Table 30-1
RISK FACTORS FOR CORONARY ARTERY DISEASE

Nonmodifiable
Age
Male sex (males are at increased risk compared with premenopausal women)
Positive family history (first-degree relative with coronary artery disease before the age of 50 years)
Modifiable
Major
Hyperlipidemia (high low-density lipoprotein and low high-density lipoprotein are the most important abnormalities)
Cigarette smoking
Hypertension
Diabetes mellitus
Minor
Obesity
Physical inactivity
Alcohol
Homocystinemia
Type A personality

causes **critical narrowing of the lumen** with the subsequent clinical presentation of **unstable angina or myocardial infarction.** In myocardial infarction, because there is **myocardial necrosis, cardiac enzymes are elevated.** Typical clinical features, ECG changes, and elevated cardiac enzymes are considered in arriving at the diagnosis. In all the different types of angina, cardiac enzymes are not elevated and ECG changes are seen only during the episodes of chest pain. Thus, a good history is key for a proper diagnosis.

Atherosclerosis primarily affects elastic arteries and large- and medium-sized muscular arteries. The most common locations of atherosclerosis, in descending order of frequency, are the abdominal aorta, coronary arteries, popliteal arteries, the descending thoracic aorta, internal carotid arteries, and circle of Willis.

Atherosclerotic plaques have three principal components: (1) cells, including smooth muscle cells and macrophages, (2) connective tissue extracellular matrix, including collagen, elastic fibers, and proteoglycans, and (3) intracellular and extracellular lipids.

Subsequent changes that may take place in these plaques include calcification, hemorrhage, superimposed thrombosis, ulceration, and erosion. Also, weakness of the underlying media may result in aneurysmal dilation.

Myocardial ischemia occurs when the supply of oxygen to the myocardium fails to meet the demand. The broad categories for myocardial ischemia are the following:

1. **Coronary artery atherosclerosis.** The atheromas itself can result in impairment of coronary perfusion. The degree of stenosis can be compromised further by superimposed thrombosis. Other causes of superadded narrowing include vasospasm.
2. **Decreased coronary artery flow** of oxygenated blood resulting from anemia or hypotension.
3. **Increased demand for oxygen** whenever there is increased cardiac output (e.g., due to thyrotoxicosis) or as a result of myocardial hypertrophy.

Congestive Heart Failure

Congestive heart failure is the most common manifestation of heart failure. Heart failure may be left heart failure, right heart failure, or "biventricular" heart failure.

Left Heart Failure

Left-sided congestive heart failure is most often due to **ischemic heart disease, hypertension, mitral and aortic valvular disease,** and **myocardial diseases.** With left heart failure, cardiac output is reduced. As renal perfusion is reduced, there is increased production of renin and angiotensin, which stimulates aldosterone secretion. Sodium and water retention takes place, and excess fluid accumulates in the interstitium.

Back pressure into the pulmonary vasculature results in pulmonary congestion and leakage of fluid into the alveolar air spaces (pulmonary edema). Engorged vessels may leak red blood cells. The iron from the red cells is taken up by macrophages. These cells are known as hemosiderin-laden macrophages or heart failure cells.

Right Heart Failure

Usually right heart failure occurs as a **consequence of left heart failure.** Pure right heart failure most often occurs with cor pulmonale. This is right ventricular hypertrophy with or without heart failure resulting from primary disease of the lungs or the lung vasculature.

In right heart failure, pulmonary congestion is minimal. Instead, the systemic and portal systems are engorged. Peripheral edema, ascites, and pleural effusions are thus evident. Congestive hepatosplenomegaly also is seen.

COMPREHENSION QUESTIONS

[30.1] A 53-year-old man presents with recurrent chest pain that has gotten progressively worse over the last several weeks. He says that approximately a year ago the pain would occasionally occur when he was mowing his yard but now the pain sometimes occurs while he is sitting in a chair at night reading a book. The pain, which is localized over the sternum, lasts much longer now than it did a few months ago. What type of angina does this individual have at present?

A. Atypical angina
B. Heberden angina
C. Prinzmetal angina
D. Stable angina
E. Unstable angina

[30.2] Prinzmetal angina (atypical angina) is characterized clinically by chest pain that occurs at rest rather than with exercise. Which of the following is the most likely cause of this type of angina?

A. Atherosclerosis of a coronary artery
B. Dissection of a coronary artery
C. Embolism of a coronary artery
D. Thrombosis of a coronary artery
E. Vasospasm of a coronary artery

[30.3] Sections of lung tissue obtained during an autopsy of a 66-year-old woman reveal numerous hemosiderin laden macrophages within the alveoli. Which of the following is the basic pathologic cause of this abnormality?

A. Bacterial infection
B. Diabetes mellitus
C. Heart failure
D. Pulmonary hypertension
E. Viral infection

Answers

[30.1] **E.** Angina pectoris is a clinical term that describes episodes of chest pain caused by myocardial ischemia. Classic angina (exertional angina or Heberden angina), which is the most common form, is characterized by retrosternal pain that occurs with exercise, stress, or excitement. In contrast, unstable angina (preinfarct angina or crescendo angina) is characterized by increasing frequency of pain, increased duration of pain, or less exertion necessary to produce the chest pain. This type of angina is important to recognize clinically because it indicates that a myocardial infarction may be near.

[30.2] **E.** In contrast to classical angina, which is caused by atherosclerosis of the coronary arteries, variant angina (Prinzmetal angina) is caused by vasospasm of the coronary arteries. In patients with variant angina, it is important to avoid β-blockers because they may cause unopposed α-stimulation and precipitate coronary vasospasm. Unstable angina is caused by fissures and hemorrhage into areas of coronary atherosclerosis, but no infarction has occurred.

[30.3] **C.** Heart failure cells are hemosiderin laden macrophages that are present within the alveoli of the lung. They are called heart failure cells because they are commonly seen in patients with congestive heart failure. Left ventricular failure increases the pressure in the lungs, which leads to increased fluid within the alveoli (pulmonary edema). Microscopic examination at this time will reveal pale pink fluid within the alveoli. Hemorrhage into the alveoli may also occur. The erythrocytes will then be phagocytized by alveolar macrophages, which will digest the red blood cells leaving behind granules of hemosiderin within their cytoplasm.

PATHOLOGY PEARLS

- Myocardial ischemia may result in angina pectoris, myocardial infarction, cardiac arrhythmias, or congestive heart failure.
- Coronary atherosclerosis is characterized by the accumulation of lipids, macrophages, and smooth muscle cells in the intima of the coronary arteries.
- When 75 percent of the cross-sectional area of the major epicardial artery is obstructed and there is a moderate increase in myocardial oxygen demand, compensatory vasodilation is inadequate to meet this increase in demand.
- The most common locations of atherosclerosis, in descending order of frequency, are abdominal aorta, coronary arteries, popliteal arteries, descending thoracic aorta, internal carotid arteries, and circle of Willis.
- In myocardial infarction, because there is myocardial necrosis, cardiac enzymes are elevated.

REFERENCES

Schoen FJ. The heart. In: Kumar V, Assas AK, Fausto N, eds. Robbins and Cotran Pathologic Basis of Disease, 7th ed. Philadelphia, PA: Elsevier Saunders, 2004: 575–82.

Schoen FJ. The heart. In: Mitchell RN, Kumar V, Abbas AK, et al., eds. Pocket Companion to Robbins and Cotran Pathologic Basis of Disease, 7th ed. Philadelphia, PA: Saunders, 2006:294–300.

❖ CASE 31

A 50-year-old male alcoholic is seen in the clinic for complaints of difficulty breathing, particularly at night when he is lying down. He has not had chest pain or diaphoresis. Physical examination reveals that the cardiac point of maximal impulse (PMI) is laterally displaced on the lungs. Bilateral basilar rales are heard. A chest radiograph shows an enlarged heart and bilateral pleural effusions. An echocardiogram is performed and reveals a markedly low ejection fraction.

◆ **What is the most likely diagnosis?**

◆ **What is the likely underlying cause of this condition?**

ANSWERS TO CASE 31: CARDIOMYOPATHY (ALCOHOL-INDUCED)

Summary: A 50-year-old male alcoholic is seen in the clinic for symptoms and signs of congestive heart failure and cardiomegaly. A chest radiograph shows an enlarged heart and bilateral pleural effusions. An echocardiogram revealed a markedly low ejection fraction.

- **Most likely diagnosis:** Congestive heart failure secondary to dilated cardiomyopathy.
- **Most likely cause:** Probably from chronic alcohol consumption. The most common cause of dilated cardiomyopathy is atherosclerotic coronary artery disease.

CLINICAL CORRELATION

This patient's symptoms are consistent with dilated cardiomyopathy resulting from chronic alcohol consumption. Alcoholic dilated cardiomyopathy is seen most frequently in males 35 to 55 years old. Typically, there is a long history of excessive alcohol consumption; usually, drinking more than 90 g (eight standard drinks) per day for over 5 years is associated with dilated cardiomyopathy, which may be asymptomatic. Alcohol may have a direct toxic effect on the heart, or cardiac signs may be secondary to vitamin deficiency from alcoholism. In dilated cardiomyopathy, the heart shows areas of hypertrophy with an increase in mass usually of 600 g or more in the adult heart. Other areas of the heart may show myofibril thinning and myofiber loss, presumably through alterations in gene expression and apoptosis. Evidence of damage with interstitial and endocardial fibrosis is seen frequently. Heart failure results from ventricular dysfunction. Left ventricular (LV) function can be measured by the LV ejection fraction (LVEF), which is the volume of blood ejected (volume at the end of diastole minus the volume at the end of systole) divided by the volume at the end of diastole, expressed as a percentage. The normal ejection fraction is 50 percent or higher and congestive failure usually is seen with an LVEF of 40 percent or less. Signs and symptoms of heart failure are the result of reduced cardiac output or reduced venous drainage or a combination of both. Congestion in the lungs can lead to dyspnea, which can manifest sometimes as orthopnea (dyspnea when lying down), or orthopnea that is worse at night: paroxysmal nocturnal dyspnea (PND). Congestion not uncommonly involves the liver, spleen, kidneys, and brain. Fluid accumulation in the pleural spaces, pericardial spaces, and subcutaneous tissue may occur, leading to edema or, when generalized and massive, anasarca.

APPROACH TO ALCOHOLIC CARDIOMYOPATHY

Objectives

- Describe the classifications of the various cardiomyopathies.
- Describe the causes of the various cardiomyopathies.
- List the effects of alcohol on the heart.

Definitions

Cardiomyopathy: Disease of the myocardium with associated clinical signs and symptoms of cardiac dysfunction.

Dilated cardiomyopathy: Damaged myocardium that results in increased ventricular mass and size, with dilation of the chambers and thinning of the ventricle walls.

Congestive heart failure: The result of left ventricular dysfunction with resultant organ congestion and edema.

Beriberi heart disease: Heart failure as a result of a high-output state secondary to thiamine deficiency from chronic alcoholism. Clinically, it may not be distinguishable from alcoholic dilated cardiomyopathy.

DISCUSSION

Classification of Cardiomyopathies

Cardiomyopathies are a group of disorders that entail **myocyte injury,** resulting in **cardiac dysfunction.** They can be classified broadly into **three categories—dilated, hypertrophic,** and **restrictive** cardiomyopathies—reflecting the resultant condition or function of the chambers of the heart (see Table 31-1). These terms do not denote specific mechanisms or etiologies but describe the state of the myocardial dysfunction. **Dilated cardiomyopathy** is by far the **most common form** and results from enlargement and dilation of the ventricles. Patients with hypertrophic cardiomyopathy have decreased diastolic filling with loss of ventricular volume, usually associated with outflow obstruction without attendant dilation of the ventricles. In about half these cases of hypertrophic cardiomyopathy, there is a familial inherited basis. Restrictive cardiomyopathy usually is due to an infiltrative process. Patients tend to have impaired ventricular compliance with decreased diastolic filling.

Causes of Dilated Cardiomyopathies

Coronary artery disease, endocrine disorders, alcohol, myocarditis, drugs, and **toxins** are common causes of dilated cardiomyopathy. Among them, the most common cause in the United States is **coronary artery disease.** Direct damage or ischemia to the myocytes results in loss of injured myocytes

Table 31-1
CLASSIFICATION AND CAUSES OF CARDIOMYOPATHIES

TYPE OF CARDIOMYOPATHY	CAUSES
Dilated	Ischemic Alcohol, toxic Pregnancy induced Coxsackie B virus Chronic cocaine use Doxorubicin Chagas disease Endocrine disorders Myocarditis, infectious Genetic
Hypertrophic	Genetics Storage disease Pheochromocytoma
Restrictive	Infiltrative process Sarcoid Amyloidosis Hemochromatosis Radiation fibrosis

with attendant fibrosis and scarring. There is hypertrophy of residual myocytes, which can lead to an overall increase in myocardial mass. With dilation, there is usually thinning of the ventricular wall thickness, and eventually this can lead to congestive heart failure.

Signs and symptoms of heart failure include dyspnea on exertion, easy fatigability, edema involving the extremities and lungs, and abnormalities in heartbeat. Ventricular dilation also can lead to arrhythmias and thromboembolus formation. Additional studies that can aid in the diagnosis include chest x-rays, chest computed tomography (CT), and cardiac function studies, including echocardiography and electrocardiography (ECG). Endomyocardial biopsy may be performed for diagnosis and exclude other causes.

Alcohol and Its Effects on the Heart

The normal myocardium is composed of myocytes and the interstitium, which is highly vascular. Myocytes are specialized striated muscle that are rich in mitochondria and depend on aerobic metabolism. Cardiac function requires the transmission of neural signals, which is mediated through the specialized smooth endoplasmic reticulum known as the sarcoplasmic reticulum. The contractile ability of myocytes requires the functioning of the sarcomeric unit, which is formed from actin and myosin units. Intercalated disk and gap junctions allow the connection and communication of individual myocytes into an organized synchronized contractile unit. The fact that alcohol has a deleterious effect on the heart has been known for over 100 years. Current studies suggest that the effect of alcohol on the heart may occur through a toxic metabolite: **acetaldehyde.** The cellular site of the effect may be the **myocyte mitochondria.** Additionally, alcohol has been shown to be responsible for **thiamine deficiency,** which in severe cases can lead to beriberi heart disease and may not be distinguishable from other causes of dilated cardiomyopathy. Noncardiac effects of alcohol include fatty liver (steatosis), cirrhosis, pancreatitis, and central nervous system syndromes (Korsakoff and Wernicke syndromes).

Treatment

Treatment of dilated cardiomyopathy includes removing the toxic insult (i.e., stopping alcohol consumption). This can lead to improvement in cardiac function. Symptomatic relief for heart failure may be achieved by means of restricting fluids and salt intake, diuretics, angiotension-converting enzyme (ACE) inhibitors, and β-blockers. Vitamins are required in patients with vitamin deficiencies. Coumadin sometimes is required for patients at risk of thromboembolic disease. In cases of end-stage heart failure, patients have received cardiac transplants.

COMPREHENSION QUESTIONS

[31.1] A 45-year-old man is admitted to the hospital for symptoms of severe congestive heart failure, including dyspnea on exertion, swelling in the legs, and difficulty lying down flat in bed. Which of the following would be most consistent with chronic alcohol consumption?

A. Restrictive cardiomyopathy
B. Valvular stenosis
C. Pericardial effusion
D. Dilated cardiomyopathy

[31.2] The toxic effect of alcohol is probably mediated through which of the following?

A. Activation of oncogenes
B. Production of toxic aldehydes
C. Deficient fluid intake
D. Yeast

[31.3] A 47-year-old male alcoholic presents with numbness and tingling in his lower legs and feet. Physical examination finds marked peripheral edema and further workup finds changes consistent with a high-output cardiac failure. These symptoms are most consistent with a deficiency of which of the following substances?

A. Pyridoxine
B. Riboflavin
C. Vitamin C
D. Vitamin D
E. Thiamine

Answers

[31.1] **D.** Alcohol usually is associated with dilated cardiomyopathy (DCM). It is probably the second most common cause of DCM after coronary artery disease.

[31.2] **B.** The toxic effect of alcohol probably is mediated through its metabolic product acetaldehyde.

[31.3] **E.** Beriberi results from a deficiency of thiamine (vitamin B_1), which may be seen in chronic alcoholics or individuals with diets high in polished rice or white flour. There are two basic forms of beriberi: wet beriberi and dry beriberi. Wet beriberi results from signs of cardiovascular involvement. Peripheral vasodilation may cause AV (arteriovenous) shunting and lead to "high output" cardiac failure (systolic dysfunction). The heart will become flabby (dilated cardiomyopathy) and subsequent heart failure will lead to generalized edema (hence the name "wet"). Dry beriberi results from peripheral nerve involvement (polyneuropathy), the signs of which include numbness and tingling in the feet and lower legs.

PATHOLOGY PEARLS

❖ Excessive alcohol use can result in dilated cardiomyopathy and probably is mediated through the effect of acetaldehyde on the myocardium.

❖ Excessive alcohol consumption affects not only the heart but also the liver, pancreas, and central nervous system. Some of the effects of alcoholism result from nutritional and vitamin deficiencies.

❖ Treatment of congestive heart failure resulting from alcoholic dilated cardiomyopathy includes discontinuing alcohol consumption as well as medical therapy, with some patients requiring a heart transplant.

REFERENCES

Schoen FJ. The heart. In: Kumar V, Assas AK, Fausto N, eds. Robbins and Cotran Pathologic Basis of Disease, 7th ed. Philadelphia, PA: Elsevier Saunders, 2004: 601–5.

Schoen FJ. The heart. In: Mitchell RN, Kumar V, Abbas AK, et al., eds. Pocket Companion to Robbins and Cotran Pathologic Basis of Disease, 7th ed. Philadelphia, PA: Saunders, 2006:307–13.

Silver MD, Gotlieb AI, Schoen FJ. Cardiovascular Pathology, 3rd ed. Philadelphia, PA: Churchill Livingstone, 2001.

CASE 32

A 52-year-old woman develops fatigue and dyspnea that have been worsening over approximately 6 months. She also complains of occasional palpitations. She describes a serious illness she had as a child, with fever, rash, joint pain, and difficulty controlling her movements. She recovered after approximately a month. Cardiac examination reveals a loud S_1, an opening snap, and a diastolic rumble. A chest radiograph shows an enlarged left atrium.

- **What is the most likely diagnosis?**
- **What is the underlying mechanism for these findings?**
- **What are the complications and prognosis for this disorder?**

ANSWERS TO CASE 32: RHEUMATIC HEART DISEASE

Summary: A 52-year-old woman with a history of probable rheumatic fever as a child develops worsening fatigue and dyspnea and palpitations over 6 months. Cardiac examination reveals a loud S_1, an opening snap, and a diastolic rumble. A chest radiograph shows an enlarged left atrium.

- **Most likely diagnosis:** Mitral stenosis
- **Underlying mechanism for these findings:** Rheumatic heart disease
- **Complications and prognosis for this disorder:** Pulmonary edema, atrial fibrillation, and intracardiac thrombosis; prognosis is good with repair of the mitral valve

CLINICAL CORRELATION

This 52-year-old woman has symptoms of cardiac insufficiency, with decreased blood pumped into the systemic circulation as a result of the stenotic mitral valve. Also, the stenotic mitral valve has led to increased left atrial volume and pressure. This may lead to pulmonary edema because of the increased hydrostatic pressure in the pulmonary vessels. The cardiac examination is also consistent with mitral stenosis. Confirmation is accomplished with echocardiography.

Almost all cases of mitral stenosis are due to rheumatic heart disease, although other causes include congenital mitral stenosis, carcinoid syndrome, Lutembacher syndrome, acquired mitral stenosis, and atrial septal defect (ASD). With rheumatic heart disease, the mitral valve is involved 90 percent of the time. The disease process results in valve thickening and cusp fusion, resulting in a narrowed valve orifice and immobile valve cusps, the so-called fish-mouth appearance when viewed from the left ventricle. The normal mitral valve orifice is approximately 5 cm^2. Symptoms typically start when the valve orifice is 2 cm^2, and these symptoms are severe when the valve orifice is 1 cm^2. With mitral stenosis, left atrial pressure increases with subsequent left atrial hypertrophy and dilation. Pulmonary venous and arterial pressure increases. Pulmonary congestion and pulmonary edema develop. With time, there is right ventricular hypertrophy and right-sided heart failure. It is important to note that in mitral stenosis the left ventricle is not affected. Treatment when the mitral valve is critical includes surgical replacement.

APPROACH TO RHEUMATIC FEVER AND RHEUMATIC HEART DISEASE

Objectives

- Describe the etiology of rheumatic fever.
- Know the criteria used for the diagnosis of rheumatic fever.
- List the key features of auscultation found in the various heart murmurs.

Definitions

Palpitation: Awareness of the beating of the heart (whether it is too slow, too fast, irregular, or normal).

Arthralgia: Joint pain.

Sydenham chorea: Also known as St. Vitus dance, is a disease characterized by rapid, uncoordinated jerking movements, primarily affecting the face, feet, and hands.

Holosystolic murmur: Also known as pansystolic, a heart murmur heard throughout systole.

DISCUSSION

Rheumatic fever is an inflammatory condition that occurs as a result of **group A β-hemolytic streptococcal infection.** It typically affects children and young adults. Initially, there is a pharyngeal infection with group A streptococci. **Antibodies** directed against the **M protein** of the bacteria are thought to **cross-react with cardiac myosin** and **laminin,** resulting in a full-blown picture of rheumatic fever. Rheumatic fever is diagnosed on the basis of Duckett Jones criteria. The diagnosis is made on the basis of at least two major criteria or one major criterion and at least two minor criteria (see Table 32-1).

With carditis, all three layers of the heart may be involved. With endocarditis, small vegetations may develop on the endocardium, especially the heart valves. Mitral valvulitis may result in a diastolic murmur (Carey Coombs murmur). If the myocardium is involved, patients may develop arrhythmias or heart failure. **Aschoff bodies,** which are granulomatous lesions with central necrotic areas, typically are seen in the involved myocardium. Pericarditis results in an effusion.

Migratory polyarthritis is characterized by fleeting arthritis of large joints such as the knee, elbow, and ankle. The involved joints exhibit all the signs of inflammation; that is, they are red, hot, and tender. As inflammation in one joint improves, another joint becomes affected.

Individuals with chorea have involuntary quasi-purposive movements and appear "fidgety." **Erythema marginatum** manifests as a pink rash with raised edges, typically involving the trunk. **Subcutaneous nodules** are painless nodules that are seen over tendons, joints, and bony prominences.

Table 32-1
CRITERIA FOR RHEUMATIC FEVER AND RHEUMATIC HEART DISEASE

Major criteria Carditis Migratory polyarthritis Sydenham chorea (Saint Vitus' dance) Erythema marginatum Subcutaneous nodules Of these the first two are the most often seen
Minor criteria Fever Arthralgia Elevated erythrocyte sedimentation rate or C-reactive protein Leucocytosis Prolonged PR interval on ECG Plus evidence of streptococcal infection (e.g., positive throat swab, raised antistreptolysin O titer, scarlet fever)

Rheumatic fever has a tendency to recur, and recurrences are most common when persistent cardiac damage is present. More than 50 percent of those with acute rheumatic carditis eventually develop chronic rheumatic valvular disease. The mitral and aortic valves are the ones most commonly affected.

Other Valvular Diseases

Other valvular diseases include **aortic stenosis,** which is the most common valvular disease (see Table 32-2 for auscultatory findings). It may be caused by rheumatic heart disease, senile calcific aortic stenosis, or calcification of a congenital deformed valve. Age-related calcifications, or "wear and tear," is the most common cause of aortic stenosis. Clinical symptoms include **angina, congestive heart failure, and sudden death.**

The mitral valve can be affected by calcification, leading to a fibrotic annulus that leads to regurgitation or even stenosis. Myxomatous degeneration of the mitral valve or mitral valve prolapse is estimated to occur in up to 3 percent of adults in the United States, especially women. **Mitral regurgitation** typically results in a **holosystolic murmur.**

Infections affecting the heart valves include **endocarditis,** primarily affecting the aortic and mitral valves when ***"viridans" streptococci*** are involved. However with **IV drug users,** ***Staphylococcus aureus*** is commonly encountered

Table 32-2
HEART MURMURS

Aortic stenosis	Crescendo-decrescendo systolic ejection murmur
Aortic regurgitation	High-pitched "blowing" diastolic murmur
Mitral stenosis	Rumbling late diastolic murmur following an open snap
Mitral regurgitation	Holosystolic "blowing" murmur
VSD	Holosystolic murmur
PDA	Continuous machine-like murmur

and usually **right-sided valves** are affected, such as the tricuspid and pulmonary valves. Individuals with **systemic lupus erythematosus** may develop **small sterile vegetations** on the mitral or tricuspid valves that are called **Libman-Sacks syndrome.** These **verrucous** lesions usually have a fine granular appearance.

COMPREHENSION QUESTIONS

[32.1] Which of the following types of infection, precedes by several weeks, the development of acute rheumatic fever?

A. Group A β-hemolytic streptococcal infection of the pharynx
B. Group D α-hemolytic streptococcal infection of the heart
C. *Staphylococcus aureus* infection of the lungs
D. *Streptococcus pyogenes* infection of the skin
E. *Treponema pallidum* infection of the abdominal aorta

[32.2] A 6-year-old boy develops fever, joint pain, and a diffuse skin rash approximately 3 weeks after recovering from a sore throat. Physical examination finds several small skin nodules, and laboratory examination finds an elevated erythrocyte sedimentation rate along with an elevated antistreptolysin O titer. Which of the following abnormalities is most characteristic of this boy's disease?

A. Anitschkow cells within the epidermis
B. Aschoff bodies within the myocardium
C. Langhans giant cells within the dermis
D. Psammoma bodies within the endocardium
E. Virchow cells within the nasopharynx

[32.3] A 44-year-old woman presents with worsening fatigue and dyspnea. The pertinent medical history is that she had rheumatic fever during childhood. Physical examination finds an early diastolic opening snap with a rumbling late diastolic murmur. A chest radiograph shows an enlarged left atrium. Which of the following is the most likely diagnosis?

A. Aortic regurgitation
B. Aortic stenosis
C. Mitral regurgitation
D. Mitral stenosis
E. Pulmonary stenosis

Answers

[32.1] **A.** Acute rheumatic fever is an inflammatory disorder that classically occurs in children and young adults 1 to 4 weeks after infection of the pharynx by group A β-hemolytic streptococci (*Streptococcus pyogenes*). Rheumatic fever is an autoimmune disorder that results from the development of antistreptococcal antibodies, such as those directed against the M protein of the bacteria, that cross-react with portions of the heart such as cardiac myosin and laminin.

[32.2] **B.** Carditis, an inflammation involving any of the three layers of the heart, is a major feature of acute rheumatic fever. With myocarditis, Aschoff bodies are found within the myocardium. Aschoff bodies are granulomatous lesions with central necrotic areas. Bacteria are not present in these lesion, but Anitschkow cells, which are modified monocytes (possibly myocytes), are seen. These cells histologically look like "caterpillar cells."

[32.3] **D.** The cardiac valve most often affected by chronic rheumatic fever is the mitral valve. With healing, fibrosis will result in stenosis of the valve, which grossly has an appearance described as being a "fish mouth" or "buttonhole." Clinically, mitral stenosis produces a rumbling late diastolic murmur with an opening snap (an early diastolic opening snap is characteristic of mitral stenosis).

PATHOLOGY PEARLS

- Acute rheumatic fever is an inflammatory condition that occurs as a result of group A streptococcal infection. It typically affects children and young adults.
- Rheumatic fever is diagnosed on the basis of Duckett Jones criteria. The diagnosis is made on the basis of at least two major criteria or one major criterion and at least two minor criteria.
- Almost all cases of mitral stenosis are due to rheumatic heart disease. Stenosis of the mitral or aortic valve develops as the acutely inflamed valve leaflets heal, becoming fibrotic and resulting in thickened, less pliable valves.
- It is important to note that in mitral stenosis the left ventricle is not affected.
- Aschoff bodies typically are seen in the involved myocardium; they are granulomatous lesions with central necrotic areas.
- Rheumatic fever has a tendency to recur, and recurrences result in progressively increasing cardiac damage.

REFERENCES

Schoen FJ. The heart. In: Kumar V, Assas AK, Fausto N, eds. Robbins and Cotran Pathologic Basis of Disease, 7th ed. Philadelphia, PA: Elsevier Saunders, 2004: 592–600.

Schoen FJ. The heart. In: Mitchell RN, Kumar V, Abbas AK, et al., eds. Pocket Companion to Robbins and Cotran Pathologic Basis of Disease, 7th ed. Philadelphia, PA: Saunders, 2006:301–3.

CASE 33

An 8-year-old boy is brought to the pediatrician's office with a 2-day history of malaise, fever of 38.8°C (102°F), nausea, and vomiting. His mother reports that he has decreased urine output and that his urine is a dark, smoky color. His blood pressure is slightly elevated, and there is some swelling of his hands and feet and around his eyes. He has been in good health except for a sore throat a week or so ago.

- **What is the most likely diagnosis?**
- **What mechanism is involved?**
- **What is the usual clinical course?**

ANSWERS TO CASE 33: GLOMERULONEPHRITIS (ACUTE POSTSTREPTOCOCCAL)

Summary: An 8-year-old male has oliguria, hematuria, proteinuria, hypertension, edema, and impaired renal function. His past history includes a sore throat.

- **Most likely diagnosis:** Nephritic syndrome, most likely caused by poststreptococcal glomerulonephritis (GN).
- **Mechanism:** Immunologic reaction against nephritogenic β-hemolytic streptococci leading to immune complexes in the glomeruli.
- **Usual clinical course:** Excellent prognosis for recovery.

CLINICAL CORRELATION

This 8-year-old child had a sore throat approximately 1 week before the acute onset of the current symptoms. This is a very typical history of poststreptococcal GN. There is usually a latent time from pharyngitis to the systemic and urinary symptoms as a result of the immune response time. Antibodies are produced to the β-hemolytic streptococci, and the antibody-antigen complexes are deposited in the glomerulus, leading to the clinical findings. Diagnosis is made by the classic history, hematuria on urinalysis, elevation of the antistreptococcal antibody (ASO) titers, and a decline in the serum complement levels. Nearly all children recover without complications. Adults do not have such a uniformly good prognosis and may develop rapidly progressive kidney disease. If a **renal biopsy** were performed it most likely would show diffuse proliferative glomerulonephritis. The glomeruli would be swollen and packed with cells, and capillary lumens would be obliterated. There would be proliferation of endothelial and mesangial cells. Polymorphonucleocyte (PMN) would be present. These changes are expected to be uniformly present in all the glomeruli seen.

APPROACH TO GLOMERULONEPHRITIS

Objectives

- Describe the pathology of glomerulonephritis.
- List the different types of glomerulonephritis and their respective presentations.
- Know the differences between nephritic and nephrotic syndrome.

Definitions

Glomerulonephritis: Inflammation of the glomeruli.

Nephritic syndrome: A clinical syndrome of oliguria, hematuria, edema, and hypertension resulting from glomerulonephritis.

Nephrotic syndrome: A clinical syndrome of massive proteinuria, edema, hypoalbuminemia, and hyperlipidemia resulting from glomerulonephritis.

DISCUSSION

Glomerulonephritis is a general term for a group of disorders in which there is a primarily **immunologically mediated glomerular injury** followed by secondary mechanisms of injury. Table 33-1 is a selective list of causes of immune-complex–mediated glomerulonephritis.

The pathogenic mechanism of the primary immunologic injury is thought to have one of two basic forms:

1. Injury resulting from deposition of **circulating soluble immune complexes.** The nature of the antigen involved in the complex may be exogenous (e.g., Lancefield group A streptococcus) or endogenous (e.g., DNA is systemic lupus erythematosus)

Table 33-1

SELECTIVE CAUSES OF IMMUNE-COMPLEX–MEDIATED GLOMERULONEPHRITIS

Viruses
Mumps
Measles
Hepatitis B and C
Epstein-Barr virus
Human immunodeficiency virus
Bacteria
Lancefield group A β-hemolytic streptococcus
"viridans" group of streptococci
Staphylococci
Parasites: *Plasmodium malaria*
Endogenous antigens
DNA
Cryoglobulin
Malignant tumors
Drugs
Penicillamine

2. Injury by **antibodies reacting with antigens within the glomerulus.** These antigens may be intrinsic glomerular antigens or antigens planted within the glomerulus from the circulation. Antibody directed against the α-3 chain of type IV collagen present in the basement membrane of the glomerulus is an example of intrinsic antigens. This antibody also reacts with alveolar basement membrane. This **anti-GBM** (glomerular basement membrane) antibody is the basis of **Goodpasture syndrome (see Figure 33-1).**

After the initial immunologic insult, several secondary events are triggered that result in further glomerular injury. These events include complement activation, platelet aggregation, fibrin deposition, and inflammation.

The clinical presentation of all the various types of glomerulonephritis can take one of six forms:

1. **Nephritic syndrome:** characterized by oliguria, hematuria, edema, and hypertension
2. **Nephrotic syndrome:** characterized by massive proteinuria, edema, hypoalbuminemia, and hyperlipidemia
3. **Acute renal failure**
4. **Chronic renal failure**
5. **Isolated proteinuria**
6. **Isolated hematuria**

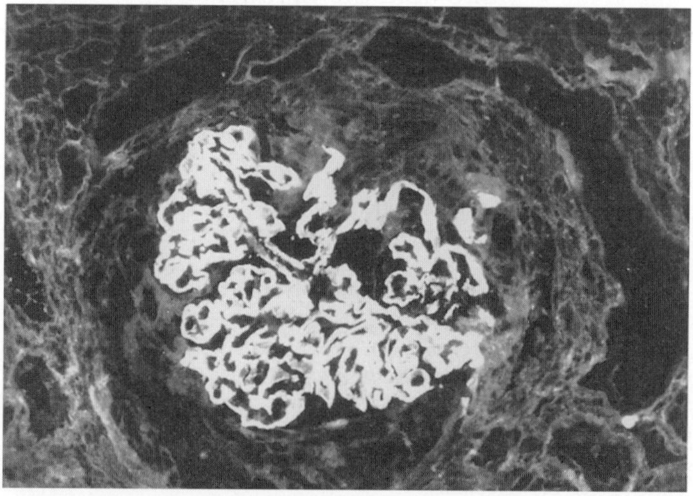

Figure 33-1. Glomerulonephritis resulting from antiglomerular basement membrane antibody. *(Reproduced with permission, from Kasper DL, Braunwald E, Fauci AS, et al., eds.* Harrison's Principles of Internal Medicine, 16th ed. *New York: McGraw-Hill, 2004:1681.)*

Initial urine analysis should show evidence of glomerulonephritis, including red cells and red cell casts. Renal function may be compromised.

Renal biopsy is not always performed in patients with glomerulonephritis. However, if biopsy is performed, the renal tissue is examined by the following processes:

1. Light microscopy.
2. Electron microscopy. The exact site of immune-complex deposition is visualized with this method.
3. Immunofluorescence. The type of immunologic injury is assessed by this method.

There is not a complete correlation between the histologic types of glomerulonephritis and the clinical presentation. Table 33-2 shows the most common associations.

In proliferative glomerulonephritis, proliferation of endothelial, mesangial, or epithelial (in the Bowman capsule) cells may take place. Capillary lumina are occluded. In diffuse GN, infiltration of PMNs usually is seen. With excessive proliferation of the epithelial cells, crescents may form. This is referred to as crescentic GN; because the crescents clinically progress rapidly to acute renal fever (ARF), this form of GN also is known as rapidly progressive GN (RPGN).

Immunofluorescent (IF) testing depicts the type of immunologic injury. Most often it is immunoglobulin G (IgG) that is detected. In IgA nephropathy, there is mesangial deposition of IgA. In Goodpasture syndrome, there is linear deposition of IgG.

Electron microscopy (EM) helps locate the site of immune-complex deposition. The possible sites include subepithelial, intramembranous, subendothelial, and mesangial. Most often the deposition of immune complexes is

Table 33-2

GLOMERULONEPHRITIS AND CLINICAL PRESENTATION

HISTOLOGIC TYPE	CLINICAL PRESENTATION
Proliferative glomerulonephritis	Nephritic syndrome
Diffuse	Hematuria, proteinuria
Focal segmental	Acute renal failure
Crescentic	Nephrotic or nephritic syndrome
Membranoproliferative (mesangiocapillary)	
Nonproliferative	Nephrotic syndrome in children
Minimal change	Nephrotic syndrome in adults
Membranous	Proteinuria or nephritic syndrome
Focal segmental glomerulosclerosis	Hematuria
IgA nephropathy	

subepithelial. In membranoproliferative cases, the complexes are found in a subendothelial location. In minimal lesions and focal segmental glomerulosclerosis (FSGS), immune complexes are absent.

Acute Diffuse Glomerulonephritis

Acute diffuse glomerulonephritis occurs mostly in children and typically follows (1 to 4 weeks) a **group A β-hemolytic streptococcal infection.** The serum complement is transiently low for several weeks. Histology reveals diffuse proliferative GN. A granular lumpy-bumpy pattern of IgG and C3 is seen on IF. EM has subepithelial electron deposits often described as dense humps.

Crescentic Glomerulonephritis

In crescentic glomerulonephritis, usually **at least 50 percent of the glomeruli** are involved. There are focal disruptions of the glomerular basement membrane with formation of crescents. A crescent is defined as at least three layers of cells between the visceral and parietal epithelium.

Crescentic GN is divided broadly into three categories: pauci-immune, immune-complex mediated, and antibasement membrane disease.

In the pauci-immune type, Wegener granulomatosis and polyarteritis nodosa are the principal examples. The immune-complex–mediated type can involve any GN that is due to immune-complex deposition and may present as crescentic GN. Systemic lupus erythematosus (SLE) is an important cause of this group.

Anti-GBM disease (Goodpasture disease) involves anti-GBM antibodies, which also cross-react with **alveolar basement membrane.** Patients present with massive hemoptysis and ARF. Studies show linear deposition of IgG in the glomerular basement membrane. Patients with crescentic GN present with acute renal failure with high morbidity and mortality.

Membranoproliferative (Mesangiocapillary) Glomerulonephritis

Membranoproliferative (mesangiocapillary) glomerulonephritis (MPGN) may present with either nephritic or nephrotic syndrome and is associated with hypocomplementemia. There are three types of MPGN, types I, II, and III.

Type I is the most common type; complement is activated by the classical pathway. **Type II** is characterized by the presence of **C3 nephritic factor** (an IgG antibody), which binds to and prevents inactivation of C3 convertase and results in persistent activation of complement by the alternate pathway. Histology shows that the glomeruli are diffusely enlarged with marked intracapillary hypercellularity and lobular accentuation. The capillary walls are thickened. Immunofluorescence shows large, granular confluent glomerular capillary walls and mesangial deposits of C3 with IgG. EM shows subendothelial deposits in types I and III. In type II the deposits are intramembranous, resulting in a diffuse electron-dense glomerular basement membrane (dense deposit disease). **Glomerulonephritis and low complement levels include** acute diffuse GN, MPGN, lupus nephritis (any GN that is due to SLE), and cryologlobulinemic GN.

COMPREHENSION QUESTIONS

[33.1] A 6-year-old boy presents with a new onset of oliguria and hematuria shortly after he has recovered from an untreated sore throat. Additional workup finds hypertension, periorbital edema, and impaired renal function with slightly increased amounts of protein in the urine. A renal biopsy most likely would reveal electron-dense deposits in which of the following sites?

A. Between the basement membrane and endothelial cells of the glomeruli
B. Between the basement membrane and epithelial cells of the glomeruli
C. Between the basement membrane and epithelial cells of the proximal tubules
D. Within the mesangium of the glomeruli
E. Within the juxtaglomerular apparatus

[33.2] Which of the following is the histologic hallmark for the diagnosis of rapidly progressive glomerulonephritis?

A. Crescents within the glomeruli
B. Fibrinoid necrosis of the efferent arterioles
C. Fibromuscular hyperplasia of the afferent arterioles
D. "Spike and dome" appearance of the glomerular basement membrane
E. "Tram-track" splitting of the glomerular basement membrane

[33.3] A renal biopsy from an adult who presented with progressive renal failure and hematuria reveals linear deposits of IgG within the glomeruli. Which of the following types of autoantibodies is most likely to be present in this individual?

A. Anti-basement membrane antibodies
B. Anticentromere antibodies
C. Anti–double-stranded DNA antibodies
D. Antimitochondrial antibodies
E. Anti–smooth muscle antibodies

Answers

[33.1] **B.** Acute diffuse proliferative glomerulonephritis most commonly presents in children after a group A β-hemolytic streptococcal infection; this explains the other name of this disorder: acute poststreptococcal glomerulonephritis. Children develop signs of the nephritic syndrome with hematuria, mild periorbital edema, and increased blood pressure. This disorder is characterized by irregular larger subepithelial (between the basement membrane and epithelial cells) electron-dense deposits.

[33.2] **A.** Rapidly progressive glomerulonephritis is characterized histologically by the presence of crescents within glomeruli (crescentic glomerulonephritis). A crescent, which is defined as having at least three layers of cells between the visceral and parietal epithelium, is composed of visceral and parietal epithelial cells, inflammatory cells, and fibrin. The three basic types of RPGN, defined by the immune pathomechanism, are anti-GBM disease (linear immune deposits), immune-complex–mediated disorders (granular immune deposits), and the pauci-immune type (very few immune deposits).

[33.3] **A.** Type I rapidly progressive glomerulonephritis is characterized by the finding of linear deposits of IgG and C3 within the glomerular basement membrane using immunofluorescence. Patients usually present with massive hemoptysis and acute renal failure. Most patients are found to have Goodpasture disease, in which autoantibodies to the glomerular basement membrane are present. These autoantibodies are directed against the noncollagenous portion of type IV collagen.

PATHOLOGY PEARLS

- Glomerulonephritis is due to a primarily immunologically mediated glomerular injury followed by secondary mechanisms of injury.
- The clinical presentation of the various types of glomerulonephritis can be one of the following six: nephritic syndrome, nephrotic syndrome, acute renal failure, chronic renal failure, isolated proteinuria, and isolated hematuria.
- Renal biopsy is examined by light microscopy, electron microscopy, and immunofluorescence.
- Acute diffuse GN typically is seen in children after a streptococcal infection and has an excellent prognosis.
- Crescentic GN or RPGN is associated with pauci-immune complex, immune complex, or anti-GBM antibody mechanisms. It has a high mortality.
- MPGN is a type of proliferative GN that can present clinically as nephritic syndrome or nephrotic syndrome. EM deposits are characteristically subendothelial (type I).

REFERENCES

Alpers CE. The kidney. In: Kumar V, Assas AK, Fausto N, eds. Robbins and Cotran Pathologic Basis of Disease, 7th ed. Philadelphia, PA: Elsevier Saunders, 2004: 963–72.

Alpers CE. The kidney. In: Mitchell RN, Kumar V, Abbas AK, et al., eds. Pocket Companion to Robbins and Cotran Pathologic Basis of Disease, 7th ed. Philadelphia, PA: Saunders, 2006:488–99.

CASE 34

A 42-year-old woman who has had proteinuria for approximately 5 years develops renal failure. She also has developed hypertension and has had several bacterial and vaginal yeast infections over the last 10 years. Her two pregnancies were uncomplicated, although she required cesarean deliveries for large babies of 9 lb and 9.5 lb. A kidney biopsy reveals increased mesangial matrix and acellular periodic acid-Schiff (PAS)-positive nodules.

- **What is the most likely diagnosis?**
- **What is the underlying mechanism?**

ANSWERS TO CASE 34: NEPHROTIC SYNDROME (DIABETIC)

Summary: A 42-year-old woman has a history of hypertension, vaginal candidiasis, proteinuria, and large babies. She presents with renal insufficiency. The renal biopsy is consistent with diabetic nephropathy.

- **Most likely diagnosis:** Nephrotic syndrome resulting from diabetic glomerulosclerosis.
- **Underlying mechanism:** Diabetic microangiopathy causing injury to the glomerulus.

CLINICAL CORRELATION

Diabetes is a leading cause of renal insufficiency in the United States. This 42-year-old woman probably has a long history of diabetes mellitus, as evidenced by her history of large babies and bacterial and vaginal candidal infections. Uncontrolled hyperglycemia can lead to microangiopathic changes, which can affect the glomerulus. The first clinical finding in diabetic nephropathy is microalbuminuria. The use of an angiotensin-converting enzyme inhibitor, control of hypertension, and tight control of the blood sugars can delay the development of renal failure. Unfortunately, this patient's renal disease has progressed to renal failure. This patient undergoes a renal biopsy that shows diffuse and nodular glomerulosclerosis with thickened basement membranes. Immunofluorescent stains would show granular deposits of immunoglobulin G (IgG) and C3. Electron microscopy (EM) would reveal prominent subepithelial immune-complex deposits. Complications related to nephrotic syndrome include hypercoagulability, sepsis (possibly related to loss of immunoglobulin in the urine), oliguric renal failure, and hypercholesterolemia, putting the patient at risk for coronary artery disease and peripheral vascular disease.

APPROACH TO NEPHROTIC SYNDROME

Objectives

- Describe the causes of nephrotic syndrome.
- List the most common cause of nephrotic syndrome in children
- Know the conditions associated with focal segmental glomerulosclerosis

Definitions

Nephrotic syndrome: A kidney disease affecting the glomerulus, leading to proteinuria higher than 3.5 g/day, hypoalbuminemia, generalized edema, and hyperlipidemia.

Primary glomerular disease: A condition of the kidney that leads to nephrosis, such as membranous glomerulopathy, minimal change disease, and focal segmental glomerulosclerosis.

Secondary glomerular disease: Conditions that are systemic, infectious, and toxic and affect the kidney, leading to nephrosis. Some of the causes are diabetes, systemic lupus erythematosus (SLE), penicillamine, and chronic hepatitis B infection.

DISCUSSION

Nephrotic syndrome consists of **massive proteinuria, hypoalbuminemia, edema, and hyperlipidemia.** Patients with nephrotic syndrome usually have heavy proteinuria. There is also increased catabolism of protein in the kidney with subsequent hypoalbuminemia. Hypoalbuminemia causes a reduction in oncotic pressure, and fluid shifts to the extravascular space. Reduction in circulating blood volume activates the renin-angiotensin system, causing increased salt and water retention. These mechanisms are thought to play a principal role in the pathogenesis of edema. Table 34-1 lists some causes of nephrotic syndrome.

Primary Glomerular Nephrotic Syndrome

Minimal lesion is the **most common cause of nephrotic syndrome** in **children.** In fact, in a child younger than 5 years old with nephrotic syndrome,

Table 34-1
CAUSES OF NEPHROTIC SYNDROME

Glomerulonephritis
Minimal
Membranous
Focal segmental glomerulosclerosis
Mesangiocapillary glomerulonephritis: may present as nephritic or nephrotic syndrome
Secondary
Diabetic nephropathy
Systemic vasculitis (e.g., systemic lupus erythematosus)
Drugs (gold, penicillamine, heroin)
Infections (HIV, malaria, syphilis, hepatitis B)
Malignancy (carcinoma, melanoma)
Allergies Amyloidosis

renal biopsy usually is not performed because minimal change is considered the underlying cause. Minimal lesion is the only type of glomerulonephritis (GN) that presents with **selective proteinuria.** This means that the protein loss is due mainly to albumin, not to high-molecular-weight proteins such as immunoglobulins. If renal biopsy is performed, light microscopy does not reveal any significant changes. Immunofluorescence (IF) studies are generally negative. EM studies do not demonstrate any immune-complex deposition. However, **loss of foot processes** of **visceral epithelial cells** can be documented. However, this EM finding is seen with any GN with proteinuria. Minimal lesion responds well to steroids and does not progress to chronic renal failure.

Membranous GN is the leading cause of nephrotic syndrome caused by primary glomerular disease in **adults.** Secondary causes of membranous GN always should be considered and ruled out. In membranous GN, there is **thickening of the basement membrane,** which is visible with light microscopy. Basement membrane **spikes** are seen usually. These spikes are well highlighted with special stains such as silver stains. IF studies demonstrate **deposition of IgG and C3.** EM shows subepithelial deposition of immune complexes. EM helps grade the disease. Membranous GN may progress to chronic renal failure (CRF).

Secondary causes of membranous GN include infections such as hepatitis B or C and syphilis; neoplasia such as carcinoma of the lung, gastrointestinal system, and breast; drugs and toxins such as gold and mercury; penicillamine; and SLE.

Focal segmental glomerulosclerosis (FSGS) is a condition associated with **HIV infection, obesity, heroin abuse, and hypertension.** Here the involvement is **focal** (not all glomeruli are involved) and **segmental** (not the entire glomerulus is involved). If the renal biopsy does not include an adequate number of glomeruli, FSGS can be missed easily. This is another GN in which immune complexes are not demonstrated on EM. Patients usually present with **nonselective proteinuria** that is heavy enough to cause nephrotic syndrome. This condition is typically resistant to steroids and is slowly progressive. Patients may end up with CRF, thus requiring a renal transplant. However, it may recur in the transplanted kidney.

Secondary Glomerular Nephrotic Syndrome

Nephrotic syndrome resulting from **diabetic glomerulopathy** is the **most common cause** of nephrotic syndrome in adults. It occurs several years after the onset of diabetes mellitus.

Diabetic glomerular disease consists of the following:

1. Nodular glomerulosclerosis **(Kimmelstiel-Wilson lesion)**
2. Diffuse glomerulosclerosis
3. Capsular drop
4. Fibrin caps

The first two lesions are seen commonly. Nodular glomerulosclerosis is the most specific lesion for diabetes mellitus. Diabetic nephropathy initially presents with microalbuminuria that is reversible with good diabetic control and angiotensin-converting enzyme inhibitors. Overt proteinuria and nephrotic-range proteinuria are subsequent events.

COMPREHENSION QUESTIONS

[34.1] Which of the following combinations of signs and symptoms is most consistent with a diagnosis of nephrotic syndrome?

A. Hematuria, hypertension, and proteinuria
B. Massive proteinuria, edema, and hyperlipidemia
C. Oliguria, hydronephrosis, and abdominal rebound tenderness
D. Painful hematuria, flank pain, and palpable abdominal mass
E. Painless hematuria, polycythemia, and increased skin pigmentation

[34.2] A 30-year-old female patient presents with a new onset of peripheral edema. Physical examination finds hypertension and bilateral pedal edema. Urinalysis finds massive proteinuria, and evaluation of her serum finds elevated levels of cholesterol. A silver stain of a renal biopsy specimen reveals a characteristic "spike and dome" pattern, and electron microscopy finds a uniform deposition of small electron-dense deposits in a subepithelial location. Which of the following immunofluorescence patterns is most characteristic of this patient's renal disease?

A. Granular pattern of IgA and C3
B. Granular pattern of IgG and C3
C. Linear pattern of IgD and C4
D. Linear pattern of IgE and C4
E. Linear pattern of IgM and C3

[34.3] A 45-year-old woman with a long-term history of poorly controlled diabetes mellitus is found to have proteinuria. A renal biopsy reveals hyaline arteriosclerosis of the afferent and efferent arterioles along with Kimmelstiel-Wilson lesions in a few of the glomeruli. Which of the following is the most likely diagnosis for these glomerular abnormalities?

A. Diffuse proliferative glomerulonephritis
B. Focal segmental glomerulosclerosis
C. Membranoproliferative glomerulonephritis
D. Membranous glomerulonephropathy
E. Nodular glomerulosclerosis

Answers

[34.1] **B.** The two basic glomerular clinical syndromes are the nephrotic syndrome and the nephritic syndrome. The nephrotic syndrome is characterized by massive proteinuria, which leads to hypoalbuminemia and widespread peripheral edema. Importantly, these patients also can develop hyperlipidemia (hypercholesterolemia), which is a risk factor for coronary artery disease and peripheral vascular disease. In contrast, the nephritic syndrome is characterized by hematuria. These patients also can develop proteinuria, but it is not as massive as the proteinuria seen with the nephrotic syndrome.

[34.2] **B.** The most common primary cause of the nephrotic syndrome in adults is membranous glomerulonephritis. This type of nonproliferative glomerulonephritis is characterized by small subepithelial electron-dense deposits. Light microscopy will reveal thickened basement membrane forming a "spike and dome" pattern, and immunofluorescence will be positive for granular deposits of IgG and C3. This granular pattern is characteristic of a type III hypersensitivity reaction.

[34.3] **E.** The most common cause of the nephrotic syndrome in adults is renal disease secondary to diabetic glomerulopathy. There are several manifestations of diabetic renal disease, but perhaps nodular glomerulosclerosis is the most specific. This abnormality, which also is known as Kimmelstiel-Wilson disease, is characterized by nodular eosinophilic deposits within the glomeruli. In contrast to deposits of amyloid, which may appear histologically similar, the deposits with diabetes do not stain with a Congo-red stain.

PATHOLOGY PEARLS

- Nephrotic syndrome consists of massive proteinuria, hypoalbuminemia, edema, and hyperlipidemia.
- Minimal lesion is the most common cause of nephrotic syndrome in children.
- In minimal lesion, light microscopy and IF do not reveal any significant changes. On EM, there is loss of foot processes without any immune-complex deposition.
- Minimal lesion responds well to steroids and does not progress to chronic renal failure.
- Membranous GN is the leading cause of nephrotic syndrome resulting from primary glomerular disease in adults.
- Light microscopy in membranous GN reveals thickened basement membrane with spikes. IF is positive for IgG, and EM shows subepithelial immune-complex deposits.
- FSGS is a condition associated with HIV infection, obesity, heroin abuse, and hypertension, and it may recur in a transplanted kidney.
- The most common cause of nephrotic syndrome in adults is diabetic glomerulopathy.
- Nodular glomerulosclerosis is the most specific lesion seen in diabetes mellitus.
- Diabetic nephropathy initially presents with microalbuminuria that is reversible with good diabetic control and angiotensin-converting enzyme inhibitors.

REFERENCES

Alpers CE. The kidney. In: Kumar V, Assas AK, Fausto N, eds. Robbins and Cotran Pathologic Basis of Disease, 7th ed. Philadelphia, PA: Elsevier Saunders, 2004: 972–84.

Alpers CE. The kidney. In: Mitchell RN, Kumar V, Abbas AK, et al., eds. Pocket Companion to Robbins and Cotran Pathologic Basis of Disease, 7th ed. Philadelphia, PA: Saunders, 2006:483–4.

CASE 35

A 55-year-old man presents to his primary care physician complaining of gross hematuria and right loin pain. Physical examination reveals a flank mass. The complete blood count (CBC) reveals a hemoglobin level of 21 g/dL and polycythemia. Ultrasound shows a 6.0-cm mass at the upper pole of the right kidney.

- **What is the most likely diagnosis?**

- **Where do these tumors arise from?**

- **What is the most likely explanation for this patient's polycythemia?**

ANSWERS TO CASE 35: RENAL CELL CARCINOMA

Summary: A 55-year-old man presents with hematuria, loin pain and renal mass, and polycythemia.

- **Most likely diagnosis:** Renal cell carcinoma.
- **Origin of cells:** Renal cell carcinomas arise from the proximal tubular epithelium.
- **Reason for polycythemia:** Up to 5 percent of renal cell carcinoma patients have **polycythemia.** This is due to inappropriate secretion of **erythropoietin** by the neoplastic cells.

CLINICAL CORRELATION

Renal cell carcinomas account for approximately 1 percent of all malignant tumors. They are the most common renal tumors in adults, with a peak incidence at age 55 years. They arise from the proximal tubular epithelium. **Bilateral renal cell carcinomas** are associated with **von Hippel-Lindau** disease. Deletion of the short arm of chromosome 3 is the most consistent cytogenetic abnormality in renal cell carcinomas.

The typical presentation includes hematuria, loin pain, and a flank mass. Up to 5 percent of patients exhibit polycythemia resulting from inappropriate secretion of erythropoietin. Fever may be present in a minority of patients. Renal cell carcinoma is one of the diagnoses that should be considered in a middle-aged adult with pyrexia of undetermined origin.

The tumor may be solitary or multiple. The cut surface is usually yellow. The tumor may extend beyond the capsule or extend into the ureter or renal vein. Involvement of the left renal vein may result in left-sided varicocele because the left testicular venous drainage is into the left renal vein. Involvement of lymph nodes and distant metastases naturally are associated with a poor outlook for the patient. There are several histologic types of renal cell carcinoma, but **conventional (clear cell) renal cell carcinoma** is the one that is encountered most frequently. Here the cytoplasm of the tumor cells is clear because of the presence of glycogen, which does not pick up on hematoxylin and eosin (H&E) stains. This type of tumor can be graded further according to the nuclear features, from grade 1 to grade 4 (**Fuhrman nuclear grade**). Nuclear size, irregularity, and presence of nucleoli are taken into account. Various imaging methods are used to arrive at a diagnosis.

Definitive treatment consists of surgical removal of the kidney (nephrectomy). Radiotherapy is of no proven value.

APPROACH TO RENAL CELL CARCINOMA

Objectives

- Describe the most common renal tumors found in adults.
- Know the association between renal cell carcinoma and von Hippel-Lindau syndrome.
- Know the presenting features seen in Wilms tumor.
- List the pathology and features of polycystic kidney disease.

Definitions

von Hippel-Lindau syndrome: It is a rare inherited genetic condition involving the abnormal growth of tumors in parts of the body which are particularly rich in blood supply.

Polycythemia: It is a condition in which there is a net increase in the total number of red blood cells in the body. The overproduction of red blood cells may be due to a primary process in the bone marrow (myeloproliferative syndrome), or it may be a reaction to chronically low levels of oxygen or, rarely, a malignancy.

Hematuria: Presence of blood in the urine.

Erythropoietin: A glycoprotein hormone secreted mainly by the kidney. The erythropoietin acts on the bone marrow stem cells to stimulate red blood cell production (erythropoiesis).

DISCUSSION

Pathology of Renal Cysts and Renal Tumors

Cystic renal diseases may be broadly categorized as follows:

Congenital: Cystic renal dysplasia, autosomal dominant and autosomal recessive polycystic kidney disease, and nephronophthisis

Acquired: Simple cysts, acquired renal cystic kidney disease (dialysis-associated), and medullary sponge kidney

In **cystic renal dysplasia** there is abnormal metanephric differentiation. This leads to the presence of abnormal structures in the kidney, such as cartilage, undifferentiated mesenchyme, and immature collecting ductules. Cystic renal dysplasia frequently is associated with obstruction of the ureters.

Autosomal dominant polycystic kidney disease is seen in 1 in 700 live births and contributes to 10 percent of chronic renal failure in patients requiring transplantation and/or dialysis. The implicated genes are *PKD1* and *PKD2,* which are located in chromosomes 16 and 4, respectively. The *PKD2* gene, however, is responsible for a milder form of the disease. In this condition, cysts are formed from any part of the nephron and typically less than 20 percent of the nephrons become cystic. With time the cysts enlarge and cause compression and damage of the remaining nephrons. The cysts may become hemorrhagic and develop nephrolithiasis. Patients usually present with hypertension with flank pain and mass and are at risk of developing renal cell carcinoma. Autosomal dominant polycystic kidney disease is associated with extrarenal manifestations that include hepatic cysts, intracranial aneurysms, colonic diverticula, and cardiac valvular abnormalities.

Autosomal recessive polycystic kidney disease manifests at birth, and the infant may die from renal failure. Patients who survive infancy develop congenital hepatic fibrosis, which is characterized by periportal fibrosis and bile ductular proliferation.

Nephronophthisis

Nephronophthisis is a group of progressive renal disorders that usually have their onset in childhood. Cysts typically located at the corticomedullary junction and associated tubular atrophy and interstitial fibrosis are features of this condition. **Simple cysts** typically are confined to the cortex; they are usually 1 to 5 cm in size and filled with clear fluid. They are common autopsy findings. Patients with end-stage renal disease who undergo dialysis may develop cortical and medullary **dialysis-associated cysts.** Uncommonly, carcinomas may be present in the wall of such cysts.

In **medullary sponge kidneys,** multiple cystic dilations of the collecting ducts in the medulla are found. The pathogenesis is not clear.

Renal Neoplasms in Adults

These tumors are subdivided into benign and malignant etiologies. **Benign** causes include papillary adenoma (small papillary neoplasm <0.5 cm and grade 1 nuclei) and oncocytoma, which is a well-circumscribed tumor with cells that have granular eosinophilic cytoplasm as a result of abundant mitochondria. **Malignant etiologies include the spectrum of renal cell carcinomas.** Conventional renal cell carcinoma includes clear cell carcinoma. Chromophobe renal cell carcinoma is characterized histologically by a perinuclear halo (clearing) and a prominent cytoplasmic border. It has a better prognosis than does conventional renal cell carcinoma.

Papillary (chromophil) renal cell carcinoma is the second most common malignant neoplasm and may be multifocal and bilateral. Papillary structures lined by tumor epithelium are seen. Collecting duct carcinoma is characterized by a high-grade tumor with significant fibrosis.

Renal Neoplasms in Children

Approximately **80 to 85 percent of renal tumors of children** are **Wilms tumors.** They are usually seen in children of ages 2 to 6 years and may be bilateral in 5 to 10 percent of the cases. The typical clinical presentation includes abdominal mass or pain and hematuria. Renin secretion may produce hypertension. Wilms tumor may be associated with Wilms tumor, aniridia, genitourinary anomaly, and mental retardation (WAGR) syndrome, a deletion of the *WT1* gene at 11p13; Denys-Drash syndrome (gonadal dysgenesis and nephropathy), a missense mutation of the *WT1* gene; and Beckwith-Wiedemann syndrome, which involves the *WT2* gene at 11p15.5. Nephroblastomatosis, which consists of multifocal or diffuse immature nephrogenic elements, also may be seen. Grossly, the tumor is a solitary, well-circumscribed soft mass with occasional foci of necrosis and hemorrhage. Histology exhibits three major components (most Wilms tumors show all three components): **undifferentiated blastema** (resembles blue cells, that is, cells with minimum of cytoplasm), **mesenchymal** (stromal) tissue (represented by spindle cells or smooth or skeletal muscle), and **epithelial tissue** (represented by tubular structures recapitulating developing tubules and glomeruli) (see Figure 35-1).

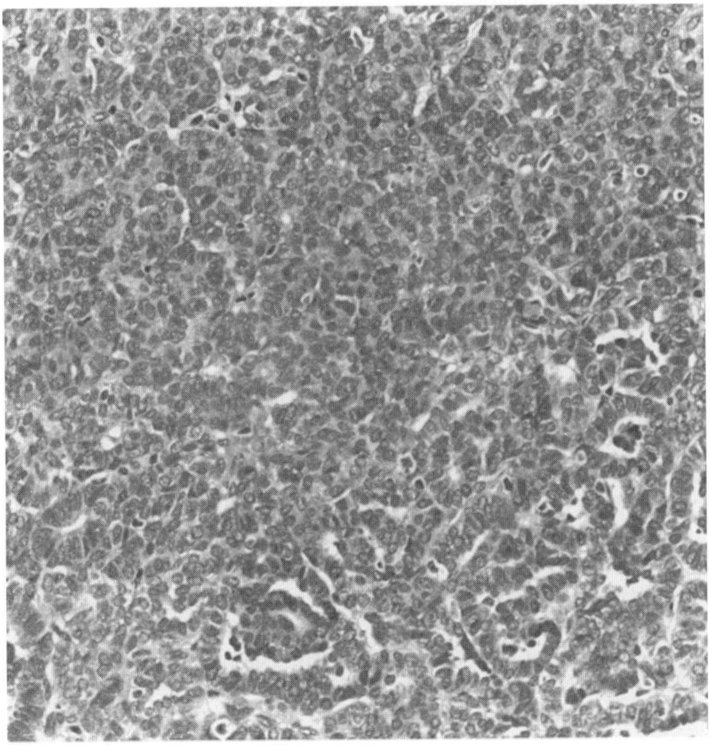

Figure 35-1. Wilms tumor with characteristic tubular/glomeruloid structures and blastema (original magnification, 40×). *(Reproduced, with permission, from Tanagho EA, McAninch JW:* Smith's General Urology, 16th ed. *New York: McGraw-Hill, 2004:359)*

COMPREHENSION QUESTIONS

[35.1] A 54-year-old man presents with worsening pain on the left side accompanied by gross hematuria. Workup finds a 4.5-cm mass in the upper pole of the left kidney. What is the characteristic histologic appearance of the conventional type of malignancy in this location?

A. Disorganized groups of immature tubules
B. Sheets of transitional epithelial cells
C. Small cells forming numerous papillary structures
D. Undifferentiated cells demonstrating abortive glomerular formation
E. Uniform cells with clear cytoplasm resulting from glycogen

[35.2] Which of the following abnormalities is most likely to be associated with the adult form of polycystic renal disease?

A. Berry aneurysms arising from the circle of Willis
B. Multiple schwannomas arising from cranial nerve VIII
C. Solitary rhabdomyomas within the heart
D. Vascular malformations within the eye
E. von Meyenburg complexes within the liver

[35.3] Histologic sections from an abdominal mass that was removed from a 13-month-old female reveal undifferentiated mesenchymal cells, immature tubules, and abortive glomerular formation. Which of the following is the most likely diagnosis for this tumor?

A. Dupuytren tumor
B. Ewing tumor
C. Ollier tumor
D. Warthin tumor
E. Wilms tumor

Answers

[35.1] **E.** The classic clinical signs produced by a renal cell carcinoma are hematuria, flank pain, and a palpable abdominal mass. Renal cell carcinomas are located in the cortex of the renal parenchyma and arise from the proximal tubular epithelium. The most common histologic type of renal cell carcinoma is the conventional type, in which the tumor cells have clear cytoplasm (clear cell carcinoma) because of the presence of glycogen and lipid in the cytoplasm of the tumor cells.

[35.2] **A.** The adult form of polycystic kidney disease is an autosomal dominant disorder that is associated with mutations of the *PKD1* gene, which is located on chromosome 16. Patients usually present with flank pain, hematuria, hypertension, and progressive renal failure. It is important to note that the autosomal dominant (adult) form of polycystic kidney disease also is associated with extrarenal manifestations such as multiple cysts in the liver and berry aneurysm of the circle of Willis. A berry aneurysm can rupture and produce a subarachnoid hemorrhage.

[35.3] **E.** Wilms tumor (nephroblastoma) is the most common primary tumor of the kidney found in children. The classic clinical presentation of a nephroblastoma, which is associated with a deletion involving the *WT1* gene on chromosome 11, is a child with an enlarging abdominal mass. Histologic sections of the tumor will reveal undifferentiated blastema and mesenchymal cells, immature tubules, and immature (abortive) glomeruli formation.

PATHOLOGY PEARLS

- ❖ Renal cell carcinoma is the most common renal tumor in adults, arising from the proximal renal tubular epithelium.
- ❖ Typically unilateral, bilateral tumors are associated with von Hippel-Lindau disease.
- ❖ Hematuria, abdominal pain, and an abdominal mass are the usual presenting features. Fever and polycythemia are established but uncommon findings.
- ❖ Conventional renal cell carcinoma with cells with clear cytoplasm remains the most commonly seen histologic type.
- ❖ Individuals with autosomal dominant polycystic kidney disease have enlarged cystic kidneys. They present with hypertension and progress to chronic renal failure. The condition is associated with intracranial aneurysms. Renal cell carcinoma (RCC) is a recognized complication.
- ❖ Wilms tumor manifests at birth, and the infant may die from renal failure. Patients who survive infancy develop congenital hepatic fibrosis.
- ❖ Eighty to eighty-five percent of renal tumors in children are Wilms tumors.

REFERENCES

Alpers CE. The kidney. In: Kumar V, Assas AK, Fausto N, eds. Robbins and Cotran Pathologic Basis of Disease, 7th ed. Philadelphia, PA: Elsevier Saunders, 2004:1015–520.

Alpers CE. The kidney. In: Mitchell RN, Kumar V, Abbas AK, et al., eds. Pocket Companion to Robbins and Cotran Pathologic Basis of Disease, 7th ed. Philadelphia, PA: Saunders, 2006:508–9.

CASE 36

A 62-year-old woman complains of fatigue and numbness of her arms and legs for 1 month. She has a history of hypothyroidism and takes thyroid replacement therapy. A complete blood count (CBC) shows white blood cells (WBC) 4000/mm^3 (normal: 4800 to 10,800/mm^3), hemoglobin (Hgb) 9 g/dL (normal: 12 to 16 g/dL), hematocrit (Hct) 27 percent (normal: 36 to 46 percent), mean corpuscular volume (MCV) 120 fL (femtoliter) (normal: 80 to 100 fL), and platelets 150,000/mm^3 (normal: 150,000 to 400,000/mm^3). A peripheral blood smear is shown in Figure 36-1.

- **What is the most likely diagnosis?**
- **What is the likely biochemical basis for this type of anemia?**

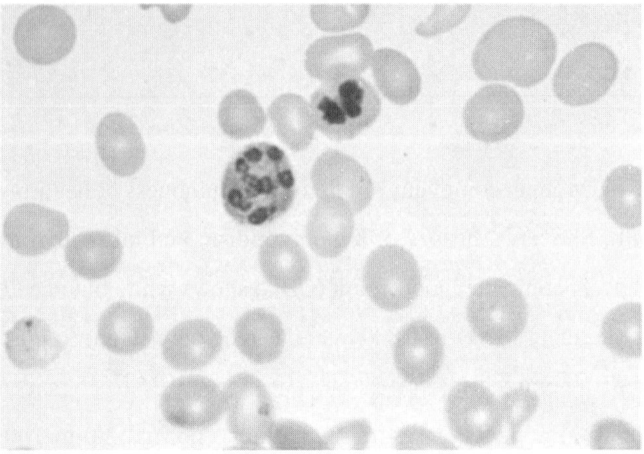

Figure 36-1. Peripheral blood smear. *(Reproduced, with permission, from Kasper DL, Braunwald E, Fauci AS, et al., eds.* Harrison's Principles of Internal Medicine, 16th ed. *New York: McGraw-Hill, 2004:605.)*

ANSWERS TO CASE 36: PERNICIOUS ANEMIA

Summary: A 62-year-old woman with a past history of thyroid disease presents with fatigue and peripheral neuropathy. Anemia is noted with oval macrocytes and hypersegmented polymorphonucleocytes (PMNs) in the peripheral smear.

◆ **Most likely diagnosis:** Pernicious anemia

◆ **Biochemical basis for anemia:** Vitamin B_{12} deficiency leading to megaloblastic anemia

CLINICAL CORRELATION

This 62-year-old woman has a history of thyroid disease and presents with findings of megaloblastic anemia with enlarged erythrocytes with **hypersegmented neutrophils** (see Figure 36-1). The two possibilities are folate and vitamin B_{12} deficiencies; both of these vitamin deficiencies can lead to defective DNA synthesis, specifically thymidine synthesis. Abnormally large red blood cells result from defects in cell maturation and division, whereas RNA synthesis and cytoplasm growth are not affected. Folate deficiency is particularly common in individuals who abuse alcohol. Vitamin B_{12} stores usually last for several years, but deficiencies may occur in patients with inadequate intrinsic factor, which is needed for vitamin B_{12} absorption in the ileum. Intrinsic factor is secreted by the parietal cells of the gastric fundus. Various autoantibodies can lead to pernicious anemia, including those which target gastric mucosa, intrinsic factor, and the intrinsic factor–vitamin B_{12} complex, leading to poor absorption of the needed vitamin. Individuals with vitamin B_{12} deficiency also may develop neurologic symptoms, specifically degeneration of the myelin in the dorsal and lateral tracts of the spinal cord. This patient has symptoms of a peripheral neuropathy, and a history of hypothyroidism suggests an autoimmune process. This would be consistent with pernicious anemia, and the diagnosis would be confirmed with a Schilling test to assess the ability to absorb radiolabeled cyanocobalamin (vitamin B_{12} complex). The treatment would be exogenous vitamin B_{12} administration.

APPROACH TO MEGALOBLASTIC ANEMIA

Objectives

- Describe the most common cause of anemia.
- List the causes of microcytic anemia.
- Know the causes of iron deficiency.
- List the causes of macrocytic anemia.
- Describe how to differentiate between vitamin B_{12} deficiency and folate deficiency.

Definitions

Anemia: A reduction in the concentration of hemoglobin, taking into account the age and sex of the individual.

Microcytic red cells: Red blood cells (RBCs) with low mean corpuscular volume (MCV; smaller than normal red cells).

Hypochromic red cells: RBCs with low mean corpuscular hemoglobin concentration (MCHC) (cells with increased central pallor).

Macrocytic red cells: RBCs with high MCV (larger than normal red cells).

Normocytic red cells: RBCs with normal MCV.

Normochromic red cells: RBCs with normal one-third central pallor.

Anisocytosis: Variation in the size of red cells. The red diameter width (RDW) is increased.

Poikilocytosis: Variation in the shape of red cells.

DISCUSSION

Iron deficiency is the most common cause of anemia in general. Only 10 percent of the daily dietary intake of iron is absorbed in the duodenum and jejunum. Absorption may be increased in iron deficiency and pregnancy. Once absorbed, the **iron is transported** by **transferrin.** Normally, one-third of the transferrin binding sites are occupied by iron. Iron is **stored** as either **ferritin** or **hemosiderin.** Serum ferritin serves as a good reflection of store status. As ferritin is an acute-phase reactant, high levels do not necessarily mean that an

Table 36-1
CAUSES OF MICROCYTIC HYPOCHROMIC ANEMIA

Iron deficiency
Anemia of chronic disease (typically presents as normocytic normochromic anemia)
Sideroblastic anemia
Thalassemia and some hemoglobin disorders (e.g., HbC, not HbS)

individual has excess stores of iron. **Iron deficiency** typically presents with **microcytic hypochromic anemia,** whereas **vitamin B_{12}- and folate-deficient** patients present with **macrocytic anemia** (see Table 36-1 for a listing of microcytic anemias and Table 36-2 for causes of iron deficiency).

Laboratory findings in iron deficiency include microcytic hypochromic anemia, anisocytosis (i.e., RDW is high), **poikilocytosis** (occasional pencil-shaped cells may be seen), occasional target cells, **low serum iron and serum ferritin,** and **elevated serum total iron-binding capacity (TIBC).** Although not specific for iron deficiency, bone marrow findings include erythroid hyperplasia with ragged cytoplasm of red cell precursors (normoblasts), and iron stains (Prussian blue) will reveal reduced or absent iron stores. See Table 36-3 for classification of the causes of anemia in general.

Macrocytic Anemias

Macrocytic anemias can be divided broadly into two categories: **megaloblastic** and **normoblastic.** Megaloblastic macrocytic anemias consist of red cells that are larger than normal (raised MCV, typically greater than 120 fL), and the red cell precursors in the bone marrow are also abnormal and large (megaloblasts). In contrast, individuals with normoblastic macrocytic anemia

Table 36-2
CAUSES OF IRON DEFICIENCY

Dietary deficiency
Chronic blood loss
Increased demands (e.g., growth, pregnancy)
Decreased absorption

Table 36-3
CLASSIFICATION OF ANEMIA

Morphologic classification
- Normocytic normochromic anemia
- Microcytic hypochromic anemia
- Macrocytic anemia

Etiologic classification
- Anemia caused by blood loss (acute or chronic)
- Anemia caused by decreased production of red cells
  - Deficiency or erythropoietic factors (e.g., iron, vitamin B_{12}, and folate)
  - Anemia of chronic disease
  - Anemia caused by bone marrow infiltration (e.g., fibrosis or malignancy)
  - Aplastic anemia
- Anemia caused by increased red cell destruction (hemolytic anemia)
  - Hemolytic anemia caused by intrinsic red cell defect
    - Red cell membrane defects (e.g., hereditary spherocytosis)
    - Red cell enzyme defects (e.g., glucose 6-phosphate deficiency)
    - Structural hemoglobin defects (hemoglobinopathies, e.g., HbS, C, E)
    - Reduced rate of globin chain synthesis (thalassemia, alpha and beta)
    - Paroxysmal nocturnal hemoglobinuria
- Hemolytic anemia resulting from extrinsic causes
  - Immune mechanisms
    - Autoimmune hemolytic anemia
    - Hemolytic anemia caused by mismatch transfusion
    - Hemolytic disease of the newborn
- Nonimmune mechanisms
  - Microangiopathic hemolytic anemia (e.g., disseminated intravascular coagulation, thrombotic thrombocytopenic purpura, hemolytic uremic syndrome)
  - Malaria
  - March- or karate-induced

have red cells that are larger than normal (although they are usually smaller than the macrocytes seen in megaloblastic macrocytic anemia, with MCV typically 100–110 fL), but the red cell precursors in the bone marrow are normal. See Table 36-4 for a listing of the causes of macrocytic anemias.

Deoxythymidine monophosphate is one of the four nucleotides present in DNA. It is synthesized from deoxyuridine monophosphate by the addition of a methyl group that is transferred from methylenetetrahydrofolate. Deficiency of folate reduces the supply of methylenetetrahydrofolate. Methylenetetrahydrofolate in turn is derived from tetrahydrofolate, which is generated from methyltetrahydrofolate. The demethylation of methyltetrahydrofolate to tetrahydrofolate is done with the help of vitamin B_{12}. Thus, a deficiency of vitamin B_{12} leads to low levels of tetrahydrofolate and methylenetetrahydrofolate, with

Table 36-4
CAUSES OF MACROCYTIC ANEMIA

Megaoblastic macrocytic anemias
Vitamin B_{12} deficiency or abnormal B_{12} metabolism
Folic acid deficiency or abnormal folate metabolism
Other defects in DNA synthesis, such as drugs that interfere with DNA synthesis (e.g., azathioprine, azidothymidine) and congenital deficiencies in DNA synthesis (e.g., orotic aciduria)
Myelodysplasia caused by dyserythropoiesis
Normoblastic macrocytic anemias
Alcohol excess
Liver disease
Reticulocytosis
Hypothyroidism

subsequent impaired conversion of deoxyuridine monophosphate to deoxythymidine monophosphate.

This results in defective nuclear maturation and the nuclear chromatin is more finely dispersed than normal and has an open stippled appearance. The synthesis of RNA and protein is unaffected. Thus, cytoplasmic enlargement is not matched by DNA synthesis, and there is a delay or block in mitotic division. This is the basis of the nuclear-to-cytoplasmic dyssynchrony.

After ingestion, vitamin **B_{12} binds with intrinsic factor** (derived from the parietal cells of the stomach) and R binder (derived from the saliva and stomach). Vitamin B_{12} bound to R binder is released by pancreatic enzymes and then binds to intrinsic factor (IF). Vitamin B_{12} is **absorbed at the terminal ileum,** and the intrinsic factor remains in the lumen. The absorbed vitamin B_{12} is transported to the various sites of function by transcobalamin (TC). In plasma, vitamin B_{12} is bound mainly to TC I, but its function is not clear. Vitamin B_{12} bound to TC II is readily available to the bone marrow and tissues.

The **most common cause of vitamin B12 deficiency in adults is pernicious anemia (see Table 36-5).** Pernicious anemia is considered an **autoimmune disease** with **antibodies** against **intrinsic factor and parietal cells.** The antibodies against intrinsic factor are more specific for the diagnosis and are of two types: blocking antibodies, which block the attachment of B_{12} to IF, and binding antibodies, which prevent the absorption of B_{12} in the ileum. Antiparietal cell antibodies, although found in up to 90 percent of patients, are less specific. Gastric biopsy shows gastric atrophy with a lymphoplasmacytic infiltrate. **Destruction of the parietal cells** results in **achlorhydria,** which typically is a disease of females over age 60 years. It is **associated with other autoimmune disorders,** particularly thyroid disease, Addison disease, and vitiligo.

Table 36-5

LABORATORY FINDINGS IN PERNICIOUS ANEMIA

Peripheral Blood

Macrocytic anemia

Mean corpuscular volume is typically greater than 120 fL; oval macrocytes are typically present

Moderate to marked anisopoikilocytosis: teardrop cells, schistocytes, and spherocytes

Basophilic stippling and Howell-Jolly bodies may be seen

With severe anemia, nucleated red blood cells may be present

Normal or low reticulocyte count

Hypersegmented polymorphonucleocytes (more than five lobes)

Pancytopenia

Bone Marrow

Hypercellular marrow with increased number of erythroblasts

Megaloblastoid changes with finely dispersed chromatin

Features of dyserythropoiesis (e.g., nuclear budding or lobulation)

Giant bands and metamyelocytes

Vitamin B_{12} and folate levels

Serum B_{12} levels: decreased

Serum folate level: normal or high

Red cell folate: normal or reduced because of inhibition of normal folate synthesis

The average adult stores of **vitamin B_{12}** are approximately 2 to 3 mg, mainly in the liver, and it **takes 2 years or more** before features of the deficiency are apparent. As the stores of vitamin B_{12} become depleted, the patient develops features of anemia, which usually has an insidious onset. It is not uncommon for patients to present with marked anemia (Hgb in the range of 3 to 4 g/dL). In such situations, the patient exhibits features of hyperdynamic circulation, and **high-output cardiac failure** is a potential threat. In the bone marrow, nuclear cytoplasmic dyssynchrony may be evident in all cell lines. However, the changes in the red cell series are the most striking. Abnormal maturation leads to intramedullary destruction of all cell lines. This is referred to as ineffective erythropoiesis. Intramedullary red cell destruction may result in mild hyperbilirubinemia and increased levels of LDH. Significant intramedullary destruction also may result in pancytopenia.

Vitamin B_{12} also is required for myelin synthesis. Vitamin B_{12} deficiency may result in neurologic changes that may be irreversible if left untreated. The **neurologic changes** include **peripheral neuropathy, subacute degeneration of the spinal cord** (damage to the pyramidal tract and dorsal column), **dementia,** and **optic atrophy.**

Megaloblastic anemias are a group of disorders characterized by a reduced rate of DNA synthesis. However, RNA transcription and translation are not affected. Nuclear maturation lags behind cytoplasmic maturation and is referred to as nuclear cytoplasmic dyssynchrony, which is the morphologic hallmark of megaloblastic anemias. Vitamin B_{12} and folic acid deficiency remain the two most common causes of megaloblastic anemia.

Treatment of pernicious anemia includes hydroxocobalamin, which needs to be given intramuscularly for the rest of the patient's life. Clinical improvement is expected within days. Peripheral neuropathy may improve over a period of 6 to 12 months. Spinal cord damage may be irreversible.

Folate Deficiency

Folates are present in food as polyglutamates in the reduced dihydrofolate or tetrahydrofolate form. The polyglutamates are broken down to monoglutamates in the upper gastrointestinal tract. During absorption they are converted to methyltetrahydrofolate monoglutamate, which is the main form in the serum. Vitamin B_{12} converts methyltetrahydrofolate to tetrahydrofolate, from which methylenetetrahydrofolate is synthesized. The hematologic features of folate deficiency are indistinguishable from those of vitamin B_{12} deficiency. Neurologic changes are not a feature of folate deficiency. Serum and red cell folate levels are low. Folate deficiency can be corrected by oral folate replacement.

COMPREHENSION QUESTIONS

[36.1] A 39-year-old woman who presented with increasing fatigue and muscle weakness is found have a microcytic and hypochromic anemia. Which of the following is the most likely cause of her anemia?

A. Folate deficiency
B. Iron deficiency
C. Viral infection
D. Vitamin B_{12} deficiency
E. Vitamin C deficiency

[36.2] Which of the following autoantibodies is most likely to be present in a patient with pernicious anemia?

A. Anticentromere antibodies
B. Antigliadin antibodies
C. Anti-intrinsic factor antibodies
D. Antimitochondrial antibodies
E. Antismooth muscle antibodies

[36.3] A 61-year-old woman with pancytopenia, mild jaundice, and peripheral neuropathy is found to have decreased serum levels of vitamin B_{12}. Which of the following abnormal cell morphologies is most likely to be present in a smear made from her peripheral blood?

A. Hypersegmented PMNs
B. Large granular lymphocytes
C. Oval microcytes
D. Pelger-Huët neutrophils
E. Plasmacytoid lymphocytes

Answers

[36.1] **B.** The most common causes of microcytic hypochromic anemia are iron deficiency, anemia of chronic disease, thalassemia, and sideroblastic anemia. Among these conditions, the **most common cause of a microcytic hypochromic anemia is a deficiency of iron.** Causes of iron deficiency include a dietary deficiency of iron, decreased intestinal absorption of iron, increased demand for iron, and chronic blood loss.

[36.2] **C.** In contrast to iron deficiency, which causes a microcytic hypochromic anemia, vitamin B_{12} deficiency produces a macrocytic anemia. The most common cause of vitamin B_{12} deficiency in adults is pernicious anemia, which is an autoimmune disease characterized by the formation of autoantibodies against intrinsic factor and parietal cells of the stomach. A gastric biopsy from an individual with pernicious anemia will show chronic inflammation with atrophy (chronic atrophic gastritis).

[36.3] **A.** The two most common causes of megaloblastic anemia are deficiencies of vitamin B_{12} or folate. These deficiencies decrease the synthesis of DNA, which results in nuclear-cytoplasmic asynchrony in maturation, which is the hallmark of megaloblastic anemias. This abnormal maturation will produce characteristic histologic changes in the cells in the peripheral blood, including oval macrocytes and hypersegmented PMNs, which are neutrophils with more than five lobes to their nuclei.

PATHOLOGY PEARLS

- Anemias may be classified on a morphologic basis and an etiologic basis.
- Iron deficiency typically presents with microcytic hypochromic anemia, whereas vitamin B_{12}- and folate-deficient patients present with macrocytic anemia.
- Megaloblastic anemias are characterized by a reduced rate of DNA synthesis.
- Vitamin B_{12} deficiency and folate deficiency are the two leading causes of megaloblastic anemias.
- Pernicious anemia is the most common cause of vitamin B_{12} deficiency in adults.
- Megaloblastic anemias are characterized by oval macrocytes and hypersegmented PMNs in the peripheral blood. In the bone marrow, there is erythroid hyperplasia with megaloblastoid changes and giant myelocytes and giant bands. Pancytopenia is one of the presenting features of megaloblastic anemias.
- The features of vitamin B_{12} deficiency and folate deficiency are indistinguishable except for the neurologic changes that may be seen in vitamin B_{12} deficiency.

REFERENCES

Aster JC. Red blood cell and bleeding disorders. In: Kumar V, Assas AK, Fausto N, eds. Robbins and Cotran Pathologic Basis of Disease, 7th ed. Philadelphia, PA: Elsevier Saunders, 2004:620–46.

Aster JC. Red blood cell and bleeding disorders. In: Mitchell RN, Kumar V, Abbas AK, et al., eds. Pocket Companion to Robbins and Cotran Pathologic Basis of Disease, 7th ed. Philadelphia, PA: Saunders, 2006:317–29.

❖ CASE 37

A 48-year-old man who works as an accountant complains of weakness, fatigue, and bleeding from the gums when he brushes his teeth. A complete blood count (CBC) shows severe pancytopenia with white blood cells (WBC) 1000/mm^3 (normal: 4800 to 10,800/mm^3), hemoglobin (Hgb) 8 g/dL (normal: 13 to 17 g/dL), hematocrit (Hct) 24 percent (normal: 41 to 53 percent), mean corpuscular volume (MCV) 10 fL (normal: 80 to 100 fL), and platelets 30,000/mm^3 (normal: 150,000 to 500,000/mm^3). A bone marrow biopsy is shown in Figure 37-1.

◆ **What is the most likely diagnosis?**

◆ **What other tests need to be done?**

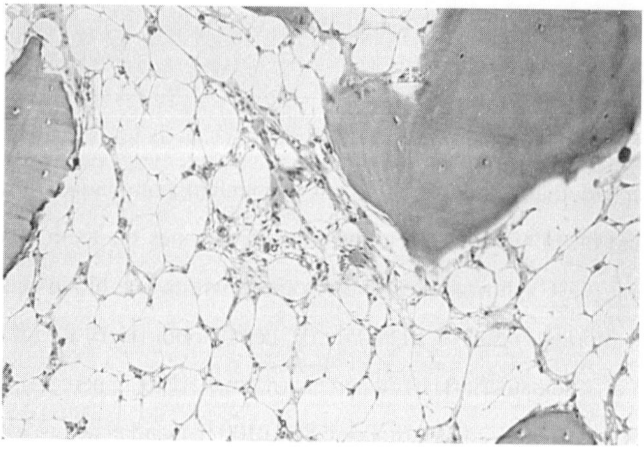

Figure 37-1. Bone marrow aspirate. *(Reproduced, with permission, from Kasper DL, Braunwald E, Fauci AS, et al., eds.* Harrison's Principles of Internal Medicine, 16th ed. *New York: McGraw-Hill, 2004:620.)*

ANSWERS TO CASE 37: APLASTIC ANEMIA

Summary: A 48-year-old man presents with symptomatic pancytopenia. The bone marrow aspirate shows a paucity of cells.

- **Most likely diagnosis:** Aplastic anemia
- **Further tests:** Review of the peripheral smear, a reticulocyte count, and a bone marrow examination

CLINICAL CORRELATION

This 48-year-old man has manifestations of pancytopenia. He has fatigue from the anemia and bleeding from the gums as a result of the thrombocytopenia. A pancytopenia (all three blood cell lines are affected) usually points to a bone marrow process. The bone marrow aspirate is the best diagnostic test and in this case reveals a paucity of cells, which is consistent with aplastic anemia. Other etiologies include drugs that may affect the bone marrow, megaloblastic anemia, bone marrow infiltration by a malignancy such as leukemia, lymphoma, carcinoma, fibrosis, and hypersplenism.

APPROACH TO APLASTIC ANEMIA

Objectives

- List the causes of aplastic anemia.
- Describe the findings seen in the bone marrow of patients with aplastic anemia.
- Know the findings seen in patients with hypersplenism.

Definitions

Pancytopenia: Presence of anemia, leukopenia, and thrombocytopenia.

Aplastic anemia: Reduction of erythroid, granulocytic/monocytic, and megakaryocytic cell lines and their progeny in the bone marrow, with resultant pancytopenia in the peripheral blood.

DISCUSSION

Aplastic anemia is defined as **pancytopenia** with **marked hypocellularity of the bone marrow** (see Table 37-1 for etiologies). Pancytopenia also is seen with certain medications, including **chemotherapeutic agents,** disease-modifying antirheumatic agents, and antithyroid drugs. Pancytopenia is an unusual mode of presentation in **megaloblastic anemia.** In megaloblastic anemia, there is **macrocytosis** of red cells and **hypersegmented polymorphonucleocytes (PMNs)** are seen in the peripheral blood. **Bone marrow infiltration** with fibrosis or tumor cells may result in pancytopenia and is referred to as myelophthisic anemia. In this condition, the peripheral smear reveals teardrop red cells and red cell and white cell precursors (leukoerythroblastic blood picture). **Hypersplenism** can cause destruction of red blood cells (RBCs), WBCs, and platelets by the splenic macrophages. The most common preceding infection is hepatitis. The **bone marrow in this condition is actually hypercellular,** and the reticulocyte count is elevated. The reticulocyte count in aplastic anemia is low. **Paroxysmal nocturnal hemoglobinuria (PNH)** is an acquired condition in which the patient's complement destroys his or her red cells, resulting in hemolytic anemia. Rarely, complement may destroy WBCs and platelets, resulting in pancytopenia.

The pathogenesis of aplastic anemia is poorly understood. The **majority of cases** are **acquired idiopathic** in nature. In these cases, it is thought that two major mechanisms play a role in the pathogenesis. In the first mechanism, stem cells are antigenically altered by an exogenous agent, followed by a T-cell immune response against the altered stem cells. The other mechanism is thought to result from genetically abnormal stem cells. RBCs survive for approximately 120 days, platelets survive for 10 days, and PMNs survive in the circulation for approximately 10 hours. With bone marrow failure, features

Table 37-1
CAUSES OF APLASTIC ANEMIA

Congenital
Fanconi anemia (autosomal recessive)
Pure red cell aplasia (Diamond-Blackfan syndrome)
Acquired
Idiopathic
Drugs and chemicals
Dose-dependent mechanism (e.g., chemotherapeutic agents)
Idiosyncratic mechanism (e.g., chloramphenicol)
Benzene
Ionizing radiation
Infections
Hepatitis virus
Parvovirus B19 (may cause transient red cell aplasia in chronic hemolytic patients)

related to neutropenia (i.e., infections) are seen first, followed by other features, such as thrombocytopenia and anemia.

The clinical course of aplastic anemia is variable. Some cases remit spontaneously. Therapy consists of transfusion of red cells, platelets, and antibiotics. Immunosuppressive therapy with antithymocyte globulin (ATG) may be tried. Bone marrow transplantation may be the required treatment for some patients.

COMPREHENSION QUESTIONS

[37.1] A 35-year-old woman with a history of hepatitis C infection presents with increasing fatigue. Physical examination finds pallor of the skin and conjunctiva and multiple petechial hemorrhages on the skin. No hepatomegaly or splenomegaly is present. A complete blood cell count finds pancytopenia. Which of the following bone marrow findings is most consistent with a diagnosis of aplastic anemia?

A. Absolute erythroid hyperplasia
B. General lymphoid hyperplasia
C. General marrow hypoplasia
D. Relative erythroid aplasia
E. Relative granulocytic hypoplasia

[37.2] A 66-year-old man presents with signs and symptoms of anemia. Examination of his peripheral blood smear reveals the abnormal presence of nucleated red blood cells and myelocytes. Which of the following is the most likely diagnosis?

A. Aplastic anemia
B. DiGeorge syndrome
C. Fanconi anemia
D. Myelophthisic anemia
E. Potter syndrome

[37.3] Which of the following laboratory tests would best differentiate hypersplenism from aplastic anemia as being the cause of peripheral pancytopenia?

A. Direct Coombs test
B. Ham test
C. Metabisulfite test
D. Reticulocyte test
E. Sugar water test

Answers

[37.1] **C.** Aplastic anemia is characterized by marked hypoplasia of all the cells in the bone marrow. The decrease in the erythroid, granulocytic, and megakaryocytic cell lines in the bone marrow will decrease all the cell lines (pancytopenia) in the peripheral blood.

[37.2] **D.** The term *myelophthisic anemia* refers to anemia caused by a space-occupying lesion within the bone marrow. Causes of myelophthisic anemia include metastases to the bone marrow, granulomas, and fibrosis (myelofibrosis). With myelophthisic anemia, the peripheral blood smear will show both immature RBCs (nucleated red blood cells) and immature WBCs (myelocytes). This abnormality of the peripheral blood also is known as leukoerythroblastosis.

[37.3] **D.** Hypersplenism can cause destruction of RBCs, WBCs, and platelets within the spleen by the splenic macrophages. With hypersplenism, the bone marrow will be hypercellular and the peripheral blood reticulocyte count will be elevated. This is in contrast to aplastic anemia, in which the bone marrow will be hypocellular and the reticulocyte count will be low.

PATHOLOGY PEARLS

- ❖ Aplastic anemia is pancytopenia with marked hypocellularity of the bone marrow; the reticulocyte count is very low.
- ❖ The majority of cases of aplastic anemia are acquired and idiopathic.
- ❖ Pancytopenia caused by bone marrow infiltration is referred to as myelophthisic anemia.
- ❖ Pancytopenia caused by hypersplenism has a high reticulocyte count.

REFERENCES

Aster JC. Red blood cell and bleeding disorders. In: Kumar V, Assas AK, Fausto N, eds. Robbins and Cotran Pathologic Basis of Disease, 7th ed. Philadelphia, PA: Elsevier Saunders, 2004:647–54.

Aster JC. Red blood cell and bleeding disorders. In: Mitchell RN, Kumar V, Abbas AK, et al., eds. Pocket Companion to Robbins and Cotran Pathologic Basis of Disease, 7th ed. Philadelphia, PA: Saunders, 2006:317–29.

CASE 38

A 4-year-old boy is seen by his pediatrician for easy bruising, joint pain, and leg pain; red dots on the skin that do not blanch; and hepatosplenomegaly. The complete blood count (CBC) reveals an elevated white blood cell count (50,000/mm^3), a low hemoglobin level (anemia), and thrombocytopenia (low platelet count). Examination of the peripheral smear of the blood shows numerous cells with a high nuclear to cytoplasmic ratio, and fine chromatin; the complete blood count shows anemia and thrombocytopenia.

- **What is the most likely diagnosis?**
- **What other investigations need to be done?**

ANSWERS TO CASE 38: ACUTE LYMPHOCYTIC LEUKEMIA

Summary: A 4-year-old boy has easy bruising, petechiae, and hepatosplenomegaly. The CBC reveals leukocytosis, anemia, and thrombocytopenia, and the peripheral smear shows cells with a high nuclear-to-cytoplasmic (N/C) ratio and fine chromatin.

- **Most likely diagnosis:** Acute leukemia, most likely acute lymphoblastic leukemia.
- **Additional studies that should be performed:** Bone marrow examination with flow cytometry and cytogenetics for the aspirate obtained from the bone marrow.

CLINICAL CORRELATION

This child has many of the clinical manifestations of acute lymphocytic leukemia: leg and joint pain, fever, enlarged spleen and liver, and petechiae. These manifestations usually are due to infiltration of the bone marrow with malignant cells or malignant proliferation cells in the liver and spleen. Leukemia is the most common malignancy of childhood, accounting for approximately one-third of childhood cancers, with acute lymphocytic leukemia (ALL) being more common than acute myelogenous leukemia (AML). Adults also can be affected, usually by AML. Children with Down syndrome and those exposed to radiation are at increased risk. This patient's peripheral blood smear reveals the classic description of "blast" cells typical of ALL; however, the diagnosis is best established by bone marrow aspirate because a peripheral smear may not reveal the blast cells.

APPROACH TO LEUKEMIA

Objectives

- Describe the clinical presentation of leukemia.
- List the different types of leukemia and their respective "key" features.
- Know the common patient populations seen in each type of leukemia.

Definitions

Leukemia: The leukemias are malignant neoplasms of the hemopoietic stem cells characterized by diffuse replacement of the bone marrow by neoplastic cells.

Blasts: Very immature cells that are medium to large in size with a large nucleus, typically with fine chromatin.

Myeloblasts: Typically larger than lymphoblasts, with a variable number of nucleoli. They may contain fine azurophilic granules, and condensation of these granules may result in distinctive red-staining rodlike structures (Auer rods). Auer rods are present in 60 to 70 percent of cases of AML and are diagnostic.

Lymphoblasts: Usually smaller than myeloblasts, with scant cytoplasm and more often without nucleoli. Nuclear foldings may be present. Typically do not have granules and certainly do not have Auer rods.

DISCUSSION

The **leukemias** are **malignant neoplasms of the hemopoietic stem cells** characterized by **diffuse replacement of the bone marrow by neoplastic cells.** They are divided broadly into two groups: **acute** and **chronic leukemias (see Table 38-1).** The **acute leukemias** are characterized by replacement of the marrow with **very immature cells (called blasts)** and a paucity of mature cells. **Blasts,** which are **lymphoid** in origin, are called **lymphoblasts**. Most **other blasts** are referred to as **myeloblasts.** Acute leukemia thus can be subclassified into **acute myelogenous leukemia (AML)** and **acute lymphocytic leukemia (ALL).** In acute leukemia, abnormal blasts accumulate as a result of prolonged survival time and also fail to mature to functional end cells.

Table 38-1
LEUKEMIA

LEUKEMIA	CELL TYPE	PATIENT POPULATION	"KEY" FEATURES
AML	Myeloblasts	Adults: median age of 60	Auer rods; positive myeloperoxidase; retinoic acid receptor t(15;17) → can treat with all-trans retinoic acid
CML	Myeloblasts	Adults: peak incidence at 40–60 years	Philadelphia chromosome t(9;22)
ALL	Lymphoblasts	Children: 75% of cases in children <6 years	Responsive to therapy; positive TdT marker; poor prognosis with Philadelphia chromosome t(9;22) or Burkitt t(8;14)
CLL	Lymphoblast	Elderly	Slow course

Worldwide, the overall incidence of acute leukemia is approximately 4 per 100,000 populations per year. Approximately 70 percent of these cases are AML. The remainder is ALL. **The vast majority of cases of AML occur in adults,** with a median age of 60 years. ALL however is predominantly a disease of children, and 75 percent of the cases of ALL occur in individuals less than 6 years of age.

The etiology of acute leukemia is unknown, but genetic, environmental, and occupational factors are thought to contribute in some cases. Individuals with **Down syndrome** are at an increased risk of developing acute leukemia, as are those with exposure to **benzene** and **radiation.** Chemotherapeutic agents, especially alkylating agents, increase the risk of developing AML.

As the leukemic blasts accumulate in the marrow, they suppress normal hemopoietic cells. This results in a paucity of normal red cells (anemia), platelets (thrombocytopenia), and white cells (neutropenia). The blasts usually overflow into the circulating blood, and because these blasts are counted as white cells, the total white cell count usually is elevated. These circulating blasts may accumulate in other tissues, including lymph nodes, liver, and spleen. Patients usually present with weakness, bleeding, and infections. Septicemia may result in widespread coagulation in the microcirculation (capillaries) known as disseminated intravascular coagulation (DIC). Physical examination may reveal hepatosplenomegaly and lymphadenopathy.

Diagnostic Approach

At presentation, a complete blood count and examination of the peripheral blood smear reveal the diagnosis in many patients. The **blasts** are **medium- to large-size cells** with a **large nucleus with fine to clumped chromatin.** Variable numbers of prominent **nucleoli** are present within the nuclei. **Myeloblasts** may contain fine azurophilic granules, and condensation of these granules may result in distinctive red-staining rodlike structures (Auer rods). The Auer rods are present in 60 to 70 percent of cases of AML and are diagnostic for AML.

The treatments of AML and ALL differ significantly from each other. Subclassification of AML and ALL also provides prognostic and therapeutic insights. A **bone marrow examination** nearly always should be performed when a diagnosis of acute leukemia is considered. Multiple smears are made from the bone marrow aspirate. Some of the smears are stained with routine stains (Wright-Giemsa), whereas others are used for special stains. Portions of the aspirate are submitted for flow cytometry and cytogenetic studies. A core biopsy of bone is obtained, and touch preparations are made from this biopsy specimen.

The smears obtained from the aspirate are assessed. A differential count of the cells is performed, and the morphology of the cells is evaluated. A minimum of 20 percent blasts is required to fulfill the criteria for the diagnosis of acute leukemia. The morphology of the blasts or other neoplastic hemopoietic precursors is evaluated to differentiate between AML and ALL as well as to categorize the two leukemias further. Till recently the two acute leukemias were subclassified according to the French-American-British (FAB) classification. However, recently a new classification system has been proposed by the World Health Organization (WHO). This classification system has more clinical and prognostic relevance than does morphology. It is not possible in many instances to differentiate between AML and ALL on the basis of morphology alone. Even if this is possible, further subclassification may be difficult. This is where special stains and immunophenotypic studies by flow cytometry play a role.

Cytochemistry for Acute Leukemia

A variety of **cytochemical stains** are available, and there is a cytochemical profile for each hemopoietic cell lineage. Myeloperoxidase (MPO), which is present in primary granules are reactive in cells in the neutrophil lineage, and variable in other granulocytic cells, and nonreactive in lymphoblasts.

Immunophenotyping

Immunophenotyping leukemic blasts are important in distinguishing AML from ALL, especially when the morphologic and cytologic profile is not definitive. The WHO classification of ALL is based on immunophenotype in recognition of its prognostic significance. Flow cytometry is the preferred method of immunophenotyping acute leukemias. If flow cytometry cannot be performed, immunophenotyping can be performed using immunohistochemical methods.

Cytogenetics

Cytogenetic studies supplement the morphologic, cytochemical, and immunophenotypic studies in the characterization of AML and may contribute to the distinction between AML and ALL in selected cases. As cytogenetic studies provide the most reliable independent indicators of prognosis, they are incorporated in the WHO classification of AML.

Molecular Studies

Molecular studies are valuable in bone marrow diagnosis for several reasons. They may establish clonality, detect specific chromosome translocations and other cryptic structural rearrangements, identify virus genomes associated with neoplasms, and detect minimal residual disease.

Electron Microscopy

With the current immunophenotyping methods and the array of antibodies available, the role of electron microscopy has been diminished greatly. It still may be useful in the characterization of acute leukemia when the blasts fail to manifest differentiating features on morphologic or cytochemical examination.

Chronic Leukemias

The **two main types** of **chronic leukemias** are **chronic myelogenous leukemia (CML)** and **chronic lymphocytic leukemia (CLL). CML** is seen almost exclusively in **adults,** with a **peak incidence at 40 to 60 years of age.** There are three phases to the disease: chronic (which may last for several years), accelerated (variable duration), and blast crises. During the chronic phase, patients typically have organomegaly (hepatosplenomegaly with or without lymphadenopathy) with very high white cell counts (as high as 100,000 to 200,000 or more). The full spectrum of white cells at the different stages of maturation is seen in the peripheral blood. Blast count is typically low (usually less than 10 percent). Basophilia and eosinophilia are characteristic. With time, the patient progresses through the accelerated phase to the final blast crisis. The vast majority of patients (75 percent) develop AML, and the remainder develops ALL. These acute leukemias are resistant to standard chemotherapy and hard to treat.

CML is characterized by the **Philadelphia chromosome.** This is due to translocation of an oncogene from chromosome 9 to chromosome 22 (the Ph chromosome), that is, t(9;22). The oncogene is referred to as *c-abl,* and the area where chromosome 22 breaks to incorporate the translocated oncogene is referred to as BCR (breakpoint cluster region). Sometimes CML patients may be negative for the *Ph* chromosome. These individuals, however, always show the *BCR-ABL* fusion gene on more sophisticated tests such as fluorescent in situ hybridization (FISH) and polymerase chain reaction (PCR).

CLL is a proliferative disorder of **mature B cells.** As in CML, patients usually present with organomegaly with lymphadenopathy and a very high white cell count. The lymphocytes are small cells with condensed chromatin with a narrow rim of cytoplasm. Damaged lymphocytes (during the process of making the smear) are plentiful and are referred to as smudge cells. CLL sometimes is associated with autoimmune hemolytic anemia, and in such cases spherocytes are evident in the smear. There is no diagnostic cytogenetic abnormality for this condition. Flow cytometry on the peripheral blood or bone marrow shows a neoplastic clone of B cells (by virtue of producing exclusive kappa or lambda light chains, referred to as light chain restriction) with abnormal expression of T-cell markers (CD5 and CD23 in this case). The disease is not an aggressive one, and typically patients maintain a good quality of life for several years, often dying from an unrelated cause. For some, overwhelming involvement of the bone marrow and subsequent bone marrow failure leads to death.

COMPREHENSION QUESTIONS

[38.1] Which of the following tests is necessary to make the diagnosis of acute leukemia?

A. Chromosomal analysis of cells obtained from a bone marrow biopsy
B. Chromosomal analysis of cells obtained from a lymph node biopsy
C. Cytochemical staining of cells obtained from a bone marrow biopsy
D. Examination of smears made from a bone marrow aspiration
E. Examination of smears made from the peripheral blood

[38.2] A 24-year-old man presents with increasing fatigue, easy bruising, and the diffuse formation of petechiae. His peripheral leukocyte count is increased, and multiple immature cells are present. A bone marrow biopsy is markedly hypercellular as a result of a diffuse proliferation of immature cells. The presence of which of the following abnormalities in these immature cells favors the diagnosis of AML rather than ALL?

A. Auer rods
B. Howell-Jolly bodies
C. Pappenheimer bodies
D. Reinke crystals
E. Russell bodies

[38.3] A 38-year-old woman presents with increasing weakness and lethargy. Her peripheral white cell count is markedly elevated, and her leukocyte alkaline phosphatase score is markedly decreased. Which of the following chromosomal translocations is most consistent with a diagnosis of chronic myelocytic leukemia?

A. t(8;14)
B. t(9;22)
C. t(11;14)
D. t(14;18)
E. t(15;17)

Answers

[38.1] **D.** The leukemias are malignant neoplasms that arise from developing hemopoietic cells. There are two basic types of leukemias: acute leukemias and chronic leukemias. The acute leukemias are characterized by replacement of the marrow with very immature cells (blasts). These immature cells have fine nuclear chromatin and nucleoli. Examination of the bone marrow is necessary to make the diagnosis of acute leukemia. A differential cell count is performed on smears made from an aspiration of the bone marrow. A minimum of 20 percent blasts is required to make the diagnosis of acute leukemia.

[38.2] **A.** The two basic types of acute leukemias are AML and ALL. It is important to differentiate between these two malignancies because their therapies are different. AML is characterized by the proliferation of myeloblasts, whereas ALL is characterized by the proliferation of lymphoblasts. Myeloblasts may be larger than lymphoblasts, but the key distinguishing cytologic feature is the presence in myeloblasts of Auer rods, which are distinctive red-staining rodlike structures within the cytoplasm. Auer rods are a feature of AML but not of ALL.

[38.3] **B.** The two main types of chronic leukemias are CML and CLL. CML is characterized by the presence of the Philadelphia chromosome, which is an abnormal chromosome formed by the translocation of an oncogene (*c-abl*) from chromosome 9 to chromosome 22: t(9;22).

PATHOLOGY PEARLS

❖ AML is more common in adults, and ALL is more common in children.

❖ The therapies for AML and ALL differ, and it is important to distinguish between the two.

❖ Acute leukemia is characterized by the presence of blasts in the blood and bone marrow.

❖ Auer rods are a feature of AML but not ALL.

❖ Examination of bone marrow, along with flow cytometry, cytochemistry, cytogenetics, and if necessary electron microscopy, is a very useful diagnostic tool for acute leukemia.

❖ Currently two classifications of AML and ALL are being used: the FAB and WHO classifications.

❖ The two main types of chronic leukemias are CML and CLL.

❖ Individuals with CML have a *Ph* chromosome or *BCR-ABL* fusion gene.

❖ The phases of CML are chronic, accelerated, and blast crisis.

❖ Patients with CLL have B cells with abnormal expression of CD5 and CD23.

REFERENCES

Aster JC. Diseases of white blood cells, lymph nodes, spleen and thymus. In: Kumar V, Assas AK, Fausto N, eds. Robbins and Cotran Pathologic Basis of Disease, 7th ed. Philadelphia, PA: Elsevier Saunders, 2004:680–9.

Aster JC. Diseases of white blood cells, lymph nodes, spleen and thymus. In: Mitchell RN, Kumar V, Abbas AK, et al., eds. Pocket Companion to Robbins and Cotran Pathologic Basis of Disease, 7th ed. Philadelphia, PA: Saunders, 2006:344–52.

CASE 39

A 16-year-old girl has a sore throat, enlarged tender cervical lymph nodes, and low-grade fever for 3 days. In addition to erythematous pharyngeal mucosa and cervical lymphadenopathy, physical examination reveals mild splenomegaly. A complete blood count (CBC) shows an increased number of white blood cells with a lymphocytosis and many reactive lymphocytes.

- **What is the most likely diagnosis?**
- **What laboratory tests would be helpful in confirming the diagnosis?**

ANSWERS TO CASE 39: INFECTIOUS MONONUCLEOSIS

Summary: A 16-year-old girl has a sore throat, enlarged tender cervical lymph nodes, and low-grade fever for 3 days. She has mild splenomegaly, lymphocytosis, and many reactive lymphocytes.

- **Most likely diagnosis:** Infectious mononucleosis.
- **Confirmatory laboratory tests:** (1) Specific antibodies for Epstein-Barr virus (EBV) antigens (viral capsid antigens, early antigens, or Epstein-Barr nuclear antigen), (2) a positive heterophil reaction (monospot test), and (3) lymphocytosis with the characteristic atypical lymphocytes in the peripheral blood.

CLINICAL CORRELATION

Infectious mononucleosis is a benign, self-limited lymphoproliferative disease caused by the Epstein-Barr virus, a herpesvirus. Infectious mononucleosis is characterized by fever, generalized lymphadenopathy, splenomegaly, sore throat, and the appearance in the blood of atypical activated T lymphocytes (mononucleosis cells). The disease occurs principally in older adolescents and young adults, particularly college students, in the upper socioeconomic classes in developed nations. In the rest of the world, primary infection with EBV occurs in childhood, is usually asymptomatic, and confers immunity to subsequent reinfection. In the great majority of patients, resolution occurs within 4 to 6 weeks, but occasionally the fatigue lasts longer. Treatment is primarily symptomatic and supportive. It includes bed rest and analgesics such as aspirin to relieve the fever, headache, and sore throat. In severe pharyngotonsillitis, corticosteroids are given to reduce inflammation.

Complications may involve virtually any organ or system in the body. The most common is marked hepatic dysfunction with jaundice, elevated hepatic enzyme levels, disturbed appetite, and, rarely, liver failure. Other complications involve the nervous system, kidneys, bone marrow, lungs, eyes, heart, and spleen. Traumatic splenic rupture is a feared complication and has been fatal in some cases.

APPROACH TO EBV INFECTION AND LYMPHOMA

Objectives

- Describe the clinical presentation and etiology of infectious mononucleosis.
- List the microscopic characterization of Burkitt lymphoma.
- Know the microscopic characterization of Hodgkin disease.

Definitions

Atypical lymphocytes: Large lymphocytes characterized by an abundant cytoplasm containing multiple clear vacuolations and an oval, indented, or folded nucleus. Most bear T-cell markers (reactive CD8+ T lymphocytes).

Heterophil antibodies: Nonspecific serum antibodies directed at sheep erythrocytes, detected by the slide monospot test, a test modified to exclude cross-reactivity with Forssman antibody. However, up to 10 percent of adults and the majority of children under 4 years of age (80 percent) do not have detectable heterophil antibody. So-called heterophil-negative infectious mononucleosis most often is associated with cytomegalovirus infection.

Oncogenic virus: A virus that can induce cancer. These viruses enter a host cell and become incorporated into its chromosomal DNA or take control of the cell's machinery for the purpose of producing viral proteins. Among the recognized oncogenic viruses in humans are the human T-cell leukemia virus-1 (HTLV-1), human papillomavirus (HPV), EBV, and hepatitis B virus (HBV).

Burkitt lymphoma: An aggressive B-cell lymphoma that is closely linked to EBV infection, especially the African variety. The African form frequently involves the maxilla or mandible, whereas the American form usually involves abdominal organs. It is associated with a characteristic cytogenetic change: t(8;14).

DISCUSSION

EBV, a member of the herpesvirus family (HHV-4), has been connected with a broad and varied spectrum of clinical disease. It is **transmitted by close human contact, frequently with saliva during kissing,** or in childhood through the sharing of virally contaminated saliva and is largely asymptomatic. In economically developed areas, exposure to EBV may not occur until adolescence or adulthood, though the increased use of day care for children may be reducing the number of EBV-seronegative individuals. The major route of transmission is through the saliva, though infected cells in blood products and transplanted organs or bone marrow also may transmit the virus.

The virus undergoes a replicative cycle in the oropharyngeal epithelium and then invades the blood by **selectively infecting B cells,** a cell population that has specific surface receptors for the virus. It is shed from the oropharynx for as long as 18 months after primary infection; thereafter, it may be spread intermittently by persons who are EBV-seropositive despite the absence of clinical disease. Asymptomatic shedding of EBV by healthy persons accounts for most of the spread of infectious mononucleosis despite the fact that it is not a highly contagious disease.

The peripheral blood usually shows an **increase in the number of leukocytes,** with a white blood cell count between 12,000/μL and 18,000/μL, **95 percent of**

which are lymphocytes. Atypical lymphocytes are common, constituting more than 20 percent of the total lymphocyte count. **Heterophil antibodies** usually appear during the second or third week and decline after the acute illness has subsided. They may, however, be detectable for up to 9 months after onset of the disease.

Infectious mononucleosis usually is **diagnosed** on the basis of clinical findings, the presence of **atypical lymphocytes** in the peripheral blood, and a **positive monospot test** or other **EBV serologic studies.** Rarely, the surgical pathologist is confronted with a lymph node biopsy, a tonsil, or a ruptured spleen from a patient who has not been diagnosed by the usual means, often because the presentation of the disease was atypical or the adenopathy persisted. It is of the utmost importance to remember that infectious mononucleosis is a great imitator. Histologically, it may show nonspecific follicular and/or paracortical hyperplasia, or it may mimic and be difficult to distinguish from both Hodgkin disease and non-Hodgkin lymphoma. The histologic changes may be similar to those described in other viral disorders, such as herpes lymphadenitis and postvaccinal lymphadenitis.

The **atypical lymphocytes** seen in the peripheral blood of patients with EBV mononucleosis are **larger than normal lymphocytes** and have a **vacuolated cytoplasm.** They can be distinguished from those found in malignant diseases by their heterogeneous appearance and polyclonality. However, the clinical presentation and large number of atypical lymphocytes may mimic features of leukemia, precipitating detailed evaluation and, rarely, a tissue biopsy.

Cytomegalovirus (CMV) infections in nonimmunosuppressed individuals may resemble changes seen in infectious mononucleosis, or they may show a histologic picture that includes a pronounced follicular hyperplasia with a monocytoid B-cell proliferation with or without an interfollicular hyperplasia. Cells infected with CMV are **markedly enlarged, with large purple intranuclear inclusions surrounded by a clear halo (owl's eye appearance)** and smaller basophilic cytoplasmic inclusions. The characteristic CMV inclusions in both nucleus and cytoplasm, together with serologic, immunohistochemical, and in situ hybridization techniques, will establish a specific diagnosis of CMV infection. CMV, like EBV, is a herpesvirus that also can cause devastating systemic infections in neonates and immunosuppressed patients. CMV can be distinguished from EBV by either an EBV-negative serologic profile or the absence of EBV reactivation markers such as antibodies to early EBV antigen.

As an **oncogenic virus, EBV** has been implicated in the pathogenesis of four types of human tumors: the **African form of Burkitt lymphoma; nasopharyngeal carcinomas; B-cell lymphomas** in the immunosuppressed, particularly after HIV infection and organ transplantation; and some cases of **Hodgkin disease.**

Burkitt lymphoma is a neoplasm of B lymphocytes that is the most common childhood tumor in **central Africa and New Guinea.** More than 90 percent of African tumors carry the EBV genome. The tumor cells have **multiple small nucleoli** and a **high mitotic index.** The lack of significant variation in nuclear shape and size lends a monotonous appearance that is interrupted by pale-staining, benign tissue macrophages that impart a **"starry sky" appearance** on low magnification (Figure 39-1).

Nasopharyngeal carcinoma is endemic in southern China, in some parts of Africa, and among Arctic Eskimos. In contrast to Burkitt lymphoma, **100 percent of nasopharyngeal carcinomas** obtained from all parts of the world contain EBV DNA. Nasopharyngeal carcinomas take one of three patterns: (1) keratinizing squamous cell carcinomas, (2) nonkeratinizing squamous cell carcinomas, and (3) undifferentiated carcinomas that have an abundant nonneoplastic, lymphocytic infiltrate (lymphoepithelioma). Histologically, the keratinizing and nonkeratinizing squamous cell lesions resemble well-differentiated and poorly differentiated squamous cell carcinomas arising in other locations.

The undifferentiated variant is composed of large epithelial cells with oval or round vesicular nuclei, prominent nucleoli, and indistinct cell borders disposed in a syncytium-like array. Admixed with the epithelial cells are abundant, mature, normal-appearing lymphocytes.

In the immunosuppressed infected with EBV, **polyclonal B-cell proliferation** may lead to death. True monoclonal B-cell lymphomas also have appeared, preceded by polyclonal proliferation. These unfortunate consequences were described in a family suffering from an X-linked recessive T-cell defect, and so the condition has been designated Duncan disease or X-linked lymphoproliferation (XLP) syndrome. XLP syndrome is characterized by the development of symptoms of infectious mononucleosis and acquired

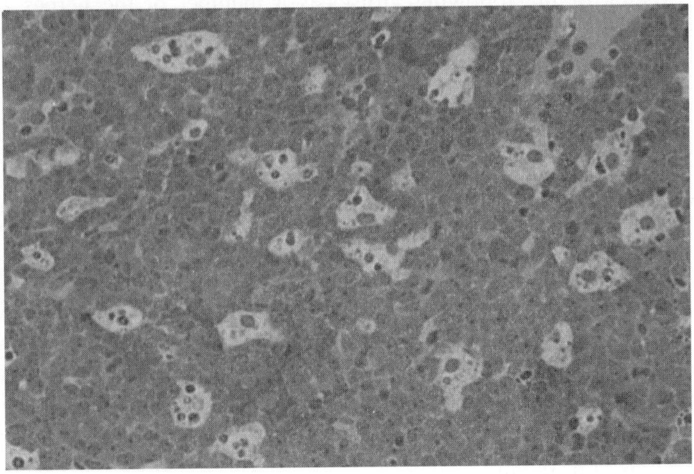

Figure 39-1. Burkitt lymphoma: Note the starry sky appearance as a result of the interspersed macrophages. *(Reproduced, with permission, from Lichtman MA, Beutler E, Kipps TJ, et al.* Williams Hematology, 7th ed. *New York: McGraw-Hill, 2006:Color plate XIV-7.)*

agammaglobulinemia, with the subsequent proliferation of B and T lymphocytes leading to non-Hodgkin lymphoma.

In **Hodgkin disease,** EBV genomes have been identified in the characteristic **Reed-Sternberg cells** in 40 to 50 percent of cases, and in some parts of the world EBV RNA can be identified in virtually all cases. Among the four subtypes of Hodgkin disease, the virus has been found most commonly in the mixed cellularity subtype (the second most common form) and almost never in the lymphocyte-predominant variant. The mixed cellularity is distinctive with its heterogeneous cellular infiltrate, which includes eosinophils, plasma cells, and benign histiocytes.

COMPREHENSION QUESTIONS

[39.1] A 20-year-old woman presents with a 4-day history of sore throat, low-grade fever, and enlarged cervical lymph nodes on her left side. Her blood is found to be positive for a heterophile antibody. A CBC finds an increased number of white blood cells, and examination of her peripheral blood smear finds numerous atypical mononuclear cells with abundant cytoplasm. These cells have peripheral condensation of their cytoplasm, giving them a "ballerina-skirt" appearance. What are these cells?

A. Atypical lymphocytes
B. Epithelioid cells
C. Immature lymphoblasts
D. Natural killer cells
E. Reactive monocytes

[39.2] Which of the following viruses is a member of the herpes family, infects B cells and epithelial cells of the oropharynx, and causes a positive heterophil reaction?

A. CMV
B. EBV
C. HBV
D. HIV
E. HSV

[39.3] A 7-year-old boy living in central Africa presents with a rapidly enlarging mass that involves his mandible. A histologic section from this mass reveals a diffuse proliferation of small noncleaved lymphocytes. In the background are numerous tingible-body macrophages that have a "starry-sky" appearance when viewed under low magnification. Which of the following is the most likely diagnosis?

A. Burkitt lymphoma
B. Hodgkin disease
C. Immunoblastic lymphoma
D. Lymphoblastic lymphoma
E. Small lymphocytic lymphoma

Answers

[39.1] **A.** Infectious mononucleosis is a benign, self-limited lymphoproliferative disorder characterized clinically by the combination of fever, generalized lymphadenopathy, and sore throat. The peripheral blood usually shows an increase in the number of leukocytes, most of which are atypical lymphocytes. These cells, which are activated cytotoxic T lymphocytes, are larger than normal lymphocytes and have abundant cytoplasm. The periphery of the cytoplasm is condensed and has a dark blue color, giving these cells a "ballerina-skirt" appearance.

[39.2] **B.** EBV is a member of the herpesvirus family (HHV-4) and has been associated with several diseases, including heterophil-positive infectious mononucleosis, Burkitt lymphoma, and nasopharyngeal carcinoma. EBV infects cells that have surface CD21, which is the receptor for EBV, such as B lymphocytes and the epithelial cells of the oropharynx. Mononucleosis caused by infection with EBV is associated with the formation of heterophil antibodies, which are nonspecific serum antibodies that are directed against sheep erythrocytes. These antibodies are detected by the slide monospot test.

[39.3] **A.** Burkitt lymphoma is an aggressive, high-grade B-cell lymphoma that is associated with infection by EBV. The African form of Burkitt lymphoma frequently involves the maxilla or mandible and is more common in children. Burkitt lymphoma is associated with a characteristic cytogenetic translocation, t(8;14), which involves the *c-myc* oncogene on chromosome 18. Histologic sections reveal a diffuse proliferation of malignant small noncleaved lymphocytes within a background of benign macrophages. These cells impart a "starry sky" appearance to the tissue when viewed under low magnification.

PATHOLOGY PEARLS

- EBV may cause infectious mononucleosis, with atypical lymphocytes and heterophil antibodies often being positive.
- Burkitt lymphoma, a neoplasm of B-lymphocytes that is the most common childhood tumor in central Africa and New Guinea, is strongly associated with the EBV genome.
- Burkitt lymphoma is characterized microscopically as tumor cells with multiple small nucleoli and a high mitotic index, along with a "starry sky" appearance.
- In Hodgkin disease, EBV genomes have been identified in the characteristic Reed-Sternberg cells.

REFERENCES

Aster JC. Diseases of white blood cells, lymph nodes, spleen and thymus. In: Kumar V, Assas AK, Fausto N, eds. Robbins and Cotran Pathologic Basis of Disease, 7th ed. Philadelphia, PA: Elsevier Saunders, 2004:690–4.

Aster JC. Diseases of white blood cells, lymph nodes, spleen and thymus. In: Mitchell RN, Kumar V, Abbas AK, et al., eds. Pocket Companion to Robbins and Cotran Pathologic Basis of Disease, 7th ed. Philadelphia, PA: Saunders, 2006:344–52.

CASE 40

A 4-year-old boy is seen by his pediatrician for a marked bruising tendency of the arms and legs. His mother says that the bruising often appeared without any apparent trauma. The mother also reports that there was no bleeding at the time of circumcision or in association with separation of the umbilical cord. At 3 years of age the patient had an episode of epistaxis that required transfusion of one unit of blood. There is a history of bleeding on the maternal side of the family. The patient's mother and maternal grandmother and great-grandmother had experienced episodes of abnormal bleeding with recurrent epistaxis and menorrhagia.

- **What types of coagulation abnormalities usually result in bruising and epistaxis?**

- **What are possible diagnoses in this patient?**

- **What laboratory studies would you use to evaluate this patient?**

ANSWERS TO CASE 40: BLEEDING ABNORMALITIES

Summary: A 4-year-old boy has marked bruising without apparent trauma and a history of epistaxis. There is a history of abnormal bleeding in the patient's mother and maternal grandmother and great-grandmother.

- **Types of coagulation abnormalities usually result in bruising and epistaxis:** Abnormalities involving platelets
- **Possible diagnoses in this patient:** Quantitative or qualitative congenital platelet abnormalities or von Willebrand disease
- **Laboratory studies you would use to evaluate this patient:** Platelet count, PT and PTT, platelet aggregation studies, and von Willebrand factor analysis.

CLINICAL CORRELATION

The strong family history of abnormal bleeding suggests an inherited condition. Since female family members are affected, hemophilias, which are X-linked, can be excluded. In addition, the type of bleeding experienced by this patient is more in keeping with an abnormality of platelet function. This would include inherited abnormalities in the number of platelets (quantitative abnormalities), abnormalities in the function of platelets (qualitative abnormalities), and abnormalities in the adhesion of platelets to endothelial surfaces (von Willebrand disease).

APPROACH TO BLEEDING ABNORMALITIES

Objectives

- Describe the clinical presentation of von Willebrand disease.
- List the pathology of von Willebrand disease.
- Know how to evaluate a patient with a bleeding disorder through the use of laboratory values.

Definitions

Primary hemostasis: The formation of a hemostatic plug composed of platelets. Endothelial cell injury exposes thrombogenic substances which results in the adherence and activation of platelets. Platelets undergo shape change and release the contents of their secretory granules. This in turn recruits more platelets and causes the platelets to aggregate.

Secondary hemostasis: The formation of a more stable hemostatic plug by the deposition of fibrin. The platelets' secretory substances, along with tissue factor synthesized in the endothelium, activate the coagulation cascade. This activates thrombin, which converts fibrinogen to fibrin. Fibrin stabilizes the clot.

Petechiae: Pinpoint-sized hemorrhages, 1 to 2 mm, often found in dependent areas where the capillary pressure is higher, typically associated with low platelet counts or defective platelet function.

Purpura: Slightly larger hemorrhages up to approximately 1 cm in size, associated with the same disorders as petechiae and may also occur secondary to trauma, vasculitis, or increased vascular fragility (e.g., in amyloidosis).

Ecchymoses: Larger, confluent areas of hemorrhage, greater than 1 cm, subcutaneous hematomas, characteristically seen after trauma.

Hemothorax, hemopericardium, hemoperitoneum, and hemarthrosis (joints): Accumulations of blood in a body cavity as indicated by the suffix.

Extrinsic coagulation pathway: Coagulation pathway activated by tissue factor, a cellular lipoprotein exposed at sites of tissue injury.

Intrinsic coagulation pathway: Coagulation pathway initiated in vitro by the activation of Hageman factor (factor XII). Although traditionally the coagulation scheme has been divided into the intrinsic and extrinsic pathways, this is an artificial division based mainly on in vitro testing. In vivo, there are interconnections between the two pathways.

Prothrombin time (PT): Tests the extrinsic and common coagulation pathways. A prolonged PT may be caused by a deficiency or dysfunction of factor V, VII, or X, prothrombin or fibrinogen.

Partial thromboplastin time (PTT): Tests the intrinsic and common coagulation pathways. A prolonged PTT may be caused by a deficiency or dysfunction of factor V, VIII, IX, X, XI, or XII, prothrombin or fibrinogen.

Disseminated intravascular coagulation (DIC): It is not a primary disease, but a thrombohemorrhagic disorder which occurs as a secondary complication to a variety of diseases. DIC is characterized by the formation of microthrombi throughout the microcirculation with consumption of platelets, fibrin, and coagulation factors and, secondarily, activation of fibrinolysis. DIC may present with signs and symptoms of tissue hypoxia or as a hemorrhagic disorder.

DISCUSSION

Abnormal bleeding may result from defects in either primary or secondary hemostasis. Abnormalities of primary or secondary hemostasis may be inherited or acquired. Bleeding which results from abnormalities of primary hemostasis often manifests as easy bruising, spontaneous petechiae or purpura, or bleeding from mucosal surfaces, such as the gums or nasal mucosa. Reproductive age females may experience unusually heavy menstrual bleeding. (See Table 40-1.) Bleeding from abnormalities of secondary hemostasis manifests as large posttraumatic ecchymoses or hematomas or prolonged bleeding after a laceration or surgical procedure. (See Table 40-2.) Some conditions,

Table 40-1
CAUSES OF PLATELET ABNORMALITIES

Inherited		
Bernard-Soulier syndrome	Defect in platelet adhesion	Deficiency of GP Ib-IX complex
Glanzmann thromboasthenia	Defect in platelet aggregation	Defect in GPIIb-IIIa
Storage pool disorders	Defect in platelet secretion	Defects in secretory granules
von Willebrand Disease	Defect in platelet adhesion	Defect or deficiency in vWF
Fanconi anemia	Congenital bone marrow failure	Thrombocytopenia
Acquired		
	Immune thrombocytopenic purpura (ITP)	
	Thrombotic thrombocytopenic purpura (TTP)	
	Infections, e.g., HIV	
	Drug-associated: aspirin, quinidine, heparin, alcohol, cytotoxic drugs	
	Bone marrow failure: acquired aplastic anemia	
	Bone marrow infiltration: metastatic cancer, leukemia	
	Disseminated intravascular coagulation	
	Uremia	

such as DIC, may involve abnormalities of both platelets and the coagulation cascade. (See Table 40-3.)

The evaluation of a patient with a bleeding disorder should include a careful medical history and family history. Most patients with a congenital bleeding disorder will have a positive family history, for example, hemophilia, von Willebrand disease (vWD), and inherited platelet abnormalities. An inherited disorder often causes symptoms from an early age, but in mild cases the symptoms may not be recognized. Any drugs that the patient is taking should be evaluated for potential effects on coagulation, particularly platelet function. The type of bleeding may provide a clue as to the underlying abnormality. For example, in the case of the 4-year-old boy, the easy bruising and epistaxis point to a defect in primary hemostasis, that is , platelet type bleeding. On the

Table 40-2
CAUSES OF ABNORMALITIES OF SECONDARY HEMOSTASIS

Inherited	
Hemophilia A	Decreased factor VIII
Hemophilia B	Decreased factor IX
von Willebrand disease (some cases)	Decreased vWF leads to decreased stability and function of factor VIII
Acquired	
Vitamin K deficiency	Impaired synthesis of factors II, VII, IX, and X and protein C
Liver disease	Impaired synthesis of factor VII and other coagulation factors
Disseminated intravascular coagulation	Multiple factor deficiencies, as well as thrombocytopenia

other hand, a patient with bleeding into a knee joint is more likely to have an abnormality of secondary hemostasis, such as hemophilia A or B.

With a frequency of approximately 1 percent in the population, vWD is believed to be one of the most common inherited disorders of bleeding. Clinically, it is characterized by spontaneous bleeding from mucous membranes, menorrhagia, or prolonged bleeding after injury. There are many variants of vWD, but most are inherited in an autosomal dominant manner. The platelet count is normal, but von Willebrand factor (vWF) is deficient or defective.

The vWF is synthesized in endothelial cells and in megakaryocytes. The vWF multimer forms a complex with factor VIII and helps to stabilize factor VIII. In patients with marked deficiency of vWF, the circulating factor VIII may be reduced, and patients may have bleeding similar to patients with hemophilia. Platelet adhesion to the extracellular matrix of an injured vessel is mediated largely through interactions with vWF. The vWF forms a bridge between receptors on the surface of platelets (GPIb) and the exposed collagen. Without sufficient and functional vWF, platelets do not adhere properly.

Laboratory Evaluation of a Patient with a Bleeding Disorder

The laboratory evaluation of a patient with a bleeding disorder will be guided by the clinical and family history. Medications and other conditions, such as uremia, should be considered before embarking on an extensive workup. The

Table 40-3
DISORDERS ASSOCIATED WITH DISSEMINATED INTRAVASCULAR COAGULATION

Obstetric complications
Abruptio placenta
Septic abortion
Amniotic fluid embolus
Toxemia
Retained dead fetus
Infections
Gram-negative sepsis
Rocky Mountain spotted fever
Meningococcemia
Histoplasmosis
Neoplasms
Carcinomas of the pancreas, prostate, lung, and stomach
Acute promyelocytic leukemia
Massive tissue injury
Trauma
Burns
Miscellaneous
Venomous snakebite
Hemolytic transfusion reaction
Vasculitis
Heat stroke
Shock
Liver disease
Giant hemagioma

starting point of the laboratory evaluation is a basic coagulation panel including a platelet count, PT and PTT. The peripheral blood smear should be reviewed for the presence of schistocytes, as seen in DIC and other microangiopathic hemolytic anemias. If the history suggests a qualitative platelet type bleeding disorder, platelet aggregation studies can be performed. In the case of vWD, the platelet aggregation studies will likely show decreased aggregation with Ristocetin. vWD can be confirmed by evaluation of vWF multimers; this can also assist in subclassifying the type of vWD.

If the PT or PTT is prolonged, a mixing study should be performed to distinguish between a factor deficiency or an inhibitor as the cause of the prolongation. Upon mixing the patient's plasma with normal plasma, a factor deficiency will be corrected and the PT or PTT will correct to the normal range. If a factor deficiency is suspected, individual factor assays can be performed. Knowledge of the coagulation cascade can assist in predicting which

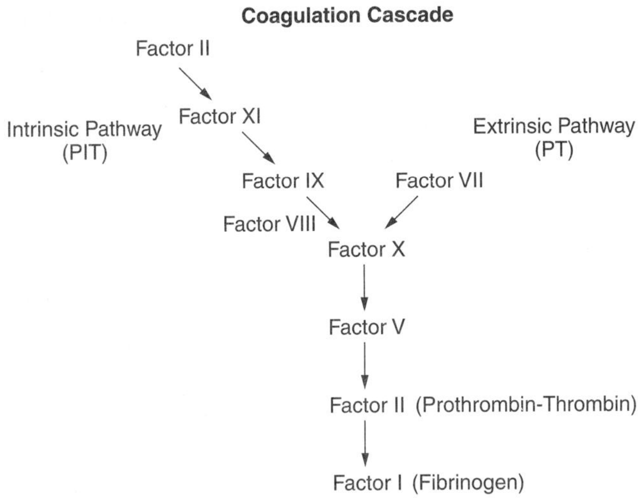

Figure 40-1. Coagulation is achieved through a series of enzymatic reactions.

factor is most likely deficient. For example, if the PT is prolonged, but the PTT is normal, then a factor VII deficiency can be confirmed by specific assay. If the PTT is prolonged, but the PT is normal, a factor VIII or IX or vWF deficiency may be present (see Figure 40-1).

COMPREHENSION QUESTIONS

[40.1] A 55-year-old woman is admitted for evaluation of worsening renal failure. She has been on renal dialysis for approximately 2 years. Over the last week or so, she noticed bruises over her arms and bleeding from her gums while brushing her teeth. On physical examination, she has numerous petichiae and ecchymotic areas over her arms and trunk. She is taking digoxin, cimetidine, and diazepam.

LABORATORY RESULTS

	PATIENT	NORMAL
PT	10.7 sec	8–11.5 sec
PTT	30 sec	24–37.5 sec
Platelet count	159,000/μL	150,000–350,000/μL
Hemoglobin	8 g/dL	12–16 g/dL
BUN	60 mg/dl	7–18 mg/dL
Creatinine	6.0 mg/dL	0.5–1.1 mg/dL

Which of the following is the most likely explanation for her abnormal bleeding?

A. von Willebrand disease
B. Immune thrombocytopenic purpura
C. Platelet dysfunction associated with uremia
D. Bone marrow failure
E. Disseminated intravascular coagulation

[40.2] A 6-year-old boy is brought to the pediatrician for gum bleeding while brushing his teeth. He is noted to have petechiae over the lower extremities. His mother says that he has been healthy other than an upper respiratory illness a couple of weeks ago. He has not had bleeding problems in the past. He is not taking any medications. There is no family history of abnormal bleeding. The peripheral blood smear shows decreased platelets, but no schistocytes or red blood cell fragments. Screening laboratory studies show:

PT:	10 sec (normal 8–11.5 sec)
PTT:	35 sec (normal 24–37.5 sec)
Platelets:	12,000/μL (normal 150,000–350,000/μL)

Which of the following is the most likely diagnosis?

A. Lupus anticoagulant
B. Factor V Leiden mutation
C. Factor VIII deficiency
D. von Willebrand disease
E. Immune thrombocytopenic purpura

[40.3] A 23-year-old electrician is seen in the emergency room with a swollen, tender right knee after falling to the ground an hour ago, while working on a power line. An emergency medical resident aspirated the knee obtaining blood. The patient has a lifelong history of knee swelling that occasionally occurred spontaneously or with minor injuries. He also had an episode of prolonged bleeding after a dental extraction. The patient had not been previously hospitalized or received blood transfusions. The patient's maternal grandfather had similar bleeding problems. The patient was taking no medication at the time of the accident.

SCREENING COAGULATION LABORATORY RESULTS

PT:	10 sec (normal 8–11.5 sec)
PTT:	57 sec (normal 24–37.5 sec)
Platelets:	450,000/μL (normal 150,000–350,000/μL)

ADDITIONAL STUDIES

PTT mixing study (50% patient plasma/50% pooled normal plasma) = 35 sec
Factor VIII:C = 120%
Factor VIIIR:Ag = 118%
Factor VIIIR:Rco = 110%
Factor IX = 20%

Which of the following is the most likely diagnosis?

A. von Willebrand disease
B. Hemophilia A
C. Hemophilia B
D. Lupus anticoagulant
E. Bernard-Soulier syndrome

Answers

[40.1] **C.** Although the pathogenesis is not fully understood, uremia is recognized as a common condition associated with acquired abnormal platelet function. The platelet count is not affected. Treatment includes dialysis and, possibly, administration of the drug DDAVP which causes the release of vWF from endothelial cells and thus facilitates platelet adhesion. Once the vWF is depleted from endothelial cells, DDAVP is no longer useful. DIC, ITP, and bone marrow failure would be associated with a decreased platelet count. Usually vWD would be associated with a prolonged PTT and would have presented earlier in life.

[40.2] **E.** In children, immune thrombocytopenic purpura (ITP) often follows an upper respiratory infection or other viral illness. In adults, ITP is more often associated with medications. In both cases, platelet destruction due to antibodies is suspected. Lupus anticoagulant and factor V Leiden mutation are associated with thrombosis, rather than bleeding. The lupus anticoagulant usually results in a prolonged PTT, even though it does not act as an anticoagulant in vivo. Factor VIII deficiency and vWD are usually associated with a prolonged PTT and would have presented earlier in life.

[40.3] **C.** The clinical history suggests an inherited coagulation abnormality. The prolonged PTT would be consistent with vWD, hemophilia A or B, or a lupus anticoagulant. However, the lupus anticoagulant would not cause abnormal bleeding. The additional laboratory studies exclude hemophilia A and vWD and confirm a factor IX deficiency, that is hemophilia B. Bernard-Soulier is an inherited abnormality of platelets and would not affect the PTT.

PATHOLOGY PEARLS

- ❖ Clinical and family histories are important in the evaluation of a patient with a bleeding disorder.
- ❖ The type of bleeding (primary versus secondary hemostasis) the patient is experiencing can guide the workup of the patient's bleeding disorder.
- ❖ Knowledge of the coagulation cascade can assist in predicting which coagulation factor(s) are deficient in a patient with abnormal coagulation studies.
- ❖ In a patient with a prolonged PT or PTT, a mixing study can distinguish between factor deficiency and inhibitor as the cause of the prolongation.
- ❖ von Willebrand disease is one of the most common bleeding disorders. There are several different subtypes of vWD with varying clinical severity.
- ❖ von Willebrand disease may present as platelet type bleeding, that is, petichiae and mucosal bleeding, or when more severe as a coagulation factor deficiency with deeper ecchymoses.

REFERENCE

Aster JC. Red blood cell and bleeding disorders. In: Mitchell RN, Kumar V, Abbas AK, et al., eds. Pocket Companion to Robbins and Cotran Pathologic Basis of Disease, 7th ed. Philadelphia, PA: Saunders, 2006:330–8.

CASE 41

An 80-year-old man who is thought to have senile dementia dies in a nursing home. Over the last several years, he developed ataxia and partial paresis. An autopsy reveals severe atherosclerosis ("tree barking") of the ascending aorta with aneurysm formation and a small liver with deep fibrous scars. Microscopically, there is a mononuclear inflammatory cell infiltrate with numerous plasma cells surrounding and within the walls of small blood vessels in most organs.

- **What is the most likely diagnosis?**
- **What is the mechanism of this condition?**
- **What other tests could be done to confirm the diagnosis?**

ANSWERS TO CASE 41: TERTIARY SYPHILIS

Summary: An 80-year-old man thought to have dementia dies in a nursing home. Over the last several years, he developed ataxia and partial paresis. Autopsy examination reveals severe atherosclerosis ("tree barking") of the ascending aorta with aneurysm formation and a small liver with deep fibrous scars. Microscopically, there is a mononuclear inflammatory cell infiltrate with numerous plasma cells surrounding and within the walls of small blood vessels in most organs.

- **Most likely diagnosis:** Tertiary syphilis affecting the central nervous system and aorta.
- **Likely mechanism:** *Treponema pallidum* infection of the aorta.
- **Confirmatory tests:** Serum treponemal antibody tests and lumbar puncture with the cerebral spinal fluid (CSF) sent for serology.

CLINICAL CORRELATION

Treponema pallidum subspecies *pallidum,* the causative agent of syphilis, is primarily a sexually transmitted disease; however, it may be transmitted vertically or through blood products.

Syphilis is a chronic systemic protean disease that can be divided clinically into primary, secondary, latent, and tertiary stages characterized by active disease followed by periods of latency. The **primary syphilis** lesion, or **chancre,** appears on the genitals or mucous membranes approximately 3 weeks after inoculation. Subsequently, the disease can progress to the bacteremic phase, or **secondary syphilis,** characterized by a subtle macular or papular skin rash that may involve the palms and soles, generalized mucosal/moist skin lesions known as **condylomata lata,** and general lymphadenopathy occurring 2 to 10 weeks after the appearance of the chancre. This is followed by a latent or subclinical phase established by a positive **specific treponemal antibody** test and the absence of CSF, clinical, or physical manifestations of the disease. **Latent syphilis** is divided into early and late latent syphilis, with early latent syphilis encompassing the first year after infection and late latent syphilis beginning 1 year after infection.

There are three possible outcomes of untreated late latent syphilis: resolution with negative serologic conversion, continued persistent infection throughout life, and progression to tertiary syphilis in approximately 30 percent of cases. Symptomatic **tertiary syphilis** is characterized by gummatous parenchymal lesions (benign tertiary syphilis) that can affect any organ. **Cardiovascular** syphilis principally affects the aorta, often resulting in aneurysms and aortic valve annulus narrowing. **Neurosyphilis** affects the central nervous system in 4 to 9 percent of untreated late tertiary syphilis patients and can range from simple CSF abnormalities to frank neurologic symptoms frequently related to the disease, such as **meningitis, general paresis, tabes dorsalis, and the Argyll Robertson pupil.** In addition, pregnant females with syphilitic infections present a profound problem because of the risk of vertical transmission to the unborn child.

This patient was thought to have senile dementia but probably had neurosyphilis. Neurosyphilis is a cause of neurologic symptoms that include confusion, memory loss, and ataxia. Thus, tertiary syphilis should be a consideration in any patient with dementia. Serology tests are usually positive, although some individuals may have negative serology but central nervous system involvement. Lumbar puncture usually reveals elevated protein and a positive nonspecific treponemal serologic test. This individual has findings of cardiac syphilitic disease. The treatment would be intravenous penicillin for several weeks.

APPROACH TO SYPHILIS

Objectives

- Describe how to diagnose syphilis.
- List the etiology of syphilis.
- Know the stages of syphilis infection.

Definitions

Primary syphilis: The initial stage of infection from the time of inoculation to approximately 6 to 8 weeks later. The chancre, a raised, painless ulcerated lesion occurring at the site of inoculation, is the lesion of primary syphilis.

Secondary syphilis: The bacteremic stage of syphilis during which the Treponema spirochetes disseminate throughout the body. This stage is marked by: condylomata lata, constitutional symptoms, and a maculopapular skin rash which frequently involves the palms and soles.

Tertiary syphilis: A late manifestation of syphilis representing chronic infection and disease, characterized by gummas. Tertiary syphilis typically involves the cardiovascular system, skin, musculoskeletal system, and liver.

Gumma: A rubbery, gray-white lesion occurring anywhere in the body composed of granulomas with central coagulative necrosis with an infiltrate of plasma cells.

Tabes dorsalis: A manifestation of neurosyphilis with demyelination of the posterior columns, dorsal roots, and dorsal ganglia.

Argyll Robertson pupil: A manifestation of tertiary syphilis, a small, irregular pupil that reacts to accommodation but not to light.

DISCUSSION

Treponema pallidum subspecies *pallidum,* the etiologic agent of syphilis, is a **spirochete** that causes a chronic systemic venereal disease with a myriad of clinical presentations. In **primary syphilis,** the skin lesion occurs on the genitals or mucous membranes as a **raised, painless erythematous ulcer** located at the site of inoculation that is known as a **chancre.** The chancre occurs approximately 3 weeks after contact with an infected individual and heals spontaneously with or without treatment within a few weeks. Histologic examination of the **chancre** reveals a **lymphocytic, histocytic, and intense plasma cell infiltrate** with **obliterative endarteritis and periarteritis** of small vessels, with the latter contributing to ulcer formation.

Secondary syphilis, or the **bacteremic** stage of syphilis, presents with grayish lesions on intertriginous moist areas of skin, including the genitals and anus, known as **condylomata lata** (not to be confused with the condylomata acuminata seen in genital warts; Figure 41-1). In addition, constitutional symptoms and a subtle maculopapular skin rash frequently involving the **palms and soles** occur 2 to 10 weeks after the appearance of the chancre. Like the chancre, the secondary syphilitic lesions (**condylomata lata**) are highly

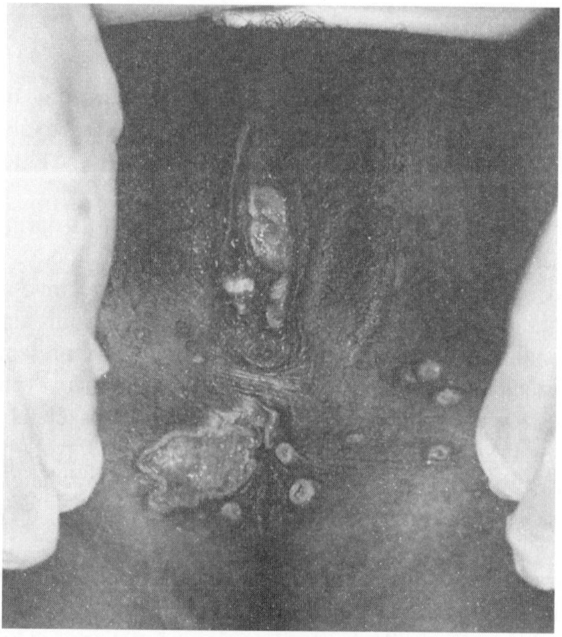

Figure 41-1. Condyloma lata. *(Reproduced, with permission, from Cunningham FG, Gant NF, Leveno KJ, et al., eds.* Williams Obstetrics, 21st ed. *New York: McGraw-Hill, 2001:1487.)*

infectious. Histologically, condylomata lata demonstrate a cellular profile and vasculitis similar to what is seen in the primary chancre.

Latent syphilis is the subclinical phase of syphilis, defined by a positive serologic test and no clinical manifestations of the disease. It is **divided into early and late latent syphilis,** with early latent syphilis defined as 1 year after infection and late latent syphilis as infection longer than **1 year.** Latent syphilis is divided temporally because early latent syphilis is much more likely to be infectious than late latent syphilis is. If it is untreated, after a variable interval of latency, approximately 30 percent of patients will progress to tertiary syphilis.

Tertiary syphilis is a late manifestation of the disease and presents with **gummatous lesions** that may occur almost anywhere in the body but most commonly affect the skin, musculoskeletal system, and liver. A **gumma** is a gray-white rubbery lesion with central coagulative necrosis surrounded by palisading macrophages and a mononuclear infiltrate rich with plasma cells. A significant number of patients develop cardiovascular syphilis and neurosyphilis.

Neurosyphilis is characterized by overt neurologic involvement or a CSF with an elevated protein, pleocytosis, and a positive CSF serology (Venereal Disease Research Laboratory). Neurosyphilis is detected in only 4 to 9 percent of patients with tertiary syphilis. However, over the course of months and even decades after infection, the symptoms can range from meningitis (usually within the first year) to overt neurologic signs (may not occur for more than a decade) such as **general paresis, tabes dorsalis, Charcot joints,** and **Argyll Robertson pupil.**

Cardiovascular syphilis or aortitis is present in up to 85 percent of patients with tertiary syphilis, although only approximately 10 percent are symptomatic. **Aortitis** demonstrates widening of the aorta with occasional linear calcifications and narrowing of the aortic annulus, resulting in **aortic regurgitation. General paresis** reflects widespread parenchymal disease that results in neurologic deficiencies.

Tabes dorsalis is the result of demyelination of the posterior column, dorsal roots, and **dorsal ganglia, causing neurosensory loss that may result in Charcot joints. Argyll Robertson pupil,** which is seen in both tabes dorsalis and general paresis, is a small, irregular pupil that reacts to accommodation but not to light.

Congenital syphilis is more readily transferred early in the maternal infection (75 to 90 percent) than in late infection (35 percent). Fetal lesions first appear around the fifth month of gestation, coinciding with fetal immunocompetence. The resulting infection frequently results in **stillbirth** and **late abortion**, although liveborn infants may be subclinical and later develop symptomatic disease. Congenital syphilis is associated with saber shins, saddle nose deformity and deafness.

Laboratory tests include **darkfield microscopy** and phase contrast microscopy, which can be used to visualize the spirochete organism in a tissue sample from a syphilitic lesion. Conventional light microscopy and hematoxylin and eosin (H&E) staining cannot detect the spirochete organism because of its thin and tightly wound structure; **silver stains** must be employed to visualize the spirochete in tissue. When darkfield microscopy is not available, **direct immunofluorescence** using a fluorescent-conjugated antitreponemal antibody directed against *T. pallidum* can be used.

Serologic testing for syphilis infection focuses on two types of detectable antibodies: **nontreponemal and treponemal. RPR** (rapid plasma reagin) and **VDRL** (Venereal Disease Research Laboratory) are screening assays that detect immunoglobulin G (IgG) and IgM cytotropic (nonspecific binding to some human cell antigens) nontreponemal antibodies directed against lipoidal antigens (cardiolipin). The VDRL assay is the only nontreponemal test approved for the CSF. **FTA-ABS** (fluorescent treponemal antibody-absorption) and **MHA-TP** (microhemagglutination assay) are both confirmatory assays that detect treponemal antibodies and have a high specificity. Many infectious and noninfectious processes can produce a **false positive** in both types of assays, such as **systemic lupus erythematosus, pregnancy, and antiphospholipid antibody syndrome.**

COMPREHENSION QUESTIONS

[41.1] Which of the following clinical signs or symptoms, if present, is most suggestive of a diagnosis of neurosyphilis?

A. Argyll Robertson pupils
B. Bitemporal hemianopia
C. Hutchinson incisor
D. Perifollicular hemorrhages
E. Retrobulbar palsy

[41.2] A 24-year-old woman presents with an "inability to urinate." She also has pain in the vulva area and physical examination finds multiple small blisters in this area, which consist of clear vesicles on a red base. Microscopic examination of a smear made from one these vesicles reveals scattered multinucleated giant cells with ground-glass nuclei. Infection with which of the following organisms is the most likely the cause of these changes?

A. *Chlamydia trachomatis*
B. *Treponema pallidum*
C. *Haemophilus ducreyi*
D. Herpes simplex virus
E. *Neisseria gonorrhoeae*
F. *Trichomonas vaginalis*

[41.3] Which of the following pathologic abnormalities is most characteristic of tertiary syphilis?

A. Apoptosis
B. Gumma
C. Karyorrhexis
D. Pannus
E. Tophus

Answers

[41.1] **A.** Neurosyphilis affects the central nervous system in a minority of individuals with untreated late tertiary syphilis. Signs and symptoms of neurosyphilis are diverse and include meningitis, general paresis, tabes dorsalis, and the Argyll Robertson pupil. Tabes dorsalis results from degeneration of the dorsal columns and dorsal roots of the spinal cord along with loss of dorsal root ganglion neurons. This results in impaired joint position sensation (proprioception), ataxia, and loss of pain sensation. Argyll Robertson pupils are pupils that constricts with accommodation, but doesn't constrict in reaction to light. This change is diagnostic for neurosyphilis.

[41.2] **D.** Herpes simplex virus is the most common infectious vulvar disease in the United States. Affected females sometimes develop urinary retention. The primary or first episode is usually systemic, and patients complain of fever, muscle aches, and joint pain. The virus then can lay dormant in the dorsal root ganglion and reactivate, leading to local symptoms. The diagnosis rests on either polymerase chain reaction (PCR) or viral culture. A Tzanck smear revealing multinucleated giant cells with ground-glass nuclei may be helpful if positive, but its low sensitivity does not make it practical as a definitive test.

[41.3] **B.** Gummata are gray-white rubbery lesions that are characteristic of symptomatic tertiary syphilis. These lesions have central coagulative necrotic areas that are surrounded by palisading macrophages and a mononuclear infiltrate composed of lymphocytes and plasma cells.

PATHOLOGY PEARLS

- The nonspecific treponemal tests should be confirmed with treponemal serology to diagnose syphilis.
- The etiologic organism that causes syphilis is *Treponema pallidum,* a spirochete.
- Because of the thinness of the spirochete, darkfield examination or special stains in biopsy specimens are required for identification; light microscopy usually is not revealing.
- The drug of choice in treating syphilis is penicillin.
- Congenital syphilis may lead to miscarriage, growth restriction, or hydrops fetalis in pregnancy. Its effects on the infant are divided into early, including nasal snuffles, skin lesions, hepatomegaly, and bony malformations, and late, including interstitial keratitis (blindness), notched central incisor teeth, and deafness.
- Tertiary syphilis most commonly involves neurosyphilis and sometimes manifests as gummata in various parts of the body, including the heart.

REFERENCES

Braunwald E, Fauci AS, Kasper DL, et al. Harrison's Principles of Internal Medicine, 16th ed. New York: McGraw-Hill, 2004.

Hook EW, Marra CM. Acquired syphilis in adults. N Engl J Med 1992;326:1060–7.

McAdam AJ, Sharpe AH. Infectious diseases. In: Kumar V, Assas AK, Fausto N, eds. Robbins and Cotran Pathologic Basis of Disease, 7th ed. Philadelphia, PA: Elsevier Saunders, 2004:381–90.

McAdam AJ, Sharpe AH. Infectious diseases. In: Mitchell RN, Kumar V, Abbas AK, et al., eds. Pocket Companion to Robbins and Cotran Pathologic Basis of Disease, 7th ed. Philadelphia, PA: Saunders:2006, 201–2.

CASE 42

A 32-year-old man is brought into the emergency department because of extensive bruising of the chest in a minor motor vehicle accident. He is known to be HIV-positive. He complains of progressive fatigue over the last 3 months and has not visited a doctor for over a year. A complete blood count (CBC) shows pancytopenia, and a bone marrow biopsy shows narrow-based budding yeast.

- **What is the most likely diagnosis?**
- **What are the usual mechanisms of HIV-induced disease?**

ANSWERS TO CASE 42: HISTOPLASMOSIS AND HIV INFECTION

Summary: A 32-year-old HIV-seropositive man develops fatigue and bruising with minor trauma. A CBC shows pancytopenia, and a bone marrow biopsy shows narrow-based budding yeast consistent with *Histoplasma capsulatum.*

- **Most likely diagnosis:** Disseminated histoplasmosis of the bone marrow.
- **Mechanism:** The human immunodeficiency virus (HIV) is a retrovirus that has a propensity for helper T-cell lymphocytes. Depletion of these helper T cells (also known as CD4 cells) leads to infections such as *Pneumocystis jiroveci* pneumonia, tuberculosis, esophageal candidiasis, and histoplasmosis.

CLINICAL CORRELATION

This 32-year-old man has an HIV infection. Involvement of the hemopoietic system is common, causing lymphadenopathy, anemia, leukopenia, and thrombocytopenia. These effects can be due to the virus itself, consequences of antiviral therapy, or opportunistic infections. Histologic studies and culture of the lymph nodes or bone marrow are often diagnostic. Bone marrow aspirates may reveal malignancy or a fungal infection such as histoplasmosis. Histoplasmosis is an opportunistic infection that is seen most frequently in the Mississippi and Ohio valleys, where *Histoplasma capsulatum* is endemic. The most common manifestation in HIV patients is reactivation after initial primary pulmonary disease has been contained. Disseminated disease after reactivation can lead to fever, weight loss, hepatosplenomegaly, and lymphadenopathy. Central nervous system involvement with a cerebral mass may be seen. Bone marrow involvement is common, with pancytopenia noted in approximately one-third of patients. Treatment is with either itraconazole or amphotericin B.

APPROACH TO HIV INFECTION

Objectives

- Describe the mechanism of HIV infection.
- List the common opportunistic infections seen in patients with HIV.
- Know the prophylaxis regimen used for patients with HIV.

Definitions

Human immunodeficiency virus (HIV): A retrovirus that causes AIDS (acquired immunodeficiency syndrome).

Retrovirus: An RNA virus that contains an enzyme, reverse transcriptase, in the virion.

ELISA: An abbreviation for an enzyme-linked immunosorbent assay. A laboratory test used to detect specific antigens or antibodies.

Western blot test: A laboratory blood test to detect the antibodies to specific antigens. It is used to check the validity of the ELISA test.

Pancytopenia: A marked reduction in the number of red blood cells, white blood cells, and platelets.

Guillain-Barré syndrome: A polyneuritis that occurs with a viral infection that causes symmetric pain and weakness in the extremities and even paralysis.

Reiter syndrome: An arthritic disorder of adult males that is associated with conjunctivitis and urethritis.

Opportunistic infection: An infection caused by normally nonpathogenic organisms in a host whose resistance has been decreased by disorders such as diabetes mellitus, HIV, and cancer or immunosuppressive drugs.

DISCUSSION

In 1981, AIDS was described in the United States. Cases were identified by diagnosing severe opportunistic infections. When the disease was found to be caused by HIV, healthy seropositive people were found at one end of the clinical spectrum and severe opportunistic infections were found at the other. The Centers for Disease Control (CDC) places AIDS into three categories.

HIV has **three modes of transmission: sexual contact, parenteral** (exposure to blood or fluids), and **vertical** (in utero). Parenteral transmission includes **intravenous drug abuse, sharing of needles, and needlesticks.** It is difficult to quantify per-contact risk because people at risk can engage in a variety of sexual practices. The risk of acquiring HIV from a needlestick with infected blood is 1 in 300. The risk of acquiring HIV infection from a needle used for intravenous drugs or from needle sharing with an infected HIV source is 1 in 150. Up to 40 percent of children born to HIV-positive infected mothers contract HIV if the mother did not receive antenatal HIV prophylaxis. In the United States, there are approximately 700,000 persons seropositive for HIV. In 2000, there were 315,000 persons living with AIDS. Females account for 24 percent of cases. An estimated 10 million persons are infected with HIV worldwide.

Etiology and Pathophysiology

AIDS is caused by the **retrovirus HIV.** Retroviruses produce the enzyme **reverse transcriptase,** which allows transcription of the viral genome into the DNA of the host cell. The major mechanism of HIV infection is continuous viral replication that causes immunodeficiency. It primarily infects the **CD4 cell count of T-helper lymphocyte** cells. The more cells infected, the lower the CD4 cell count. The CD4 cell count is a good prognostic indicator for infection. Certain infections can occur at any CD4 cell count, whereas others occur only below a certain CD4 count. These infections occur below levels of 500, 200, and 50 cells/mm^3. Histoplasmosis occurs when the CD4 cell count falls below 100 cells/mm^3.

Clinical Disease

There are complications of HIV related to infections that can affect every bodily organ. Symptoms can range from nonspecific to specific. Common symptoms are **fever, night sweats, and weight loss.** The physical examination can be normal and nonspecific initially, ending with a host of signs on physical examination once AIDS ensues. The weight loss can be multifactorial, and of course nausea and vomiting contribute to weight loss secondary to a decreased caloric intake. There is also an increased metabolic rate that exacerbates the decrease in caloric intake. A decrease in protein synthesis also makes maintaining muscle mass difficult.

Pulmonary Disease

***Pneumocystis* pneumonia,** which is caused by *P. jiroveci,* is **the most common opportunistic infection.** It can be difficult to diagnose because the symptoms are nonspecific, such as fever, cough, and shortness of breath. The cornerstone of diagnosis includes the **chest radiograph,** which reveals **diffuse or perihilar infiltrates.** Only about two-thirds of affected persons have this finding on x-ray. Up to 10 percent can have a normal chest radiograph, and the remainder of this group has atypical infiltrates. Definitive diagnosis is obtained in 50 to 80 percent by a **Wright-Giemsa stain of induced sputum.** Sputum induction is performed by having patients inhale an aerosolized solution of 3 percent saline produced by an ultrasonic nebulizer. If a patient is negative but there is still suspicion of the disease, **bronchoalveolar lavage** will establish the diagnosis 95 percent of the time.

Other pulmonary infections include bacterial, mycobacterial, and viral pneumonias. The community-acquired form is the most common pulmonary disease in HIV infected persons.

Noninfectious pulmonary diseases include **Kaposi sarcoma, non-Hodgkin lymphoma, and interstitial pneumonitis.**

Central Nervous System

Central nervous system (CNS) disease is divided into **four categories: intracerebral space-occupying lesions, encephalopathy, meningitis,** and **spinal cord processes. Toxoplasmosis** is the **most common space-occupying lesion.** These persons can present clinically with headache, focal neurologic deficits, seizures, or altered mental status. The diagnosis is made by computed tomography **(CT) scan findings** consistent with multiple peripheral contrast-enhancing lesions with a predilection for the basal ganglia. **Non-Hodgkin lymphoma** is the second most common lesion. On CT, in contrast, lymphomas are often solitary. Other diseases include **AIDS dementia complex,** which is often a diagnosis of exclusion. **Cryptococcal meningitis clinically presents with fever and headache.** The diagnosis is based on a positive latex agglutination test or a positive culture of cerebral spinal fluid. HIV myelopathy is a late manifestation of HIV. These patients have leg weakness and incontinence. **Progressive multifocal leukoencephalopathy (PML)** is a viral infection that occurs in the white matter of the brainstem that is seen in patients with very advanced HIV infection.

The **peripheral nervous system** also has clinical syndromes. **Guillain-Barré syndrome,** an inflammatory demyelinating polyneuropathy, occurs in HIV-infected persons. Peripheral neuropathy is common in HIV-infected persons. Typically present with numbness, tingling, and pain in the lower extremity. Other diseases that can cause similar symptoms are alcoholism, vitamin B_{12} deficiency, syphilis, and thyroid disease. The most common cause of peripheral neuropathy is prior antiretroviral therapy. These patients are treated with gabapentin 300 to 900 mg three times a day.

Rheumatologic and Ocular

Arthritis can involve both single and multiple joints. Large joint involvement is the most common. Common syndromes are **Reiter syndrome and systemic lupus erythematosus (SLE).** Retinitis requires immediate medical evaluation. **Cytomegalovirus (CMV)** is the most common and can be progressive.

Oral

Oral lesions are highly suggestive of HIV infection. Patients with these lesions have rapid progression to AIDS. **Hairy leukoplakia** is caused by the **Epstein-Barr virus.** On examination, a **white lesion on the lateral aspect of the tongue can be flat or slightly raised.** It also has vertical parallel lines with fine or thick "hairy" projections. **Oral candidiasis** can present with an unpleasant taste or mouth dryness. Gingival disease is due to overgrowth of microorganisms. Aphthous ulcers are painful and interfere with eating.

Gastrointestinal

Esophageal candidiasis is common in patients with AIDS infection. Liver disease is the site of infections and neoplasms. **Gastropathy** and malabsorption are common. There is a decrease in acid production in HIV-infected persons. As the acid level lowers, the risk of infection with *Salmonella* and *Shigella* increases. Enterocolitis and cholecystis are also common.

Skin

Staphylococcus is the **most common bacterial cause of skin disease in HIV-infected patients; such diseases include folliculitis. Herpes simplex and herpes zoster** also are common infections. **Kaposi sarcomas** are red or purple flat papules that occur on the skin. Seborrheic dermatitis is also common.

Malignancies

Kaposi sarcoma lesions can occur anywhere on the body. **Non-Hodgkin lymphoma** in HIV-infected persons tends to be very aggressive. Anal dysplasia and squamous cell carcinoma correlate with previous infection with human papillomavirus (HPV).

Gynecologic

Vaginal candidiasis, cervical dysplasia and/or cervical cancer, and pelvic inflammatory disease are common in HIV-infected women. There is a 40 percent incidence of cervical dysplasia in HIV-infected women. Cervical cancer is more aggressive in HIV-infected women. Most females with the cancer will die from the cancer rather than from AIDS. Cervical cancer was added to the CDC definitions of AIDS in 1993.

Diagnosis

HIV is diagnosed by using antibody and antigen testing. Screening is first done with the ELISA antibody test. The **confirmatory test is the Western blot.** Ninety-five percent of patients develop detectable antibodies by screening within 6 weeks after exposure to HIV infection. It is common before diagnosis to obtain nonspecific laboratory findings such as anemia, leukopenia, and thrombocytopenia. Other diseases can present with symptoms similar to those of HIV. The differential diagnoses include cancer, alcoholism, liver disease, chronic lung infections, thyroid disease, vitamin deficiency, gastrointestinal infections, and inflammatory bowel disease.

Table 42-1
HIV PROPHYLAXIS FOR OPPORTUNISTIC INFECTIONS

ORGANISM	CD4 COUNT	TREATMENT
Pneumocystis jiroveci (PCP)	<200/mm^3	TMP-SMX
Toxoplasma gondii	<100/mm^3	TMP-SMX
Mycobacterium avium (MAC)	<50/mm^3	Azithromycin

Treatment

HIV therapy can be divided into **four categories:** (1) treatment for opportunistic infections and malignancies, (2) antiretroviral treatment, (3) hemopoietic stimulating factors, and (4) prophylaxis of opportunistic infections. (See Table 42-1.) The goal of antiretroviral therapy is to suppress HIV replication as measured by viral load. An aggressive combination of treatments must be used. The current recommendation is to start with **three drugs** at a time. Counseling is an important part of the therapy. The patient has to be compliant with the medications. If compliance is in question, therapy should be withheld until the patient is able to comply.

The current recommendations include initiating treatment for either symptomatic HIV-positive persons or asymptomatic HIV-positive persons with a CD4 count less than 200 cells/mm^3. If a patient is asymptomatic and the CD4 count is higher than 200 cells/mm^3, the decision to initiate therapy should be individualized. It is rare to initiate therapy for a CD4 count higher than 350 cells/mm^3. If the CD4 count falls rapidly or the viral load is greater than 50,000, one should consider starting therapy.

There are three categories of drugs: **protease inhibitors, nucleoside/nucleotide analogues,** and **nonnucleoside reverse transcriptase inhibitors.** It is important to monitor patients closely for toxicity when they are taking medication. Laboratory evaluation of the patient should be done every 3 months to measure markers of efficacy: the CD4 cell count and the HIV viral load.

Resistance can occur with treatment because of the chance of mutations occurring in the virus. If therapy begins to fail, drug resistance testing should be instituted. Antiretroviral regimens may need to be changed for reasons that include intolerable adverse reactions, a rising or persistent high viral load, clinical progression of disease, and a falling CD4 cell count. If medication is changed, one should start with at least two medicines that the patient has not taken yet.

Histoplasmosis in an HIV-Positive Patient

Histoplasma capsulatum is a **dimorphic fungus** that is found in contaminated soil and bird and bat dropping. Infection occurs by inhalation of conidia. The conidia are converted into small budding cells in the lung. The organism then can proliferate and spread hematogenously to other organs. Histoplasmosis can appear clinically in three forms: acute, chronic, and disseminated disease. The severity and duration of the disease depend on the host's immunologic resistance.

The **acute form** clinically appears with **influenzalike symptoms** that can last from a few days to 14 days. Symptoms may include fever, chills, headache, myalgia, cough, and pleuritic chest pain. The examination may be without findings. A chest radiograph can show small, scattered reticulonodular infiltrates that will resolve over time and large mediastinal lymph nodes. These infiltrates, when healed, will calcify. Most cases are asymptomatic and may go unrecognized. Most resolve with bed rest and supportive measures.

The **chronic form** is mostly a diagnosis of **middle-aged men.** It can be hard to distinguish clinically from other forms of chronic obstructive lung disease. Initial symptoms can appear as a productive cough, pleuritic chest pain, fever, and weight loss. Clinically, the patient may **mimic tuberculosis.** On chest radiography, there are **interstitial pulmonary infiltrates in the apical segments of the upper lung lobes.** Without treatment, the patient will develop progressive lung failure and death. **Disseminated disease** is the **most severe and life-threatening** form and can occur in **infants,** the **elderly,** and persons who are **immunodeficient.** It can be fatal in 6 weeks if untreated.

Hematogenous dissemination results in a **very slow and progressive spread to various organs.** The patient can present clinically with fever, chill, weight loss, a productive cough, headache, drowsiness, generalized lymphadenopathy, hepatosplenomegaly, lacerations of the oropharynx and intestines, and bone marrow suppression with one or more cytopenia. Patients with AIDS can have papules on the skin and on the oral mucosa. The CD4 cell count is less than 100 cells/mm^3. The chest radiograph shows a miliary pattern (diffuse interstitial infiltrates) in 50 percent of AIDS patients and appears normal in approximately 30 percent. Mortality is greater than 80 percent without antifungal therapy.

Pathology

The **solitary nodule, or histoplasmoma,** is **round measuring 1 to 2 cm.** Cavitary lesions are usually present with reinfection. On chest radiography, this lesion appears as a **"coin" lesion** and can resemble carcinoma. *Histoplasma capsulatum* is dimorphic, having a yeast form and a mycelial form. In tissue sections, cells are yeastlike, hyaline, oval, and 2 μm in diameter and have single buds attached at the base. They usually are seen in clusters because of initial confinement to macrophages. With hematoxylin and eosin (H&E) stains, the fungal cells appear as a **"halo"** because the cytoplasm is retracted from the cell wall. In the **Gomori methenamine silver (GMS) stain,** a fungal special stain, the fungal walls are darkly stained to reveal the true size of the organism, eliminating the halo effect.

The host response varies with the number of conidia inhaled, age, and the immunologic status of the patient. In immunodeficient patients, there is a vast amount of intracellular multiplication of abundant fungal cells, multiple yeast-laden histiocytes, and widespread involvement. On tissue section, there are rapidly dividing histoplasma cell aggregates that appear as yeast lakes. In bone marrow examination, many patients can exhibit well-formed granulomas, whereas others exhibit diffuse histiocytic hyperplasia with poor granuloma formation.

Diagnosis

Disseminated histoplasmosis is diagnosed by demonstrating **yeast** in a **peripheral blood smear or a bone marrow biopsy.** A positive blood smear or bone marrow biopsy is positive more than 80 percent of the time. A urine antigen assay is sensitive more than 90 percent of the time. Rarely is a sputum culture positive in this form of the disease. Laboratory findings are consistent with a pancytopenia, an increase in alkaline phosphatase and liver enzymes, and an increase in ferritin levels.

The treatment of choice is **itraconazole 200 to 400 mg/day** for non-meningeal disease. **Amphotericin B** is reserved for patients who cannot take oral medication, have failed on itraconazole, or have meningitis. For severe disease, liposomal amphotericin B is used at 3 mg/kg/day. Patients with AIDS-related histoplasmosis require lifelong suppression with itraconazole 200 to 400 mg/day.

COMPREHENSION QUESTIONS

[42.1] A 38-year-old man has been HIV-positive for 5 years. One week ago, he began to have a fever to 39.4°C (103°F), a productive cough, and respirations of 35 per minute. He has lost 50 lb in 8 months. On examination, he has generalized lymphadenopathy and lung fields that are clear to auscultation. On chest radiography, there are bilateral diffuse pulmonary infiltrates. A CD4 count is 178 cells/mm^3. A Wright-Giemsa stain of sputum is positive. Which of the following is the most likely diagnosis?

A. Community-acquired pneumonia from *Pseudomonas aeruginosa*
B. *Pneumocystis* pneumonia
C. Interstitial pneumonia
D. Non-Hodgkin lymphoma

[42.2] A 26-year-old woman presents with a 2-week history of undulating fevers along with night sweats, weight loss, and a nonproductive cough. A chest x-rays reveal enlarged mediastinal lymph nodes and small reticulonodular infiltrates in the apices of both lungs. A bronchial biopsy is performed to obtain diagnostic material. Which of the following histologic findings is most consistent with a diagnosis of infection with *Histoplasma capsulatum*?

A. Macrophages containing multiple small yeast
B. Nonbranching pseudohyphae and blastocysts
C. Nonseptate hyphae with right-angle branching
D. Septate hyphae with acute-angle branching
E. Yeast with broad based budding

[42.3] A 32-year-old man, with AIDS for 10 years is on three medications for therapy. In March, the patient was in good spirits and was feeling well. His viral load was low, and his CD4 count was 710 cells/mm^3. Within the last 2 months, the patient has experienced a fever to 39.4°C (103°F), a 15-lb weight loss, many oral aphthous ulcers, generalized lymphadenopathy, and lethargy. Laboratory data reveal elevated liver function tests and a pancytopenia. A bone marrow biopsy reveals granulomas. Which of the following CD4 cell counts is most closely associated with his current clinical condition?

A. 550 cells/mm^3
B. 210 cells/mm^3
C. 162 cells/mm^3
D. 75 cells/mm^3

Answers

[42.1] **B.** *Pneumocystis* pneumonia is the most common opportunistic infection associated with AIDS. Symptoms can be nonspecific at the time of clinical presentation. The chest x-ray establishes the diagnosis up to 90 percent of the time. Diffuse infiltrates are the most common, but apical infiltrates also can be seen. *Pneumocystis* pneumonia commonly occurs with a CD4 cell count below 200 cells/mm^3.

[42.2] **A.** *Histoplasma capsulatum*, a dimorphic fungus that has a yeast form and a mycelial form, appears in tissue sections as multiple small, oval, hyaline structures that fill the cytoplasm of macrophages. The fungal cells may be surrounded by clear "halos" because the cytoplasm retracts from the cell wall. Infection is acquired by inhalation of soil contaminated with bird (starlings, chickens) or bat dropping in the Ohio and Mississippi valleys. Signs of histoplasmosis are: similar to tuberculosis, usually self-limited and asymptomatic but can be chronic and progressive.

[42.3] **D.** The CD4 lymphocyte cell count is a prognostic marker for opportunistic infections. Some infections occur at any CD4 cell count, whereas others rarely occur unless the CD4 cell count has dropped below a specific level. This patient has disseminated histoplasmosis. The CD4 cell count may be less than 100 cells/mm^3 for this infection to occur.

PATHOLOGY PEARLS

- ❖ HIV is a retrovirus requiring the enzyme reverse transcriptase to transcribe RNA viral genome into DNA.
- ❖ HIV primary infects CD4 helper T cells.
- ❖ *Pneumocystis* pneumonia is the most common opportunistic infection in HIV-infected individuals.
- ❖ HIV therapy consists of four parts: (1) treatment of opportunistic infection and malignancies, (2) antiretroviral therapy, (3) hemopoietic stimulating factors, and (4) prophylaxis for opportunistic infections.

REFERENCES

Connor DH, Chandler FW, Schwartz DA, et al. Pathology of Infectious Disease, vol. II. Stamford, CT: Appleton & Lange, 1997.

Foucar K. Bone Marrow Pathology, 2nd ed. Chicago, IL: American Society of Clinical Pathologists, 2001.

Nelson AM, Horsburgh CR Jr. Pathology of Emerging Infections-2. Washington, D.C: ASM Press, 1998.

Mitchell RN. Diseases of immunity. In: Mitchell RN, Kumar V, Abbas AK, et al., eds. Pocket Companion to Robbins and Cotran Pathologic Basis of Disease, 7th ed. Philadelphia, PA: Saunders, 2006:140–5.

Tierney LM, McPhee SJ, Papadakis MA. Current Medical Diagnosis and Treatment, 43rd ed. New York: McGraw-Hill, 2004.

CASE 43

A 75-year-old woman is brought to the emergency department because of massive hemoptysis. Despite appropriate measures, including volume replacement and circulatory support, she dies. Postmortem examination reveals hilar lymphadenopathy with caseous necrosis and infiltration and destruction of a large pulmonary artery by this process. The lungs show extensive consolidation with other areas of caseous necrosis.

- **What is the most likely diagnosis?**

- **What type of cells most likely would be seen on the biopsy specimen?**

- **What is the usual clinical course in patients with this condition?**

ANSWERS TO CASE 43: TUBERCULOSIS

Summary: A 75-year-old woman dies from massive hemoptysis. Postmortem examination reveals hilar lymphadenopathy with caseous necrosis and infiltration and destruction of a large pulmonary artery. Extensive pulmonary consolidation with other areas of caseous necrosis is noted.

- **Most likely diagnosis:** Pulmonary tuberculosis.
- **Cells likely to be seen on biopsy:** Epithelioid cells and Langhans-type giant cells typically surround the tuberculous granuloma (tubercle) with a central area of caseous necrosis.
- **Usual clinical course:** Initial pulmonary involvement with granuloma formation and later reactivation during times of stress or immunocompromise.

CLINICAL CORRELATION

Worldwide, tuberculosis is the leading cause of death by a single infectious agent. It is a disease of the socially disadvantaged, the elderly, and the immunocompromised. This patient probably had been exposed to tuberculosis sometime earlier and then developed secondary tuberculosis from reactivation of latent disease or reinfection. The symptoms before presentation with massive hemoptysis typically would include remittent fever, weight loss, night sweats, anorexia, general malaise, and weakness.

Hemoptysis occurs in more than 50 percent of patients with secondary tuberculosis. It is caused by the formation of a cavity between the blood vessels and the airways. This patient died from blood loss secondary to erosion of the pulmonary artery. Other causes of death in tuberculosis patients include massive destruction of the lung parenchyma, constrictive pericarditis from infection of the pericardial sac, constrictive lung disease from infection of the pleura, and infection and destruction of other organs and systems, such as the liver and kidneys.

APPROACH TO TUBERCULOSIS

Objectives

- Describe the etiology of tuberculosis.
- List the pathology and natural history of tuberculosis.
- Know the extrapulmonary manifestations of tuberculosis.

Definitions

Caseous necrosis: Destruction of cells that results in a thick cheese-like mixture of lipids and proteins.

Delayed-type hypersensitivity: An immune response that takes more than 24 hours to develop and is mediated by T lymphocytes rather than by antibodies.

Granuloma: A chronic inflammatory lesion made up of an accumulation of macrophages and giant cells into a discrete, well-formed focus.

PPD test: Purified protein derivatives (PPD) from *Mycobacterium tuberculosis* are injected into the dermis. If the body has been exposed to tuberculosis and immunity has been formed, a hypersensitivity reaction will occur within 48 to 72 hours, causing a visible wheal.

DISCUSSION

Tuberculosis is caused by members of the *M. tuberculosis* complex, with the most important member being *M. tuberculosis* itself. *Mycobacterium tuberculosis,* like all mycobacteria, is a **nonmotile, non–spore-forming aerobic bacterium.** It is covered by a hydrophobic layer made of mycolic acid and other free lipids. The lipids are **acid-fast,** meaning that once they are stained by dye, even acid alcohol cannot remove the stain, and **weakly gram-positive.** This **virtually impermeable wall,** along with other factors, gives *M. tuberculosis* the ability to **survive phagocytosis by macrophages.**

Tuberculosis usually is spread, with rare exceptions, by **person-to-person droplet spread.** A person with active disease can cough up live bacteria in tiny droplets that can remain airborne in the surrounding currents for several hours. Within this time, unsuspecting persons can **breathe in the droplets,** bringing the **bacteria into their lungs.** In an immunocompetent person with no previous exposure to tuberculosis, these invaders quickly are **engulfed by the alveolar macrophages** and carried to the **hilar lymph nodes.** This is the beginning of **primary tuberculosis,** and it usually takes place in the **middle or lower lobes of the lungs.** Unsensitized macrophages cannot fight off the infection because *M. tuberculosis* inhibits the acidification of the macrophage lysosomes, not only surviving phagocytosis but also replicating and destroying the macrophages. The bacteria then can infect other macrophages or travel through the blood or lymph to other organs and tissues. During this time, infected persons may experience what they think is a **flu-like illness or may be asymptomatic.**

Within 2 to 3 weeks, a **hypersensitivity immune response** develops. The formation of this response correlates with the **PPD becoming positive.** Through a class II major histocompatibility complex (MHC), the macrophages present a bacterial peptide to CD4 T cells. These helper cells recognize the antigen as foreign and produce cytokines such as interferon-γ. The interferon-γ activates the macrophages, causing them to produce reactive nitrogen intermediates that are able to kill the mycobacteria and cause the formation of the epithelioid granulomas. The **epithelioid cells can merge, forming the multinucleated Langhans giant cells.** $CD8^+$ T cells cause lysis of the macrophages through a granule-dependent mechanism and cause death of the mycobacteria. $CD4^-CD8^-$ T cells cause lysis of the macrophages through a Fas-dependent mechanism, but this does not kill the organisms. This causes progression of the epithelioid granuloma to a **caseous granuloma.**

The **initial parenchymal granuloma** is referred to as the **Ghon focus.** The Ghon focus and the caseated hilar lymph nodes that drain the area are called the **Ghon complex,** which subsequently may undergo **calcification,** becoming the **Ranke complex.** Mycobacteria can survive for years within this complex as latent tuberculosis. A chest x-ray of primary pulmonary tuberculosis typically shows a single calcified lesion in the parenchymal area.

With **secondary pulmonary disease,** an exposed person can be reinfected or there can be reactivation of the latent disease in times of stress. In rare cases, especially in immunocompromised individuals, primary disease can progress directly to secondary tuberculosis. *Mycobacterium tuberculosis* has a **high oxygen requirement** during reproduction. **Secondary pulmonary tuberculosis** usually occurs in the **apex** of one or both lungs because of the increased oxygen content compared with the other areas of the lungs. Because the immune system already is sensitized to the bacteria, macrophages quickly wall off the area of infection, resulting in less initial lymph node involvement. The caseous granuloma forms relatively rapidly, eroding into surrounding airways and blood vessels. When the **granuloma erodes into an airway,** the caseous material drains out of the poorly formed fibrous shell, leaving **cavitations.** If the granuloma extends into both airways and blood vessels, it creates a channel for blood to enter the airway, leading to the classic clinical symptom of **hemoptysis.** (See Figure 43-1 for an illustration of the natural history of tuberculosis.)

Drainage of the infectious material into the airways allows for localized spread through the connected parenchyma. This is the point of the disease at which a person is most **infectious.** The airways are full of mycobacteria; it is estimated that one cough from a person with active tuberculosis can produce 3000 infectious droplets. Proper antibiotic coverage can stop the progression of the disease, but the body's attempt to repair the cavitations leads to permanent damage. The **cavitations** and areas of **caseation** are repaired by **fibrous deposits, leaving open pockets or thick scars.** These open areas are walled off from the body and are highly oxygenized, creating a perfect environment for the fungus ***Aspergillus*** to proliferate. A thick ball of fungus can form that can block the few working airways the patient has left.

In some cases, the lungs may not be the only system involved. **Hematogenous, lymphatic,** and **direct spread** can cause infection in other systems. In some cases, a single organ may be involved, and dysfunction of that organ may present before the pulmonary symptoms appear. Table 43-1 displays the most common extrapulmonary manifestations of tuberculosis.

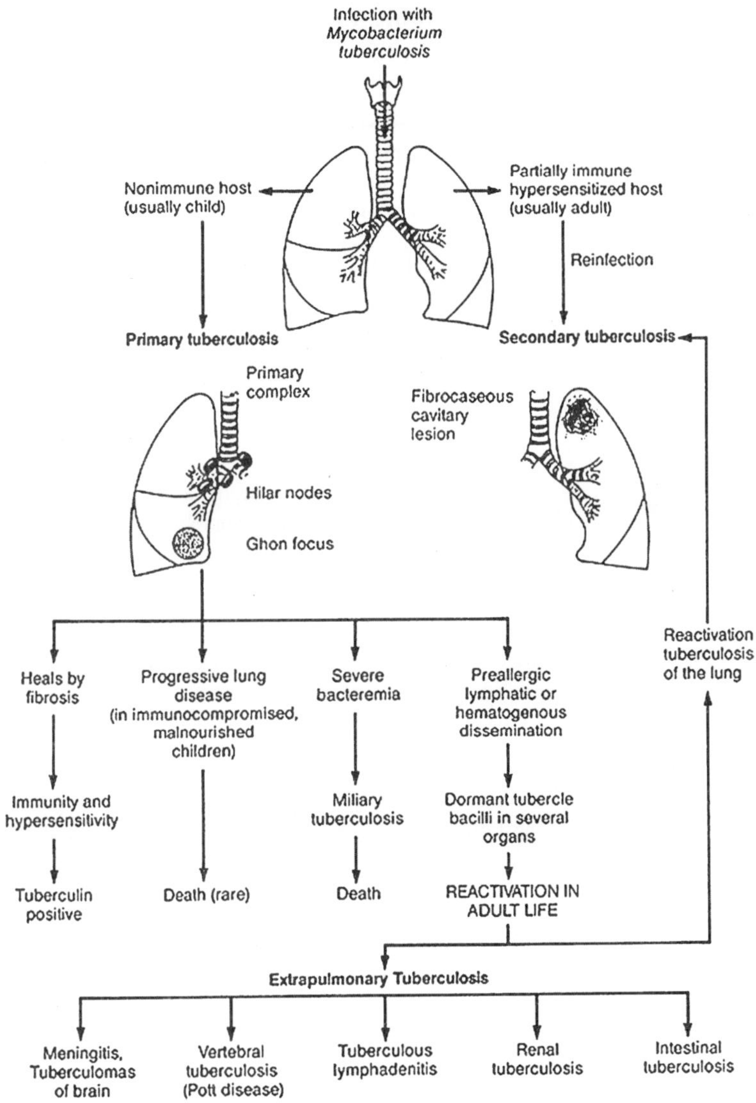

Figure 43-1. Pulmonary tuberculosis. *(Reproduced, with permission, from Chandrasoma P, Taylor CR:* Concise Pathology, 2nd ed. *Originally published by Appleton & Lange. Copyright 1995 by The McGraw-Hill Companies, Inc.)*

In developed countries, tuberculosis had been on the decline for several years until the emergence of HIV. In the United States, **HIV infection is the greatest risk factor for developing secondary tuberculosis.** A normal, immunocompetent person has a 10 percent lifetime risk of developing secondary disease, whereas an immunocompromised person has a 10 to 15 percent

Table 43-1
SELECTED LIST OF TYPES OF EXTRAPULMONARY TUBERCULOSIS (IN ORDER OF FREQUENCY)

Tuberculosis lymphadenitis	Painless lymph node swelling, most often in the cervical (scrofula) or supraclavicular nodes. Scrofula may form a fistulous tract to the skin
Pleural tuberculosis	Can be part of primary tuberculosis. Bacteria enter pleural space, causing inflammation and an effusion. The fluid usually contains >50% serum protein, normal to low glucose, pH <7.2, and detectable white blood cells. Rupture of a cavity in secondary tuberculosis can cause an empyema (much less common than an effusion), which can result in pleural fibrosis and restrictive lung disease
Tuberculosis of upper airways	Involvement of the larynx, pharynx, and epiglottis in advanced secondary disease. Symptoms: hoarseness, dysphagia, chronic productive cough
Genitourinary tuberculosis	Usually caused by hematogenous spread. Causes local symptoms in the urinary tract. Genital tuberculosis can affect the fallopian tubes and endometrium in females, causing infertility, pain, and menstrual abnormalities. In males the epididymis may be affected, producing a tender mass that may form a fistula to the skin
Skeletal tuberculosis	Hematogenous or lymphatic spread; weight-bearing joints most often affected. Spinal tuberculosis (Pott disease) may cause formation of abscesses that track along muscles and ligaments
Tuberculous meningitis and tuberculoma	Hematogenous spread or rupture of a subependymal tubercle; more common in children. Ranges between headache and altered sensorium and/or paresthesias. Tuberculoma is a mass lesion that can cause seizures and focal symptoms
Gastrointestinal tuberculosis	Swallowing infected sputum or ingestion of milk infected with *Mycobacterium bovis* (rare in industrialized countries). The bacteria are trapped in the lymphoid nodules of the intestinal mucosa causing bowel inflammation and ulceration
Tuberculous pericarditis	Caused by progression of a pericardial focus or rupture of a nearby lymph node. Symptoms are those of pericarditis or pericardial effusion. May progress to constrictive pericarditis
Disseminated (miliary) tuberculosis	Hematogenous spread to multiple organ systems. Lesions are small yellow foci of infection that may coalesce, forming large areas of consolidation. Symptoms are usually nonspecific and include night sweats, fever, and weight loss

yearly risk. A big problem comes from the fact that the presentation of tuberculosis in an HIV patient is often not the typical presentation. The T-cell-dependent mechanism for controlling *M. tuberculosis* infection is reduced in these patients.

In HIV patients with moderate immunocompromise, pulmonary tuberculosis may present as the typical cavitations, but without the lymph node involvement. The big diagnostic problem comes with **severely affected HIV patients because they may not get cavitations;** instead, they **may develop pulmonary and miliary infiltrates.** These patients do not have enough T cells to produce the needed hypersensitivity reaction; therefore, they **may not be PPD-positive.** This, combined with the atypical chest x-ray findings, may delay the diagnosis and treatment of the disease, with devastating results.

COMPREHENSION QUESTIONS

[43.1] Which of the following terms best describes a subpleural pulmonary lesion plus associated enlarged hilar lymph nodes in a patient with tuberculosis?

A. Ghon complex
B. Miliary tuberculosis
C. Pott disease
D. Progressive tuberculosis
E. Pulmonary scrofula

[43.2] A 58-year-old woman with a history of a positive PPD comes to the clinic with a complaint of lower back pain. A radiograph of the lumbar spine reveals probable involvement of the vertebral body. Which of the following is the most accurate statement regarding this patient's condition?

A. *Mycobacterium tuberculosis* most often reaches the spine through lymphatic spread.
B. Lesions often are found in multiple sites along the spine.
C. The synovium is commonly infected, and the infection spreads to the vertebral bodies.
D. The infection can track down the rectus muscle and create a "cold" abscess.

[43.3] A 27-year-old man presents with cough, fever, night sweats, and weight loss. A chest x-ray reveals a mass in the upper lobe of his right lung. Which of the following histologic findings, if seen in sections from this pulmonary mass, is most consistent with a diagnosis of tuberculosis?

A. Budding yeast, hyphae, and pseudohyphae
B. Caseating granulomas with acid-fast organisms
C. Dense deposits of granular, PAS positive, eosinophilic material
D. Multinucleate giant cells with intranuclear inclusions
E. Squamous cells covered with coccobacilli

Answers

[43.1] **A.** The initial primary lesion produced by infection with tuberculosis is the Ghon complex, which consists of a subpleural lesion near the fissure between the upper and lower lung lobes, and enlarged caseous lymph nodes that drain the pulmonary lesion. The Ghon complex is an example of a T-cell-mediated reaction.

[43.2] **C.** Pott disease is tuberculosis of the spine. There is usually only a single focus of infection unless the patient is severely immunocompromised, in which case there may be many sites of infection in the spine and other bones. The most common route of infection is hematogenous spread from the lungs. Vertebral collapse and resulting neurologic deficits are a long-term consequence of this disease. Pott disease may spread via the psoas muscle to form an abscess without the inflammatory response typical of bacterial processes.

[43.3] **B.** The classic histologic feature of tuberculosis, which is caused by infection with *M. tuberculosis*, is the presence of caseating granulomas, which are aggregates of epithelioid cells (activated macrophages) along with central caseous necrosis and Langhans-type giant cells. The classic clinical signs and symptoms of primary tuberculosis are fever, weight loss, night sweats, cough, and hemoptysis.

PATHOLOGY PEARLS

- ❖ Tuberculosis is caused by *M. tuberculosis,* an acid-fast bacterium that can survive phagocytosis by unsensitized macrophages.
- ❖ The typical tubercle is an epithelioid granuloma with central caseating necrosis and surrounding Langhans-type giant cells.
- ❖ The Ghon complex is an example of a T-cell–mediated reaction, resulting in caseous necrosis of a pulmonary focus and hilar lymph nodes in primary tuberculosis.
- ❖ T-cell–mediated hypersensitivity is responsible for the tissue destruction that causes the cavitary lesions in secondary pulmonary tuberculosis.

REFERENCES

Maitra A, Kumar V. The lung and the upper respiratory tract. In: Kumar V, Cotran R, Robbins S, eds. Robbins Basic Pathology, 7th ed. Philadelphia, PA: Saunders, 2003:453–508.

McAdam AJ, Sharpe AH. Infectious diseases. In: Kumar V, Assas AK, Fausto N, eds. Robbins and Cotran Pathologic Basis of Disease, 7th ed. Philadelphia, PA: Elsevier Saunders, 2004:381–6.

McAdam AJ, Sharpe AH. Infectious diseases. In: Mitchell RN, Kumar V, Abbas AK, et al., eds. Pocket Companion to Robbins and Cotran Pathologic Basis of Disease, 7th ed. Philadelphia, PA: Saunders, 2006:199–200.

Pfyffer GE, Brown-Elliott BA, Wallace RJ. Mycobacterium: General characteristics, isolation, and staining procedures. In: Murray PR, Baron EJ, Jorgensen JH, et al., eds. Manual of Clinical Microbiology, 8th ed. Washington, DC: AMS Press, 2003:532–5.

Rauiglione MC, O'Brien RJ. Tuberculosis. In: Braunwald E, Isselbacher KJ, Petersdorf RG, et al., eds. Harrison's Principles of Internal Medicine, 15th ed. New York: McGraw-Hill, 2001:1017–35.

❖ CASE 44

A 32-year-old woman notices an irregularly shaped, slightly raised, darkly pigmented nodule on the skin of her lower back. She vaguely recalls a smaller "mole" in the same location for several years, but because the site could not be seen easily, she did not notice the increase in the size of the mole. She does not have any other skin lesions and has no systemic symptoms. A biopsy of the nodule reveals an invasive tumor composed of pigmented cells.

◆ **What is the most likely diagnosis?**

◆ **What are the risk factors for this disorder?**

◆ **What are the most important prognostic considerations?**

ANSWERS TO CASE 44: MALIGNANT MELANOMA

Summary: A 32-year-old woman has an irregularly shaped, slightly raised, darkly pigmented nodule on the lower back. A biopsy of the nodule reveals an invasive tumor composed of pigmented cells.

- **Most likely diagnosis:** Malignant melanoma.
- **Risk factors for this disorder:** Genetic predisposition, number of nevi, sun exposure.
- **Most important prognostic consideration:** Depth of invasion.

CLINICAL CORRELATION

This 32-year-old woman has an excision of a pigmented lesion on her lower back. She sought medical attention for it and underwent surgical excision, which is the best treatment for malignant melanoma (MM). These malignancies involve melanocytes and thus are usually pigmented. Features of the lesion that were suspicious are summarized by the acronym **ABCD: asymmetry, borders** (irregular being worrisome), **color** (variation of color), and **diameter** (greater than 6 mm). These features are presented in Figure 44-1. Other characteristics include itchiness or burning, appearance in adulthood,

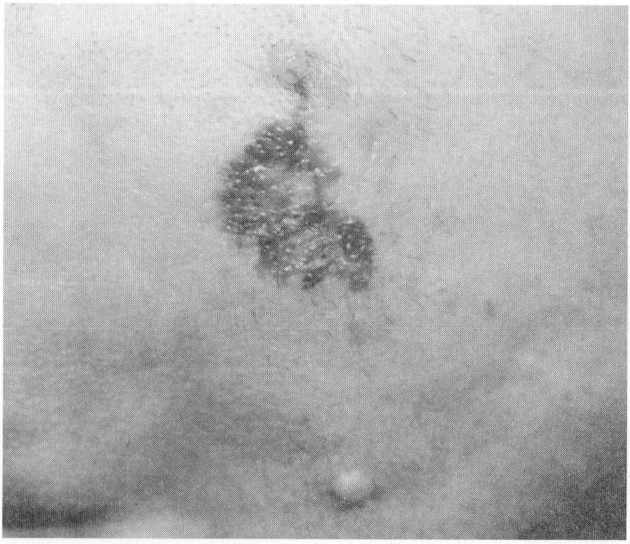

Figure 44-1. Malignant melanoma. *(Reproduced, with permission, from Brunicardi FC, Anderson DK, Billiar TR, et al., eds.* Schwartz's Principles of Surgery, 8th ed. *New York: McGraw-Hill, 2005:441.)*

and rapid growth. The back and legs have a higher incidence of these malignancies, and usually they occur in lightly pigmented individuals. Sun exposure is not necessarily a predisposing factor. Diagnosis is made by histologic analysis, and staging is determined by depth of invasion. Surgical excision is the best therapy, although adjuvant chemotherapy may play a role.

APPROACH TO MALIGNANT MELANOMA

Objectives

- Describe the ABCD criteria.
- Know the most important prognostic factor for malignant melanoma.
- List the clinical presentation of other skin neoplasms.

Definitions

Melanocytic nevi: Generally considered a benign neoplastic proliferation of melanocytes that vary considerably in clinical and histologic appearance.

Dysplastic nevi (atypical nevi): A clinical and histologic continuum between common nevi and superficial spreading melanoma. Dysplastic nevi are common, occurring in 2 to 18 percent of the population; however, patients with dysplastic nevi and two family members with melanoma have a 50 percent lifetime risk of developing melanoma.

Malignant melanoma: A malignant proliferation of melanocytes that have the potential for local invasion and metastasis.

Mucosal lentiginous melanoma: Most likely arises in mucosa, opposed to skin, in the oral and anogenital regions.

Ocular melanoma: A primary melanoma that arises in the eye; unlike cutaneous melanoma, it is associated with early hematogenous metastasis to the liver.

ABCD criteria: Clinical criteria used for differentiating benign pigment lesions from malignant melanoma: **A**symmetry (one-half does not match the other half in shape or color), **B**order irregularity, **C**olor variegation, and **D**iameter greater than 6 mm.

DISCUSSION

Normal skin consists of three layers: **epidermis, dermis,** and **subcutaneous fat.** The **epidermis** is the most superficial layer of the skin and consists of **keratinizing squamous epithelium** with regularly spaced **melanocytes** within the basal layer that are typically the origin of melanoma. The dermis interdigitates with the epidermis and provides support for the growing epidermis. Occasionally, melanomas arise within the dermis from **melanocytic nevi.**

Underlying the dermis is the subcutaneous fat with lobular septa, which anchors the skin to the deep connective tissues and provides cushioning and energy storage.

Melanoma usually arises from melanocytes in the skin; however, other sites of origin include the oral and anogenital mucosa, esophagus, meninges, and eye. Melanoma most frequently arises in chronically sun-exposed areas and commonly is associated with a **melanocytic nevus.** Although there is not always a clear clinical distinction between the different types of melanoma, there are four common histologic types of **cutaneous melanoma** with prognostic significance. Three of these—**superficial spreading melanoma, lentigo maligna melanoma,** and **acral lentiginous melanoma**—have an initial period of **radial growth** (horizontal growth within the epidermis) when the lesion increases in size without deep (vertical) invasion. It is during the radial growth phase that melanoma is most capable of being cured with total surgical excision. The fourth type, **nodular melanoma,** does not have a recognizable radial growth phase and usually presents with deep invasion that is capable of metastasis.

Superficial spreading melanoma (50 to 75 percent of cases) is the **most common form of melanoma,** occurring most frequently on sun-exposed areas of the back and extremities. Superficial spreading melanoma initially has a period of radial growth with lesion cells extending throughout all layers of the epidermis, giving it a **"Swiss cheese" appearance** known as **pagetoid spread.** During this phase of radial growth, surgical excision is generally curative.

Lentigo maligna melanoma (5 to 15 percent of cases) occurs on chronically sun-exposed skin such as the face, neck, and upper extremities in elderly patients. It has an extensive radial growth phase that typically is composed of single atypical melanocytes with occasional nesting limited to the basal layer of the epidermis. Thus, these lesions **almost never metastasize** and are cured with excision.

Acral lentiginous melanoma (5 to 10 percent of cases) occurs on the hairless skin of the **palms, soles,** and ungual and periungual regions. It is uncommon in all ethnic groups but is the predominant form of melanoma in **dark-skinned individuals.** The term ***lentiginous*** refers to the radial extension of the lesion cells along the epidermal-dermal junction. Melanoma on acral skin tends to have a worse prognosis compared with melanoma in other sites.

Nodular melanoma (15 to 35 percent of cases) by definition lacks a radial growth phase and thus directly invades (**vertical growth**) the tissue underlying the epidermis. Because of the lack of radial growth, nodular melanoma tends to be well circumscribed and have a small diameter; thus, it does not tend to follow the **ABCD** clinical criteria used to differentiate melanoma from other benign pigmented lesions. Because of the invasive nature of this lesion, it tends to have a worse prognosis.

The incidence of malignant melanoma has increased significantly in the last two decades. **Risk factors** include **habitual sun exposure, fair complexion,** and certain types of melanocytic nevi, such as **large congenital nevi** and **dysplastic nevi** (atypical nevi). The most important prognostic factor for melanoma is the stage at presentation. Fortunately, the majority of melanomas are stage I or stage II and are confined to the primary lesion without any evidence of disease elsewhere. In **stage I and stage II,** a **prognosis** gradient is based on **tumor thickness,** with tumors less than **0.76 mm** having a 96 to 99 percent cure rate using surgical resection versus a 40 percent cure rate for tumors 3.65 mm or more. The site can affect the prognosis, with acral and mucosal melanoma having a worse prognosis than cutaneous melanoma of the extremities or back. Melanoma typically spreads through the **lymphatics,** with ocular melanoma being the exception; thus, **sentinel lymph node** biopsy at the time of surgical excision of the primary lesion can provide important prognostic information.

Basal Cell Carcinoma

Basal cell carcinoma (BCC) is the **most common skin tumor** appearing in **sun-exposed older patients.** These are **slow-growing** tumors that appear in sun-exposed areas such as the face and the forearms. They appear clinically as pearly or ulcerated lesions. On histology, they have a characteristic **pearly appearance** with **nests of basal-like cells within the dermis.** Farmers and others who are exposed to sunlight are at risk. Patients who are immunocompromised, such as those who are HIV-infected, and those with defects in DNA repair, such as xeroderma pigmentosum, also have a high incidence of these cancers. Treatment consists of local excision.

Squamous Cell Carcinoma

Squamous cell carcinoma (SCC) is the **second most common skin tumor** affecting **sun-exposed areas** and has a higher incidence in **men.** Sunlight, old burn scars, certain chemical exposures, radiation, tobacco exposure (smoking and chewing), and chronic infections (ulcers) are risk factors. DNA damage from ultraviolet light is the most important etiology; individuals who are immunocompromised or have difficulty with DNA repair are at particular risk. **Precursor lesions** include squamous cell carcinoma in situ (which has not penetrated through the basement membrane) and **actinic keratosis,** which is also called a **cutaneous horn,** with marked hyperkeratosis and parakeratosis. SCC lesions are usually nodular and ulcerated and have atypical squamous epithelial cells and keratin pearls invading into the dermis. Surgical excision is the treatment of choice. Treatment of premalignant lesions with curettage, cryotherapy, or excision can prevent their progression.

COMPREHENSION QUESTIONS

[44.1] A 74-year-old woman presents with an irregular pigmented lesion covering a large portion of the right side of her face. A biopsy from this lesion reveals a proliferation of individual melanocytes throughout the basal layer of the epidermis. These melanocytes are atypical in appearance, and occasional nesting is present, although no pagetoid pattern (Swiss cheese appearance) of epidermal invasion is seen. The dermis has marked solar degeneration, and in several areas there are markedly atypical melanocytes infiltrating into the reticular dermis. Mitoses are present. Which of the following is the most likely diagnosis?

A. Acral lentiginous melanoma
B. Compound dysplastic nevus
C. Junctional dysplastic nevus
D. Lentigo maligna melanoma
E. Superficial spreading melanoma

[44.2] A 52-year-old woman presents because of an enlarging, darkly pigmented lesion on the skin of her upper back. Physical examination finds the lesion to be 1.7 cm in the greatest dimension, and a small enlarged lymph node is found in her left axilla. The skin lesion is excised, and histologic sections reveal malignant melanocytes infiltrating 1.3 mm into the dermis. Mitoses and lymphocytes are numerous, and scattered pagetoid cells are present within the epidermis. Which of the following is the most important prognostic factor for this lesion?

A. The depth of dermal invasion
B. The grade of the malignant cells
C. The number of atypical mitoses
D. The presence of lymphocytes

[44.3] A 60-year-old man presents with a slowly enlarging lesion just beneath his right eye. Physical examination finds a 7-mm pearly papule with irregular raised margins and a central depression. A biopsy from this lesion would most likely reveal which of the following histologic changes?

A. Hyperplasia of the epidermis forming numerous keratin-filled pseudocysts
B. Hyperplasia of the stratum corneum forming a central keratin-filled "crater"
C. Infiltrating groups of basaloid cells having peritumoral clefting
D. Infiltrating groups of eosinophilic cells with keratin formation
E. Infiltrating spindle-shaped cells with melanin production

Answers

[44.1] **D.** The combination of infiltrating atypical melanocytes with mitoses is diagnostic of malignant melanoma. The most common type of melanoma, superficial spreading melanoma, has a characteristic pagetoid pattern of infiltration within the epidermis that has a Swiss cheese appearance. In contrast, lentigo maligna melanoma, which is found most commonly on the sun-damaged faces of elderly individuals, lacks this pagetoid spread. Instead there is an extensive intraepidermal radial growth phase in which atypical melanocytes proliferate in a lentiginous pattern.

[44.2] **A.** The most important prognostic factor for malignant melanoma is the stage at presentation, that is, whether metastases are present. For lesions that have not yet metastasized, the most important prognostic factor is the depth of invasion of the malignant cells into the dermis, which is called the Breslow depth.

[44.3] **C.** Basal cell carcinoma is the most common type of skin cancer. These lesions, which develop on sun-damaged skin, typically have peripheral raised "pearly" margins and central ulceration ("rodent ulcer"). Histologic sections show infiltrating groups of "basaloid" cells with peripheral palisading of the tumor cells. Characteristically, there is a space between the groups of tumor cells and the adjacent stroma (peritumoral clefting). Squamous cell carcinomas are the next most common type of skin cancer. Histologic sections show infiltrating groups of atypical squamous cells with abundant pink cytoplasm that form intercellular bridges and produce keratin ("keratin pearls").

PATHOLOGY PEARLS

- ❖ In general, sunlight is the most significant risk factor for the development of skin cancers.
- ❖ The ABCD characteristics help differentiate benign nevi from malignant melanomas.
- ❖ The depth of invasion is the most significant prognostic factor in MM that has not yet metastasized.
- ❖ Actinic keratosis, a premalignant lesion to squamous cell cancer, also is known as a cutaneous horn.
- ❖ Basal cell carcinomas are the most common skin cancers, appearing on sun-exposed areas in older people.

REFERENCES

Braunwald E, Fauci AS, Kasper DL, et al., eds. Harrison's Principles of Internal Medicine, 16th ed. New York: McGraw-Hill, 2004.

Cotran RS, Kumar V, Collins T. Robbins Pathologic Basis of Disease, 6th ed. Philadelphia, PA: Saunders, 2004.

Elder D, Elenitsas R, Jaworsky C, et al. Lever's Histopathology of the Skin, 8th ed. Philadelphia, PA: Lippincott Williams & Wilkins, 1997.

Sellheyer K. The skin. In: Mitchell RN, Kumar V, Abbas AK, et al., eds. Pocket Companion to Robbins and Cotran Pathologic Basis of Disease, 7th ed. Philadelphia, PA: Saunders, 2006, 608–9.

CASE 45

A 57-year-old man complains of fatigue, weakness, and weight gain, particularly around the abdomen. On examination, he is found to have hypertension, fullness over the upper back, and abdominal striae. Laboratory studies include an elevated serum cortisol level that is not suppressed with dexamethasone. Imaging studies reveal no pituitary or adrenal masses, but a computed tomography (CT) scan of the chest shows a right lung mass arising near the hilum.

- **What is the most likely diagnosis?**
- **What other disorders may cause similar clinical findings?**
- **What are the underlying mechanisms involved?**

ANSWERS TO CASE 45: PARANEOPLASTIC SYNDROME (LUNG CANCER)

Summary: A 57-year-old man complains of cushingoid features. Laboratory studies include an elevated cortisol level that is not suppressed with dexamethasone. A CT scan of the chest shows a right lung mass arising near the hilum.

- **Most likely diagnosis:** Cushing syndrome caused by small cell carcinoma of lung through a paraneoplastic process.
- **Other disorders causing similar clinical findings:** Cancers of various origins; commonly seen in pancreatic cancer, small cell carcinoma of lung, and thymoma.
- **Underlying mechanisms:** The lung cancer cells probably are producing ectopic adrenocorticotropic hormone (ACTH), resulting in Cushing syndrome.

CLINICAL CORRELATION

The paraneoplastic syndromes are collections of symptoms that result from substances produced by a tumor, and they occur remotely from the tumor. Approximately 10 percent of malignancies manifest these syndromes. **Small cell carcinoma** is the **most common type of cancer** that causes **clinical hormone syndromes,** and it causes a number of **paraneoplastic** effects. These manifestations can result from immune reactivity to tumor and/or tissue antigens, metabolic disorders causing electrolyte abnormalities, and endocrine dysfunction. The tumor cells may produce ectopic ACTH, resulting in Cushing syndrome. The symptoms of Cushing syndrome are nonspecific and often are attributed to other factors. Another paraneoplastic hormone syndrome that commonly occurs in small cell carcinoma of lung is the syndrome of inappropriate antidiuretic hormone (SIADH), which is caused by the secretion of adrenocorticotropic hormone (ACTH) from the tumor. Symptoms are related to the plasma hypotonicity that is secondary to water retention.

APPROACH TO LUNG CANCER

Objectives

- Describe the paraneoplastic syndromes and their associated malignancies.
- List the most common malignancy responsible for paraneoplastic syndrome.

Definitions

Paraneoplastic syndromes: Clinical syndromes involving systemic effects, that accompany malignant disease, that occur "remote" from the neoplasm and are not a direct effect of the mass of the primary tumor or metastases.

Cushing syndrome: A constellation of findings that result from corticosteroid excess, such as hypertension, buffalo hump, abdominal striae, easy bruising, and weight gain.

DISCUSSION

Paraneoplastic syndromes result from substances produced by the tumor rather than from the tumor itself. The symptoms may be endocrine, neuromuscular or musculoskeletal, cardiovascular, cutaneous, hematologic, gastrointestinal, renal, or miscellaneous in nature. See Table 45-1 for a summary of the common neoplastic syndromes.

Cushing Syndrome

Cushing syndrome is a hormonal disorder caused by prolonged exposure of body tissues to high levels of the hormone cortisol. Sometimes called hypercortisolism, it is a group of nonspecific systemic symptoms and is relatively rare. It most commonly affects adults aged 20 to 50 years. An estimated 10 to 15 in every 1 million people are affected each year. Symptoms vary, but most people have upper body obesity, a rounded face, increased fat around the neck, and thinning of the arms and legs. The skin becomes fragile and thin and bruises easily and heals poorly. **Purplish-pink stretch marks (striae)** may appear on the abdomen, thighs, buttocks, arms, and breasts. The bones are weakened by **osteoporosis,** and pathologic fractures of the ribs and spinal column occur more frequently. Severe fatigue, weak muscles, high blood pressure, high blood sugar, irritability, anxiety, and depression are common. The most common cause of Cushing syndrome is excessive exogenous intake of glucocorticoid hormones for disease control, such as prednisone for asthma, rheumatoid arthritis, lupus, and other inflammatory diseases or for immunosuppression after transplantation. Others develop Cushing syndrome because of overproduction of cortisol by the body, such as in pituitary tumors and adrenal gland tumors. Ectopic production of ACTH in various neoplasms is a common initial presentation of malignancy.

Small Cell Carcinoma

Small cell carcinoma accounts for approximately **20 percent of all lung cancers. Smoking** is a well-demonstrated etiologic factor in the development of small cell tumors, and this is consistent with the predilection for the **central**

Table 45-1
PARTIAL LISTING OF PARANEOPLASTIC SYNDROMES

CLINICAL SYNDROMES	MECHANISM OF ACTION	MAJOR FORMS OF CANCER
Cushing syndrome	Adrenocorticotropic hormone (ACTH) or ACTH-like substance	Small cell carcinoma of lung; pancreatic cancer
Syndrome of inappropriate ADH secretion	Antidiuretic hormone (ADH) or atrial natriuretic hormone	Small cell carcinoma of lung; brain tumors
Hypoglycemia	Insulin or insulinlike substance	Fibrosarcoma; hepatocellular carcinoma
Hypercalcemia	Parathyroid hormone-related protein	Breast cancer; renal carcinoma; squamous cell carcinoma of the lung
Carcinoid syndrome	Serotonin, bradykinin	Bronchial adenoma; pancreatic carcinoma; gastric carcinoma
Polycythemia	Erythropoietin	Renal cell carcinoma; cerebellar hemangioma
Myasthenia (Eaton-Lambert syndrome)	Immune-mediated (autoantibodies)	Bronchogenic carcinoma; breast cancer
Venous thrombosis	Tumor products that induce thrombosis	Pancreatic cancer and others

airways and the mucosal irritation caused by smoking. Many patients who are diagnosed with small cell lung cancer are symptomatic at presentation. Small cell carcinoma is characterized by its origin in large central airways and the histologic composition of sheets of small cells with scanty cytoplasm. Small cell carcinoma is a tumor of **neuroendocrine origin,** and the tumor cells are positive for epithelial markers such as pan-cytokeratin and neuroendocrine markers such as chromogranin, synaptophysin, and N-CAM. There are multiple genetic markers associated with small cell lung carcinoma (SCLC), including p53 mutations, retinoblastoma gene mutations, and other tumor suppressor gene mutations.

Up to 15 percent of cases of small cell carcinoma include paraneoplastic syndromes. Hyponatremia, commonly resulting from **SIADH,** can be seen in up to 1 percent of cases. **Cushing syndrome** caused by **ectopic ACTH production** is seen in up to 5 percent. Antibodies to various neural tissue types produce syndromes such as **Lambert-Eaton syndrome (weakness** caused by a **myasthenic-like** syndrome), encephalomyelitis, peripheral neuropathy, and sudden bilateral blindness resulting from retinopathy, among others.

Small cell carcinoma is very aggressive and metastasizes early and often. SCLC is incurable by surgery and is well known to be highly responsive to chemotherapy and radiation; however, it also relapses quickly. Even though treatment of primary tumor is necessary for cure, symptomatic treatment of paraneoplastic syndromes also may be appropriate.

COMPREHENSION QUESTIONS

[45.1] A 57-year-old man who has smoked for 30 years presents with increasing fatigue and weakness. Physical examination finds obesity of the face, neck, and trunk, along with purple abdominal striae and hypertension. Laboratory examination reveals increased plasma cortisol and ACTH levels. The serum glucocorticoid levels are not decreased after dexamethasone administration. Which of the following is the most likely cause of these signs and symptoms?

A. Secretion of ACTH by a carcinoma of the lung
B. Secretion of ACTH by an adenoma of the anterior pituitary
C. Secretion of cortisol by a carcinoma of the liver
D. Secretion of cortisol by an adenoma of the adrenal cortex
E. Secretion of proopiomelanocortin (POMC) by an adenoma of the hypothalamus

[45.2] A 71-year-old man who is a long-term smoker presents with a persistent cough and marked weight loss over the last 3 months. A chest x-ray finds a 3.5-cm mass in the hilum of the lung. A biopsy is taken from the mass, and the diagnosis by the pathologist is "oat cell" carcinoma. Which of the following is the typical histologic appearance of this malignancy?

A. Large polygonal cells with intercellular bridges and keratin
B. Large undifferentiated cells with abundant eosinophilic cytoplasm
C. Small pleomorphic cuboidal cells arranged in a glandular pattern
D. Small undifferentiated cells with very small amounts of cytoplasm
E. Well-differentiated columnar epithelial cells that secrete mucus

[45.3] A 51-year-old man who has smoked two packs of cigarettes a day for more than 30 years presents with recent weight gain and is found to have a lung mass on a chest x-ray. Laboratory examination reveals increased serum levels of vasopressin (ADH), and the diagnosis of SIADH is made. Which of the following laboratory findings is most consistent with this diagnosis?

A. Oliguria and hyperkalemia
B. Oliguria and hyponatremia
C. Polydipsia and hypernatremia
D. Polyuria and hypernatremia
E. Polyuria and hypokalemia

Answers

[45.1] **A.** Paraneoplastic syndromes are defined as clinical signs and symptoms that result from the effects of malignant tumors and are not a direct mass effect of the primary tumor. Paraneoplastic syndromes can result from the ectopic production of hormones by malignant tumors. For example, the tumor cells of a lung cancer, particularly a small cell carcinoma of the lung, may produce ectopic ACTH and thus produce Cushing syndrome. Clinical signs of this hormonal disorder include upper body obesity, thin fragile skin, increased bruising, and stretch marks on the abdomen. In contrast to a pituitary adenoma that secretes ACTH, the ectopic production of ACTH by a lung cancer is not diminished with high-dose dexamethasone.

[45.2] **D.** Small cell carcinoma of the lung is a highly malignant tumor that accounts for approximately 20 percent of all lung cancers. This tumor is histologically composed of sheets of small undifferentiated cells with very small amounts of cytoplasm. The nuclei are small and round and rarely have nucleoli. Because of this appearance, it also is called "oat cell" carcinoma. This malignancy is a type of neuroendocrine tumor, and the tumor cells are positive for epithelial markers such as pan-cytokeratin and neuroendocrine markers such as chromogranin and synaptophysin. Electron microscopy reveals membrane-bound dense core neurosecretory granules.

[45.3] **B.** Another paraneoplastic hormone syndrome that occurs commonly with small cell carcinoma of lung is the syndrome of inappropriate antidiuretic hormone. This syndrome results from the ectopic secretion of ADH. It is characterized by excess water retention that produces oliguria and decreasing serum osmolality, increasing urine osmolality, and a decreasing serum sodium concentration (hyponatremia).

PATHOLOGY PEARLS

- Approximately 10 percent of malignancies manifest a paraneoplastic syndrome.
- Small cell carcinoma of the lung is the most common cause of paraneoplastic syndrome.
- Hyponatremia may be caused by inappropriate ADH, and hypercalcemia may be caused by a parathyroid hormone–like secretion.
- Weakness may be due to immune-mediated myasthenia (Eaton-Lambert syndrome), which is common with bronchogenic carcinomas of the lung.

REFERENCE

Kumar V, Assas AK, Fausto N, eds. Robbins and Cotran Pathologic Basis of Disease, 7th ed. Philadelphia, PA: Elsevier Saunders, 2004.

CASE 46

A 70-year-old Jewish man presents to his primary care physician with weakness. Physical examination reveals pallor and hepatosplenomegaly. A bone marrow aspiration and a biopsy are performed to evaluate the cause of his anemia. Histiocytes that appear enlarged with "wrinkled tissue paper" cytoplasm are noted in the bone marrow.

- **What is the most likely diagnosis?**
- **What is the underlying etiology of this condition?**
- **What are the other clinical features of this disease?**

ANSWERS TO CASE 46: GAUCHER DISEASE

Summary: A 70-year-old man presents with anemia, hepatosplenomegaly, and enlarged histiocytes with "wrinkled tissue paper" cytoplasm (Gaucher cells) in bone marrow.

- **Most likely diagnosis:** Gaucher disease, adult type.
- **Underlying etiology:** Insufficient glucocerebrosidase leading to accumulation of glucocerebroside in the phagocytic cells of the body and the central nervous system.
- **Other clinical features:** Hypersplenism (i.e., leukopenia and thrombocytopenia) and pathologic fractures resulting from bone involvement.

CLINICAL CORRELATION

Gaucher disease, a lysosomal storage disorder, results from mutations in the genes that encode glucocerebrosidase. As a result of insufficient enzyme, glucocerebroside accumulates in the phagocytic cells of the body and the central nervous system. Several types of disease can occur, including a chronic non-neuronopathic variety (type I) that affects the skeletal regions and the spleen and liver. Bone marrow involvement can lead to leukopenia and thrombocytopenia. Type II usually affects infants and entails cerebroside accumulation in the brain and abdominal organs. Early death is likely. The diagnosis is confirmed by decreased glucocerebrosidase levels. Treatment is with enzyme replacement. Bone marrow transplantation also is being investigated.

APPROACH TO GAUCHER DISEASE

Objectives

- Know the pathology of lysosomal storage diseases.
- Describe inborn errors of metabolism and their respective enzyme deficiencies.
- List inborn errors of metabolism and their respective clinical presentations.

Definitions

Storage disease: A general term to describe an inherited disorder in which there is a defect or deficiency in either lysosomal enzymes **(lysosomal storage diseases)** or in glycogen metabolism **(glycogen storage diseases).** The defect results in the inability to metabolize normal substrates which accumulate in macrophages (lysosomal storage diseases) or in tissues such as the heart, muscle or liver (glycogen storage diseases).

Gaucher cell: The hallmark of Gaucher disease, a lipid-filled macrophage containing the undigested glucosylceramide that accumulates in the disease. Gaucher cells may be found anywhere in the body, but are usually prominent in the liver, spleen, and bone marrow.

DISCUSSION

PATHOLOGY OF LYSOSOMAL STORAGE DISEASES

Lysosomes are considered **key components of intracellular digestion.** They contain **hydrolytic enzymes** that are capable of breaking down a variety of complex macromolecules. When one of the lysosomal enzymes is missing, complete breakdown of the molecule is not possible. This leads to the accumulation of the incompletely digested molecule within the cell. The lysosomes and subsequently the cell and the organ increase in size. Normal cellular function is compromised significantly.

Gaucher disease is the **most prevalent lysosomal storage disorder.** It is due to the deficiency of the enzyme **glucocerebrosidase,** which is a lysosomal enzyme. The disease is inherited in an **autosomal recessive** manner. Deficiency of the enzyme results in the accumulation of glucocerebroside in the cells of the reticuloendothelial system, especially in the **bone marrow, liver, and spleen.** Thus, **hepatosplenomegaly** is very common.

There are **three clinical types.** The most common is the **adult type** (type I or the chronic nonneuronopathic type), which has an insidious onset of hepatosplenomegaly. It has a high incidence among **Ashkenazi Jews** and accounts for 99 percent of all cases of Gaucher disease. Patients have reduced but detectable levels of glucocerebrosidase activity. Phagocytic cells become distended with glucocerebroside and are referred to as **Gaucher cells; these cells are enlarged with periodic acid-Schiff (PAS)-positive cytoplasm with a fibrillary appearance as a result of the stacking of the lipid bilayers in the lysosomes.** Accumulation of Gaucher cells in the bone marrow may cause bone deformity or bone destruction, ultimately resulting in pathologic fractures. Life expectancy in general is normal.

The **infantile type,** also referred to as **type II** or acute neuronopathic, is characterized by **progressive central nervous involvement** and **death at an early age.** There is virtually no detectable glucocerebrosidase activity in the tissues. The **third type (type III)** has features intermediate between those of types I and II.

Other Lysosomal Storage Diseases

Niemann-Pick disease is due to a deficiency of lysosomal sphingomyelinase. Accumulation of sphingomyelin cholesterol and glycosphingolipids in the reticuloendothelial macrophages occurs in organs such the liver, spleen, bone marrow, and lymph nodes.

Mucopolysaccharidoses are a group of disorders caused by a deficiency of the lysosomal enzymes normally required for the degradation of glycosaminoglycans (mucopolysaccharides). The glycosaminoglycans are dermatan sulfate, heparan sulfate, keratan sulfate, and chondroitin sulfate. There are 10 subtypes of this disorder, all but 1 of which are transmitted as autosomal recessive.

Tay-Sachs disease is a condition in which there is **accumulation of GM_2 gangliosides in the nervous system.** It is particularly common among Ashkenazi Jews.

Fabry disease is an X-linked recessive condition in which there is deficiency of α-galactosidase resulting in accumulation of glycosphingolipids. Neurologic and renal problems dominate the clinical features.

Inborn Errors of Carbohydrate Metabolism

Glycogen Storage Disease

In glycogen storage disease, there is a **hereditary deficiency** of one of the enzymes involved in the **synthesis or degradation of glycogen.** As in most enzyme deficiencies, the majority of the subtypes are transmitted as **autosomal recessive.** In the hepatic forms of the condition, enzyme deficiency results in organomegaly, principally **hepatomegaly,** and impaired glucose release into the circulation, leading to **hypoglycemia.** With **type I (von Gierke disease),** there is **deficiency of glucose-6-phosphatase,** an enzyme required for the conversion of glucose 6-phosphate in the liver to glucose, which then is released into the circulation. Glucose 6-phosphate accumulates within the hepatocytes, as does glycogen.

Type V (McArdle disease) is a **myopathic** form involving **muscle phosphorylase** deficiency; muscle phosphorylase breaks down glycogen, and the resultant glucose is used in the glycolytic pathway. This is normally responsible for the breakdown of muscle glycogen. Muscle cramps and myoglobinuria after exercise are typical features. A type of glycogen storage disease that is considered a **lysosomal storage disease is type II (Pompe disease),** in which **acid maltase is lacking.** Acid maltase breaks down glycogen directly to glucose.

Other inborn errors of carbohydrate metabolism are summarized in Table 46-1.

Table 46-1
SELECTED LIST OF INBORN ERRORS OF METABOLISM

NAME OF DISEASE	ENZYME DEFICIENCY	CLINICAL SYNDROME
Galactosemia	Galactose 1-phosphate uridyl transferase (interferes with conversion of galactose to glucose)	Mental retardation, failure to thrive, cataracts; hepatosplenomegaly
Hereditary fructose intolerance	Deficiency of aldolase B leading to accumulation of fructose 1-phosphate, which is toxic	Hypoglycemia, vomiting, cirrhosis
Phenylketonuria	Deficiency of phenylalanine hydroxylase	Musty body odor; mental retardation, fair skin
Albinism	Deficiency of tyrosinase (tyrosine is precursor of melanin synthesis)	Albinism; increased risk of skin cancer
Alkaptonuria	Deficiency of homogentisate oxidase, which impairs conversion of homogentisate to maleylacetoacetate	Accumulation of homogentisate leads to urine darkening on standing and deposition in cartilage, resulting in joint damage
Homocystinuria	Deficiency of cystathionine synthetase; homocysteine is converted to cystathionine by cystathionine synthetase	Mental retardation, Marfan-like habitus, and dislocation of lens
Maple syrup urine disease	Deficiency of branched-chain α-ketoacid dehydrogenase	Urine smells like maple syrup; accumulation of the corresponding α-ketoacid, leading to mental retardation and other neurologic problems
Fanconi syndrome	Two types: congenital (De Toni–Fanconi syndrome) and acquired (e.g., due to drugs, heavy metal poisoning) tubular reabsorption of amino acid, glucose, phosphate	Hypophosphatemic rickets and low bicarbonate (with resultant metabolic acidosis)

(Continued)

Table 46-1
SELECTED LIST OF INBORN ERRORS OF METABOLISM *(Continued)*

NAME OF DISEASE	ENZYME DEFICIENCY	CLINICAL SYNDROME
Cystinuria	Defective tubular reabsorption of cysteine, ornithine, arginine, and lysine (COAL)	Cysteine stones in kidneys
Hartnup disease	Defective reabsorption of tryptophan (because tryptophan is converted to niacin, low niacin results)	Pellagra (if dietary niacin is insufficient)

COMPREHENSION QUESTIONS

[46.1] A 71-year-old man presents with signs of anemia and is found to have an enlarged liver and spleen along with peripheral pancytopenia. Sections from bone marrow reveal numerous macrophages with a fibrillar appearance of the cytoplasm that resembles wrinkled tissue paper. Which of the following enzyme deficiencies does this individual most likely have?

A. Acid maltase
B. Arylsulfatase A
C. Glucocerebrosidase
D. Homogentisate oxidase
E. Phosphorylase

[46.2] A 2-year-old girl of Ashkenazi Jewish descent is being evaluated for mental retardation, seizures, and ataxia. Physical examination finds enlargement of the liver, spleen, and several lymph nodes. A bone marrow biopsy reveals aggregates of lipid-laden macrophages (foam cells). These cells contain excessive amounts of sphingomyelin and cholesterol. Further workup finds a deficiency of the enzyme sphingomyelinase. Which of the following is the most likely diagnosis?

A. Fabry disease
B. Gaucher disease
C. Niemann-Pick disease
D. Sandhoff disease
E. Tay-Sachs disease

[46.3] A familial deficiency of glucose-6-phosphatase is most likely to be associated with the abnormal accumulation of glycogen in which of the following locations?

A. Basal ganglia
B. Cardiac muscle
C. Liver cells
D. Lymph nodes
E. Skeletal muscle

Answers

[46.1] **C.** Gaucher disease is the most common lysosomal storage disorder. This autosomal recessive disorder results from a deficiency of the enzyme glucocerebrosidase. As a result, glucocerebroside accumulates in the cells of the reticuloendothelial system, such as the bone marrow, liver, and spleen. The most common type of Gaucher disease is the adult type, which has a high incidence in the Ashkenazi Jewish population. In addition to hepatosplenomegaly, features of the adult type of Gaucher disease include hypersplenism and pathologic fractures.

[46.2] **C.** Niemann-Pick disease is an autosomal recessive disorder that results from a deficiency of the lysosomal enzyme sphingomyelinase. As a result, sphingomyelin accumulates in the cytoplasm of macrophages in the liver, spleen, bone marrow, and lymph nodes. These lipid-filled macrophages are called foam cells. The most common type of Niemann-Pick disease is the infantile type, which is characterized by mental retardation, seizures, ataxia, and death by the age of 3 years.

[46.3] **C.** The glycogen storage diseases result from hereditary deficiencies involving any of the enzymes involved in the synthesis or degradation of glycogen. Type I glycogen storage disease (von Gierke disease) results from a deficiency of glucose-6-phosphatase, an enzyme that is necessary for the conversion of glucose 6-phosphate to glucose in the liver. This deficiency results in the accumulation of glycogen in the cytoplasm of hepatocytes. Symptoms of this disorder result from recurrent severe fasting hypoglycemia and include dizziness, sweating, and convulsions.

PATHOLOGY PEARLS

- Gaucher disease is the most prevalent lysosomal storage disorder and is due to a deficiency of the enzyme glucocerebrosidase.
- Type I Gaucher disease has a high incidence among Ashkenazi Jews, and affected patients have reduced but detectable levels of glucocerebrosidase activity.
- Niemann-Pick disease is due to a deficiency of lysosomal sphingomyelinase.
- In Tay-Sachs, disease there is accumulation of GM2 gangliosides in the nervous system.
- Fabry disease is an X-linked recessive condition in which there is deficiency of alpha-galactosidase, resulting in the accumulation of glycosphingolipids.
- Galactosemia is due to a deficiency of galactose 1-phosphate uridyl transferase.
- Hereditary fructose intolerance is due to a deficiency of aldolase.
- Phenylketonuria is due to a deficiency of phenylalanine hydroxylase.
- Albinism is due to a deficiency of tyrosinase.
- Alkaptonuria is due to a deficiency of homogentisate oxidase.
- Homocystinuria is due to a deficiency of cystathionine synthetase.
- Maple syrup urine disease is due to a deficiency of branched-chain α-ketoacid dehydrogenase.
- Tubular reabsorptive defects of amino acids may be generalized (De Toni–Fanconi syndrome) or specific (cystinuria, Hartnup disease).

REFERENCES

Kumar V, Assas AK, Fausto N, eds. Robbins and Cotran Pathologic Basis of Disease, 7th ed. Philadelphia, PA: Elsevier Saunders, 2004.

Husain AN. The lung. In: Mitchell RN, Kumar V, Abbas AK, et al., eds. Pocket Companion to Robbins and Cotran Pathologic Basis of Disease, 7th ed. Philadelphia, PA: Saunders, 2006:396–8.

CASE 47

A 30-year-old woman presents to the emergency department with acute abdominal pain that is colicky in nature. She has hematuria and bone pain. Physical examination reveals her to be dehydrated. Plain x-ray of the abdomen reveals a radiopaque renal calculus on the right side. Serum calcium is found to be elevated. The patient's past medical history is significant for an islet cell tumor of the pancreas (insulinoma).

- **What is the most likely diagnosis?**

- **What is the reason for her dehydration?**

- **What syndrome does this patient most likely have?**

ANSWERS TO CASE 47: PRIMARY HYPERPARATHYROIDISM

Summary: A 30-year-old woman has hypercalcemia, renal stone, and bone pain, with a past history of islet cell tumor.

- **Most likely diagnosis:** Primary hyperparathyroidism caused by an adenoma.
- **Reason for dehydration:** Primary hyperparathyroidism results in hypercalcemia. This causes impairment of the action of antidiuretic hormone (ADH) at the collecting ducts. This is thus an example of nephrogenic diabetes insipidus. These patients are expected to have polyuria and may become dehydrated, especially if water intake is not maintained.
- **Most likely syndrome:** Multiple endocrine neoplasia (MEN) type 1.

CLINICAL CORRELATION

In primary hyperparathyroidism, there is autonomous spontaneous overproduction of parathyroid hormone (PTH). The most common causes are an adenoma (>80 percent of cases) and hyperplasia of all glands. Some of these cases are caused by inherited syndromes such as MEN type 1. High levels of PTH cause bone resorption with resultant hypercalcemia. High serum calcium then leads to metastatic calcification. One of the sites is the cornea. Hypercalcemia prevents the action of ADH on the collecting ducts, resulting in nephrogenic diabetes insipidus and subsequent polyuria and polydipsia. Increased excretion of calcium through the renal tubules would result in renal stones. Hypercalcemia also is associated with peptic ulcer and pancreatitis. Psychiatric disturbances also are reported with hyperparathyroidism. All these possible features are very well put together in the phrase **bones, stones, abdominal groans, and psychic moans.**

APPROACH TO HYPERPARATHYROIDISM

Objectives

- Know the signs and symptoms of hypercalcemia.
- Describe the causes of hypercalcemia and hypocalcemia.
- List the most common cause of elevated PTH.
- List the MEN syndromes.

Definitions

Primary hyperparathyroidism: Autonomous spontaneous overproduction of PTH, most often as a result of an adenoma. Serum calcium levels are high.

Secondary hyperparathyroidism: Physiologic compensatory hypertrophy of the parathyroid glands caused by hypocalcemia. PTH levels are raised, but serum calcium is not elevated.

Tertiary hyperparathyroidism: Long-standing secondary hyperparathyroidism leads to autonomous and hyperactive parathyroids. This occurs most often in the setting of chronic renal failure.

Primary hypoparathyroidism: Parathyroid underactivity resulting from intrinsic disease of the parathyroid glands. PTH levels are low.

Pseudohypoparathyroidism: End-organ resistance to PTH. The patient has hypocalcemia, and PTH levels are elevated.

DISCUSSION

There are two pairs of parathyroid glands, the superior and the inferior, located behind the thyroid. The superior pair is derived from the fourth pharyngeal pouch, and the inferior pair is derived from the third pharyngeal pouch. The superior pair is more constant in position. Parathyroid glands may be located elsewhere in the neck or mediastinum. The **parathyroid glands secrete PTH,** which is involved in calcium metabolism.

Calcium Metabolism

The normal range of serum calcium is 8.5 to 10.5 mg/dL, of which approximately **40 to 50 percent is ionized** and is physiologically active. The remainder is bound to proteins, typically albumin. **Calcium homeostasis** is maintained by **parathyroid hormone, 1,25-dihydroxycholecalciferol (activated vitamin D_3),** and **calcitonin.** The effects of PTH and calcitonin on calcium levels are rapid. Several steps are involved in the production of 1,25-dihydroxycholecalciferol; thus, the final effect of vitamin D on calcium levels is not immediate. Table 47-1 describes some of the causes of hypercalcemia, and Table 47-2 lists the causes of hypocalcemia. **Primary hyperparathyroidism** and **malignancies** remain the **two most common causes** (>90 percent) of **hypercalcemia.**

Parathyroid Hormone Metabolism

PTH is an 84-amino acid hormone and is secreted from the **chief cells of the parathyroid** glands. PTH levels rise as serum ionized calcium levels fall. PTH increases calcium levels by activating osteoclasts, which increase bone resorption, increasing the intestinal absorption of calcium, promoting the formation

Table 47-1
SELECTED CAUSES OF HYPERCALCEMIA

Excess of parathyroid hormone (PTH) Primary and tertiary hyperparathyroidism Ectopic PTH secretion
Excess of Vitamin D: granulomatous disease (e.g., sarcoidosis)
Excess of calcium intake: "milk-alkali" syndrome
Malignancies (e.g., bone deposits, myeloma)
Drugs Thiazide diuretics Vitamin D and analogues
Miscellaneous Immobility Familial hypocalciuric hypercalcemia

of 1,25-dihydroxycholecalciferol, and increasing renal tubular reabsorption of calcium and excretion of phosphate. At the cellular level, PTH acts on cell membrane receptors, resulting in an increase of adenylate cyclase activity, with increased levels of intracellular cyclic adenosine monophosphate (cAMP).

Vitamin D Metabolism

Dietary sources are not the primary source of vitamin D; instead, the primary source is the conversion of 7-dehydrocholesterol to cholecalciferol by **sunlight. Cholecalciferol** is **converted in the liver to 25-hydroxycholecalciferol,** which subsequently is **converted to 1,25-dihydroxycholecalciferol** in the **kidney.** This is the biologically active form of vitamin D. 1,25-Dihydroxycholecalicferol is required for bone mineralization and also promotes calcium absorption from the gut.

Calcitonin

This is a **32-amino acid hormone** produced by the **parafollicular C cells in the thyroid. Calcitonin inhibits osteoclastic bone resorption** and **increases renal excretion of calcium and phosphate.** The contribution of calcitonin to calcium metabolism is unclear. States of low calcitonin (total thyroidectomy) or high calcitonin (medullary carcinoma of the thyroid) does not result in altered calcium levels.

Table 47-2
SELECTED CAUSES OF HYPOCALCEMIA

Chronic renal failure (very common cause)
Hypoparathyroidism After thyroid or parathyroid surgery (usually transient) Congenital deficiency (DiGeorge syndrome) Idiopathic (autoimmune parathyroid disease)
Vitamin D deficiency
Parathyroid hormone resistance (also known as pseudohypoparathyroidism)
Drugs (those that inhibit osteoclasts, e.g., calcitonin, bisphosphonates)
Miscellaneous Acute pancreatitis Massive transfusion (citrate in blood may cause hypocalcemia)

Hyperparathyroidism

Primary hyperparathyroidism is the most common cause of elevated PTH. Secondary hyperparathyroidism occurs as a physiologic compensatory hypertrophy of the parathyroid glands resulting from hypocalcemia. PTH levels are raised, but serum calcium is not elevated. **Tertiary hyperparathyroidism** occurs after long-standing secondary hyperparathyroidism the parathyroid becomes autonomous and hyperactive, resulting in tertiary hyperparathyroidism. This occurs most often in the setting of chronic renal failure.

Malignancies Resulting in Hypercalcemia

Hypercalcemia usually is due to **bony metastases** in certain tumors. Common examples of such tumors are **malignant tumors of the lung and breast and myeloma.** Cytokines and prostaglandins are thought to be liberated, resulting in bone resorption with subsequent hypercalcemia. Ectopic PTH secretion by tumors is rare. The tumor cells produce a PTH-related protein that exhibits homology to PTH in the amino acid sequence.

Multiple Endocrine Neoplasia

This term is used for simultaneous or metachronous occurrence of endocrine tumors. These tumors **typically are inherited as autosomal dominant.** The underlying pathogenesis is thought to be the expression of recessive oncogenic mutations. See Table 47-3 for a listing of the MEN syndromes.

Table 47-3
MULTIPLE ENDOCRINE NEOPLASIA (MEN) SYNDROMES

MEN type 1 Parathyroid adenoma Pituitary adenoma Pancreatic islet cell tumor
MEN type 2A Pheochromocytoma Medullary carcinoma of the thyroid Parathyroid hyperplasia
MEN type 2B Pheochromocytoma Medullary carcinoma of the thyroid Marfanoid habitus with mucosal and visceral ganglioneuromas

The various types of hypoparathyroidism include **primary hypoparathyroidism and pseudohypoparathyroidism.** All the forms are uncommon except transient hypoparathyroidism, which is seen after thyroid or parathyroid surgery. Idiopathic hypoparathyroidism is an autoimmune condition. Pseudohypoparathyroidism is due to end-organ resistance to PTH. The patient has hypocalcemia, and PTH levels are elevated. Certain somatic features are part of this condition, including mental impairment, short stature, and short metacarpals. The term **pseudopseudohypoparathyroidism** refers to individuals who have the somatic features of pseudohypoparathyroidism but in whom calcium and PTH levels are normal.

COMPREHENSION QUESTIONS

[47.1] Which of the following statements best describes the pathomechanism involved in producing secondary hyperparathyroidism in an individual with chronic renal failure?

A. Decreased PTH levels increase serum calcium.
B. Elevated serum phosphorus levels increase PTH levels.
C. Increased PTH levels decrease serum calcium.
D. Loss of calcium increases PTH levels.
E. Retention of calcium increases PTH levels.

[47.2] In what organs are tumors characteristically found in individuals with MEN type 1?

A. Adrenal, thyroid, and parathyroid
B. Kidneys, adrenal, and liver
C. Liver, pancreas, and small intestines
D. Parathyroid, pineal, and pancreas
E. Pituitary, parathyroid, and pancreas

[47.3] Which of the following enzymes is necessary for the final biochemical reaction involved in the activation of vitamin D?

A. 1-α-Hydroxylase in the kidney
B. 7-α-Hydroxylase in the liver
C. 17-Hydroxylase in the adrenal cortex
D. 11-Hydroxylase in the adrenal cortex
E. 25-Hydroxylase in the skin

Answers

[47.1] **D.** Secondary hyperparathyroidism refers to physiologic hyperplasia of all four parathyroid glands as a result of decreased serum levels of calcium (hypocalcemia), the most common cause of which is the loss of calcium in the urine in an individual with chronic renal failure.

[47.2] **E.** Multiple endocrine neoplasia is a term used to describe the simultaneous occurrence of endocrine tumors in multiple sites. MEN type 1 is characterized by the formation of tumors in the anterior pituitary gland (pituitary adenomas), parathyroid glands (parathyroid adenomas), and pancreas (islet cell adenomas).

[47.3] **A.** The main source of vitamin D is the conversion of 7-dehydrocholesterol to cholecalciferol by sunlight in the skin. This reaction forms previtamin D_3 (cholecalciferol), which in the liver is converted to 25-hydroxy-D_3 (calcifediol) by a cytochrome P-450 mixed-function oxidase. Calcifediol is converted in the kidney to 1,25-dihydroxy vitamin D_3 (calcitriol, the most potent vitamin D metabolite) by a renal tubular mitochondrial hydroxylase: 1-α-hydroxylase.

PATHOLOGY PEARLS

- Calcium homeostasis is maintained by parathyroid hormone, 1,25-dihydroxycholecalciferol (activated vitamin D_3), and calcitonin.
- Primary hyperparathyroidism and malignancies are the two most common causes (>90 percent of cases) of hypercalcemia.
- In primary hyperparathyroidism, there is autonomous spontaneous overproduction of PTH. The causes are an adenoma (>80 percent of cases) and hyperplasia of all glands.
- Primary hyperparathyroidism in some cases is associated with multiple endocrine neoplasia.
- PTH levels are raised but serum calcium is not elevated in secondary hyperparathyroidism.
- After long-standing secondary hyperparathyroidism the parathyroids become autonomous and hyperactive, resulting in tertiary hyperparathyroidism.
- MEN syndromes are transmitted as autosomal dominant.
- The various types of hypoparathyroidism include primary hypoparathyroidism and pseudohypoparathyroidism. All forms arc uncommon except transient hypoparathyroidism, which is seen after thyroid or parathyroid surgery.

REFERENCES

Kumar V, Assas AK, Fausto N, eds. Robbins and Cotran Pathologic Basis of Disease, 7th ed. Philadelphia, PA: Elsevier Saunders, 2004.

Maitra A. The endocrine system. In: Mitchell RN, Kumar V, Abbas AK, et al., eds. Pocket Companion to Robbins and Cotran Pathologic Basis of Disease, 7th ed. Philadelphia, PA: Saunders, 2006:580–2.

CASE 48

A 21-year-old woman college student complains of fatigue, an unintentional 10-lb weight loss, and a persistent oral ulcer. On physical examination, swelling and tenderness of the distal joints in both hands are also noted. Laboratory studies show a normocytic anemia, positive antinuclear antibody (ANA) titers, and decreased C3 complement levels.

- **What is the most likely diagnosis?**
- **What is the underlying mechanism for these findings?**
- **What additional laboratory tests would confirm the diagnosis?**

ANSWERS TO CASE 48: SYSTEMIC LUPUS ERYTHEMATOSUS

Summary: A 21-year-old female college student complains of fatigue, weight loss, and a persistent oral ulcer. Swelling and tenderness of the distal joints in both hands also are noted. Laboratory studies show a normocytic anemia, positive ANA titers, and decreased C3 levels.

- **Most likely diagnosis:** Systemic lupus erythematosus (SLE).
- **Underlying mechanism for these findings:** Autoimmune antibodies.
- **Additional studies:** Anti–double-stranded DNA antibody and anti–Smith antibodies are specific for the diagnosis of SLE.

CLINICAL CORRELATION

Systemic lupus erythematosus is an autoimmune disease in which affected patients form numbers of antibodies directed against self-constituents. Virtually any organ system can be involved. The course of the illness is characterized by periods of active disease and periods of remission. Manifestations can range from mild dermatologic symptoms to life-threatening organ failure. SLE can occur in any age group, but the most common time for the first presentation is the second, third, or fourth decade. It is found in all ethnic and racial groups but is most common and most severe in the black and Hispanic populations. Eighty percent of those affected are women.

Common presenting symptoms include fever, malaise, weight loss, joint pain, and dermatologic manifestations. The most characteristic skin manifestation is a malar rash, a flat or raised erythematous rash over the nose and malar eminences. It is described as being shaped like a **butterfly** and can be associated with photosensitivity. Painless oral or nasopharyngeal ulcers are also common.

Laboratory findings in SLE are helpful in making the diagnosis. A positive ANA is found in 99 percent of SLE patients but is not indicative of SLE because other connective tissue diseases also can result in a positive ANA. Anti–double-stranded DNA and anti–Smith antibodies are 95 percent and 99 percent specific for SLE, respectively. Serum complement often is decreased. Hemolytic anemia can be found, as well as leukopenia, lymphopenia, and thrombocytopenia. Other connective tissue disorders are listed in Table 48-1.

APPROACH TO SYSTEMIC LUPUS ERYTHEMATOSUS

Objectives

- Describe the various autoimmune diseases and their respective clinical presentations.
- Know the various autoimmune diseases and their respective antibodies.
- List the criteria used for the diagnosis of systemic lupus erythematosus.
- Know CREST syndrome.

Definitions

Antinuclear antibodies: Antibodies produced by the immune system that are self-directed. The antibodies attach to and damage the host's own natural cells. There are many different kinds, most of which are found in higher numbers in specific autoimmune diseases.

Type II hypersensitivity reaction: A reaction mediated by antibodies directed toward antigens present on the surface of cells or tissues that causes lysis of the target cell or opsonization.

Type III hypersensitivity reaction: An immune complex–mediated reaction in which antigen-antibody complexes are formed. These complexes deposit into tissues and activate the complement system, producing tissue damage.

DISCUSSION

The true cause of SLE is unknown, but the fundamental defect is a failure of the regulatory mechanisms that sustain self-tolerance. Numerous **antibodies against nuclear and cytoplasmic parts of the cell** that are not organ-specific have been identified; **antinuclear antibodies** are particularly prominent. These antibodies are responsible for the pathology seen with SLE. These antinuclear antibodies are also useful in making the diagnosis. Immunofluorescence is used to identify the presence of specific antibodies that can correlate with certain pathologies.

Genetic and nongenetic factors appear to contribute to the development of SLE. The current belief is that an individual can be born with a genetic predisposition to develop the condition. There is then an unknown type of environmental stimulus that triggers the disease, coupled with a fundamental defect in the person's immune system that ultimately leads to the development of SLE. These factors combine to cause an activation of helper T cells and B cells that results in the secretion of several species of antibodies. These antibodies are the mediators of tissue injury. Most of the **visceral lesions** are mediated by **immune complexes** resulting from a type III hypersensitivity reaction. These complexes then are deposited into various body tissues. In

Table 48-1
SELECTED CONNECTIVE TISSUE AUTOIMMUNE DISEASES

DISEASE	CHARACTERIZING PATHOLOGY	ASSOCIATED ANTIBODIES
Systemic lupus erythematosus	Injury to the skin, kidney, and serosal membranes	Anti–double-stranded DNA, anti-Smith
Diffuse scleroderma	Widespread skin fibrosis with rapid progression and early visceral involvement	Anti ScI-70
Limited scleroderma	Fibrosis of the fingers, forearms, and face; CREST syndrome and late visceral involvement	Anticentromere
Sjögren syndrome	Dry eyes and dry mouth from destruction of lacrimal and salivary glands	Anti-Ro, anti-La
Polymyositis	Symmetric proximal muscle weakness	Anti-Jo
Dermatomyositis	Symmetric proximal muscle weakness with associated rash of upper eyelids, knuckles, knees, and elbows	Anti-Jo
Mixed connective tissue disease	Coexistence of features suggestive of systemic lupus erythematosus, polymyositis, and scleroderma	Anti-RNP

addition, there are type II hypersensitivity reactions to red cells, white cells, and platelets. The most characteristic lesions result from **immune complex deposition** in **kidneys, skin, joints, and serosal membranes.**

The **kidneys** appear to be involved in **60 to 70 percent of cases of SLE.** Lupus **nephritis** is classified into four subtypes, all resulting from **DNA–anti-DNA complexes** depositing within the glomeruli. **Mesangial lupus glomerulonephritis** is the mildest of the lesions, and affected patients may present with only **mild hematuria or transient proteinuria.** The histologic changes show granular mesangial deposits of immunoglobulin and complement. This is the earliest of the lesions seen in lupus, as is evidenced by the accumulation of complexes only in the mesangium. **Focal proliferative glomerulonephritis** is, as the name implies, focal in location. Usually fewer than 50 percent of glomeruli are affected, and only portions of each glomerulus are affected. The histology shows swelling and proliferation of endothelial and mesangial cells, infiltration with neutrophils, and sometimes fibrinoid deposits. These patients have hematuria and proteinuria. This can progress to **diffuse proliferative glomerulonephritis, which is the most serious renal lesion in SLE.** Histologic changes show proliferation of endothelial, mesangial, and epithelial cells producing crescents that fill the Bowman space. Almost all the glomeruli are affected uniformly. These patients have hematuria as well as proteinuria severe enough to cause nephrotic syndrome. Hypertension and renal insufficiency are also common. **Membranous glomerulonephritis** in SLE has the same pathology as idiopathic membranous glomerulonephritis.

Skin involvement in SLE is almost universal. Skin manifestations can range from the characteristic **malar butterfly rash** on the face to **urticaria, bullae, maculopapular** lesions, and ulcers on any part of the body. Sunlight seems to exacerbate the areas of erythema. Histologic skin changes show edema in the dermis and epidermis. **Vasculitis and fibrinoid changes to blood vessels** are common. Immunofluorescence shows deposition of immunoglobulin and complement at the dermoepidermal junction.

Joint pain is a common complaint in patients with SLE. The typical lesion seen in the joints is a **nonerosive synovitis** with little deformity. In the acute phase of lupus arthritis, there is an exudate of neutrophils and fibrin into the synovium and a perivascular mononuclear cell infiltrate in the subsynovial tissue. The fact that SLE-induced **arthritis does not cause deformity** is useful in distinguishing it from rheumatoid arthritis, because these patients may present with the same clinical picture of red, swollen, painful joints.

Inflammation of the **serosal lining** of membranes may be acute, subacute, or chronic. During the acute phase, the surfaces can be covered with fibrinous exudates, later becoming thickened, opaque, and coated with a shaggy fibrinous material. This may cause partial or total occlusion of a serosal cavity. **Cardiovascular system** involvement usually is manifested as pericarditis but also can involve **myocarditis** or **valvular** abnormalities. The **heart lesion** often associated with SLE is **Libman-Sacks endocarditis,** the result of a thickened heart valve covered with **warty vegetations.** The spleen can be enlarged with capsular thickening. Lung involvement usually results in **pleuritis and pleural effusions.** Less commonly, there can be alveolar injury and interstitial fibrosis. The diagnostic criteria for SLE are listed in Table 48-2.

A typical patient with SLE will have a clinical course with flare-ups and remissions spanning the course of years to decades. Disease exacerbations are treated with **corticosteroids or other immunosuppressant drugs.** There is currently 90 percent 5-year survival and 80 percent 10-year survival. The most **common causes of death are renal failure and infection.**

Other connective tissue diseases should be considered in initially evaluating a patient suspected of having SLE. **Scleroderma** or **systemic sclerosis** is characterized by **excessive fibrosis** throughout the body. The skin is affected most commonly, but the gastrointestinal tract, kidneys, lungs, and heart also

Table 48-2
CRITERIA FOR CLASSIFICATION OF SYSTEMIC LUPUS ERYTHEMATOSUS

CRITERION*		
Malar rash	Arthritis	Hematologic disorder
Discoid rash	Serositis	Immunologic disorder
Photosensitivity	Renal disorder	Antinuclear antibody
Oral ulcers	Neurologic disorder	

*Patient should have 4 of 11 criteria present during a period of observation to make a diagnosis of SLE.

are involved commonly. The pathology seen in scleroderma is the result of excessive deposition of collagen into tissues caused by an abnormal activation of the immune system. Because of the variability in the disease, it has been divided into two categories: **diffuse scleroderma,** which is characterized by widespread skin involvement at onset with rapid progression and early visceral involvement, and **localized scleroderma,** which has limited skin involvement confined to the fingers, forearms, and face. Visceral involvement occurs late, and therefore this variant has a more benign course. These patients are said to have the **CREST syndrome:** of **calcinosis, Raynaud phenomenon, esophageal dysmotility, sclerodactyly,** and **telangiectasia.** Like most autoimmune diseases, this condition typically is found in women, but it has a later age of presentation than does SLE, usually occurring in the fifth to sixth decade.

COMPREHENSION QUESTIONS

[48.1] A patient with known SLE presents complaining of seeing blood in her urine. It is found that she has new-onset hypertension and severely impaired kidney function. A kidney biopsy is done. The pathology report comes back describing all glomeruli as having "wire loop" lesions. Which of the following is the most likely diagnosis?

A. Focal glomerulonephritis
B. Normal kidney histology
C. Mesangial lupus glomerulonephritis
D. Diffuse proliferative glomerulonephritis

[48.2] A patient presents complaining of painful joints, malaise, and fever. She denies ever having experienced those symptoms before. She has no past medical history except for a positive purified protein derivative (PPD) 1 month ago, for which she is taking isoniazid. Her laboratories reveal that she has a high level of ANAs, especially antihistone antibodies. Which of the following is the most likely diagnosis?

A. Systemic lupus erythematosus
B. Scleroderma
C. Drug-induced lupus erythematosus
D. Polymyositis

[48.3] A 30-year-old woman presents after having had some laboratory tests done. She is concerned because she tested positive for syphilis. She denies any history of syphilis or other sexually transmitted diseases (STDs). She has been married for 10 years and believes that the relationship is monogamous. Further workup finds that these results are in fact false-positive laboratory results and more tests are performed to investigate the possibility of the patient having SLE. Which of the following positive laboratory tests is most specific for a diagnosis of SLE?

A. Positive anti–double stranded DNA antibodies
B. Positive antineutrophil cytoplasmic antibodies
C. Positive antineutrophil nuclear antibodies
D. Positive antineutrophil nucleolar antibodies
E. Positive antismooth muscle antibodies

Answers

[48.1] **D.** "Wire loop" lesions often are described in biopsies of patients with diffuse proliferative glomerulonephritis. They are the result of extensive subendothelial deposits that cause a thickening of the capillary wall. These lesions can be seen with light microscopy and immunofluorescence. They reflect active disease and indicate a poor prognosis.

[48.2] **C.** A lupuslike syndrome can develop in patients who take a variety of drugs. In this patient the cause is isoniazid. The patient had a positive PPD for which she was given isoniazid for prophylactic therapy. Other drugs that may cause this syndrome are hydralazine, procainamide, and D-penicillamine. Drug-induced lupus differs from SLE by having high levels of antihistone antibodies but rarely having anti–double-stranded DNA antibodies. Patients with drug-induced lupus rarely show central nervous system or renal involvement.

[48.3] **A.** In some instances, a positive test for syphilis can be indicative of lupus, pregnancy, or antiphospholipid syndrome or be unexplained. The rapid plasma reagin test sometimes can come back positive in a patient who does not have syphilis but actually has SLE, an autoimmune disorder that is associated with the development of numerous autoantibodies. In these patients with false-positive laboratory tests, it is best to get a confirmatory syphilis test such as the FTA-ABS, and if this more specific test is positive, the patient is treated for syphilis. If the confirmatory test is negative, an ANA test may be obtained to assess for SLE. Antinuclear antibodies that are specific for SLE include anti–double-stranded DNA (rim) and anti–Smith antibodies.

PATHOLOGY PEARLS

- SLE is an autoimmune process whereby antibodies are made against numerous nuclear and cytoplasmic parts of the cell.
- The manifestations of SLE are many including skin changes, serosal ulcers or inflammation, joint inflammation, renal effects, neurological symptoms, and hematological changes.
- The clinical course of SLE is generally marked by flare-ups and remissions.
- The principal treatment of SLE is corticosteroids or other immunosuppressant agents.
- The most common causes of death to patients with SLE are renal failure and infection.

REFERENCES

Kumar V, Assas AK, Fausto N, eds. Robbins and Cotran pathologic Basis of Disease, 7th ed. Philadelphia, PA: Elsevier Saunders, 2004.

Mitchell RN. Diseases of immunity. In: Mitchell RN, Kumar V, Abbas AK, et al., eds. Pocket Companion to Robbins and Cotran Pathologic Basis of Disease, 7th ed. Philadelphia, PA: Saunders, 2006:130–4.

❖ CASE 49

A 45-year-old woman with a known history of rheumatoid arthritis presents to her primary care physician with fatigue, weight gain, and cold intolerance. Examination reveals an enlarged thyroid gland (goiter), coarse skin, and bradycardia. Her thyroid function tests show elevated thyroid-stimulating hormone (TSH) levels and low levels of total triiodothyronine (T_3) and thyroxine (T_4).

- **What is the most likely diagnosis?**
- **What is the most likely underlying etiology for this condition?**
- **What are the other symptoms and signs related to this condition?**
- **What tests would confirm the mechanism of this disorder?**

ANSWERS TO CASE 49: HYPOTHYROIDISM

Summary: A 45-year-old woman with rheumatoid arthritis complains of weakness, cold intolerance, bradycardia, and goiter and has thyroid function tests consistent with primary hypothyroidism.

- **Most likely diagnosis:** Primary hypothyroidism
- **Likely underlying etiology:** An autoimmune process such as Hashimoto thyroiditis
- **Symptoms of hypothyroidism:** Fatigue, goiter, weight gain, cold intolerance, dry coarse skin, muscle weakness, constipation, and menorrhagia or oligomenorrhea
- **Signs of hypothyroidism:** Mental slowness, change in voice, dry thin hair and skin, loss of eyebrows, bradycardia, pericardial effusion, anemia, and slowing of the relaxation phase of reflexes
- **Confirmation tests:** Antithyroglobulin and antithyroid peroxidase assays

CLINICAL CORRELATION

This patient has very typical symptoms of hypothyroidism with fatigue, weight gain, and cold intolerance. Depression is also common. Hypothyroidism is categorized broadly into two types: primary hypothyroidism and secondary hypothyroidism. With primary hypothyroidism, which is by far the more common variety, thyroid hormone production from the thyroid gland is insufficient, resulting in low levels of these hormones and subsequent elevation of TSH levels. In secondary hypothyroidism, TSH levels are low, usually as a result of hypopituitarism with subsequent hypothyroidism. Levels of thyroid hormones and TSH are low. See Table 49-1 for etiologies for hypothyroidism. The supersensitive TSH level is the best screening test for hypothyroidism.

APPROACH TO THYROID DISEASE

Objectives

- Describe the most common cause of hypothyroidism.
- Describe how to differentiate between the various causes of thyroiditis.
- List the clinical features of hyperthyroidism.

Table 49-1
SELECTED CAUSES OF HYPOTHYROIDISM

Primary
Agencies of thyroid gland
Iodine deficiency
Genetic defect of enzymes required for hormone synthesis (dyshormonogenesis)
Antithyroid drugs
Autoimmune: Hashimoto thyroiditis
After surgery
After radiation
Secondary
Hypopituitarism

Definitions

Goiter: Enlargement of the thyroid gland (see Table 49-2 for causes).

Hypothyroidism: A clinical state resulting from underactivity of the thyroid gland.

Primary hypothyroidism: Hypothyroidism caused by intrinsic pathology of the thyroid gland.

Secondary hypothyroidism: A clinical state of hypothyroidism, but the thyroid gland is normal; the cause is usually hypopituitarism with low TSH secretion.

Hyperthyroidism or thyrotoxicosis: A clinical state resulting from overactivity of the thyroid gland.

Euthyroid: State of normal thyroid activity.

Thyroid hormones: Triiodothyronine (T_3) and thyroxine (T_4). The thyroid gland synthesizes mostly T_4, which in the periphery is converted to T_3. T_3 has tenfold higher biological activity than does T_4.

DISCUSSION

The thyroid gland consists of two lobes connected by the isthmus. It consists of follicles lined by cuboidal epithelial cells with colloid in the center. Interspersed between the follicles are the calcitonin-secreting parafollicular C cells. The thyroid produces T_4 and T_3. More T_4 is produced, but T_4 is converted to the more active T_3 in the peripheral tissues. In plasma, T_4 and T_3 are mostly bound to thyroxine-binding globulin (TBG), thyroxine-binding prealbumin, and albumin. The unbound (free) fraction of the hormones is physiologically active. When T_4 and T_3 levels are routinely measured, it is the total levels that are measured. However, if the levels of the binding proteins are altered, the total values of T_4 and T_3 also will change. In such situations, free T_3 and free T_4 should be measured.

Table 49-2
SELECTED CAUSES OF THYROMEGALY

Diffuse
Physiologic (puberty, pregnancy)
Iodine deficiency
Thyroiditis (Hashimoto thyroiditis, lymphocytic thyroiditis, De Quervain thyroiditis)
Graves disease
Medications: antithyroid drugs
Nodular
Multinodular goiter
Thyroid neoplasms: adenoma (benign), carcinoma, lymphoma

Causes of increased thyroid-binding globulin include hereditary causes, **pregnancy,** and **estrogen therapy or oral contraceptive pills.** Causes of **decreased TBG** include hereditary causes, androgens, and hypoproteinemic states (nephrotic syndrome, chronic liver disease, malnutrition).

Most patients who present with thyroid disease present with a goiter, accompanied by a hyper- or hypothyroid state (Table 49-2 lists the common causes of goiters). **Iodine deficiency** is a major cause of goiter (endemic goiter) worldwide because iodine is essential for thyroid hormone synthesis.

Thyroiditis

Hashimoto thyroiditis is the **most common cause of hypothyroidism** in parts of the world where there are **sufficient levels of iodine** in the diet. It is due to gradual **autoimmune destruction of the thyroid gland.** It is associated with the presence of **other autoimmune diseases,** such as rheumatoid arthritis. There seems to be an association with the human lymphocyte antigens HLA-DR5 and HLA-DR3. The autoimmune destruction of the gland is mediated by T-cytotoxic cells and antithyroid antibodies. The **thyroid gland is diffusely enlarged.** Microscopic examination reveals **extensive mononuclear inflammatory infiltrate,** predominantly **lymphocytes.** Lymphoid follicles with germinal centers may be seen. Some of the thyroid epithelial cells have granular eosinophilic cytoplasm that is referred to as **Hürthle cell change.** With time, there is deposition of collagen. Patients develop features of hypothyroidism, requiring lifelong hormone replacement therapy. Patients with Hashimoto thyroiditis are at **increased risk for developing B-cell lymphomas.**

Lymphocytic thyroiditis, also known as subacute painless thyroiditis, is seen predominantly in **adult women,** especially during the **postpartum** period. It is considered part of the spectrum of **thyroid autoimmune diseases.** Some patients go on to hypothyroidism. Females affected by postpartum thyroiditis are at increased risk for recurrence with subsequent pregnancies. As the name implies, **lymphocytic infiltration of the thyroid gland** is the usual histologic feature. Unlike Hashimoto thyroiditis, formation of **lymphoid follicles** with germinal centers and **Hürthle cell change are not seen.**

De Quervain thyroiditis also is known as **subacute thyroiditis (granulomatous thyroiditis).** It is thought to be related to **viral infection.** The disease process is self-limiting. The thyroid gland is **painfully enlarged.** With initial destruction of the thyroid follicles and liberation of hormones into the circulation, a transient thyrotoxicosis occurs. Later on, with the catabolism of the hormones and damaged epithelial cells unable to synthesize new hormones, there is an insufficiency of hormones (hypothyroidism). With regeneration of the thyroid follicular epithelium, the patient recovers to a euthyroid state.

Common causes of hyperthyroidism are **Graves disease** and **toxic nodular/multinodular goiter. Graves disease** is the **most common cause of hyperthyroidism** (see Table 49-3 for common symptoms and signs). It is characterized by a diffusely enlarged thyroid gland, eye findings, and skin changes (pretibial myxedema). It is due to an autoimmune process in which **IgG antibodies** that **bind** to the **TSH receptors** (thyroid-stimulating immunoglobulins) are found that instead of destroying the target stimulates the receptors, resulting in thyrotoxicosis. There is an association with HLA-B8 and HLA-DR3. With time, blocking antibodies develop that block the binding of IgG antibodies to the TSH receptors, and at the same time autoimmune destruction of the gland develops with a resultant hypothyroid state.

Table 49-3
CLINICAL FEATURES OF HYPERTHYROIDISM

SYMPTOMS	SIGNS
Weight loss	Thyroid eye signs (seen only in Graves disease)
Increased appetite	Exophthalmos
Tremor	Lid lag and lid retraction
Heat intolerance	Tachycardia; atrial fibrillation
Diarrhea	Proximal myopathy
Oligomenorrhea	Hypertension

Multinodular goiter usually is seen in the setting of **persistent iodine deficiency.** Palpation of a single nodule does not rule out the presence of multiple nodules. A single nodule, however, increases the likelihood of an underlying neoplasm. Nodules may be assessed by radioactive ^{131}I uptake scan. A nodule that is **hyperfunctioning** is referred to as a **"hot"** nodule. A **nodule that fails to take up radioactive ^{131}I** is a **"cold"** nodule. It is highly **unlikely for a hot nodule to be neoplastic,** whereas **up to 10 percent of cold nodules harbor malignancies.**

An **adenoma** is an encapsulated benign neoplasm of the thyroid gland. **Follicular, papillary,** and **anaplastic** carcinomas are the main types of malignant neoplasms. All the neoplasms described above arise from the follicular epithelium. **Medullary** carcinoma arises from the **parafollicular C cells,** and can be part of the multiple endocrine neoplasia (MEN) type 2b syndrome.

COMPREHENSION QUESTIONS

[49.1] A 41-year-old woman with a history of rheumatoid arthritis presents with increasing weakness and cold intolerance. Physical examination finds a goiter, and laboratory evaluation finds her thyroid function tests to be consistent with primary hypothyroidism. Which of the following histologic findings is most consistent with a diagnosis of Hashimoto thyroiditis in this individual?

A. Amyloid deposition
B. Granulomatous inflammation
C. Lymphoid infiltrate with Hürthle cells
D. Parafollicular hyperplasia
E. Scalloping of colloid

[49.2] A 35-year-old woman presents with increasing fatigue, slight weight gain, and a low-grade fever. Approximately 3 weeks before developing these symptoms she had a 4-day upper respiratory viral infection. At present a physical examination finds a tender enlarged thyroid gland. If a biopsy specimen reveals granulomatous inflammation with giant cells, which of the following is the correct diagnosis?

A. De Quervain thyroiditis
B. Graves disease
C. Hashimoto thyroiditis
D. Plummer disease
E. Schmidt syndrome

[49.3] The clinical combination of hyperthyroidism, exophthalmos, and pretibial myxedema is most likely to be seen in an individual with which of the following types of autoantibodies?

A. Antimitochondrial antibodies
B. Antineutrophil cytoplasmic antibodies
C. Antismooth muscle antibodies
D. TSH-receptor-blocking antibodies
E. TSH-receptor-stimulating antibodies

Answers

[49.1] **C.** Hashimoto thyroiditis is an autoimmune disorder that is a common cause of hypothyroidism. Clinically, the thyroid gland is diffusely enlarged, and histologic sections characteristically reveal a lymphocytic infiltrate with Hürthle cells, which are thyroid epithelial cells that have a granular eosinophilic cytoplasm.

[49.2] **A.** De Quervain (subacute) thyroiditis is a self-limited cause of hypothyroidism. It typically follows a viral infection when patients develop the acute onset of fever with painful enlargement of the thyroid gland. Patients may develop mild hyperthyroidism early, but later they usually develop hypothyroidism. De Quervain thyroiditis also is known as granulomatous thyroiditis because histologic sections will show granulomatous inflammation with giant cells surrounding fragments of colloid.

[49.3] **E.** The clinical combination of hyperthyroidism, exophthalmos, and pretibial myxedema is most consistent with the diagnosis of Graves disease. This autoimmune disorder is the most common cause of hyperthyroidism. It is characterized by the presence of IgG autoantibodies that bind to and stimulate the TSH receptor. Patients develop diffuse uniform enlargement of the thyroid gland; this is called a diffuse toxic goiter.

PATHOLOGY PEARLS

- Alterations in levels of thyroxine-binding protein affect the total values of T_4 and T_3. In such situations free T_3 and free T_4 should be measured.
- Most patients who present with thyroid disease present with a goiter, accompanied by a hyper- or hypothyroid state.
- Hashimoto thyroiditis, lymphocytic thyroiditis, and Graves disease are the principal autoimmune thyroid diseases.
- Hashimoto thyroiditis is the most common cause of hypothyroidism in areas where iodine is sufficient.
- Individuals with Hashimoto thyroiditis are at risk for B-cell lymphomas.
- Graves disease and nodular goiters are the common causes of hyperthyroidism.
- The eye changes seen in thyrotoxicosis are exclusive to Graves disease.
- Patients with long-standing Graves disease usually convert to a hypothyroid state.
- De Quervain thyroiditis is a self-limiting condition.
- It is highly unlikely for a hot nodule to be neoplastic, whereas up to 10 percent of cold nodules are malignant.

REFERENCES

Kumar V, Assas AK, Fausto N, eds. Robbins and Cotran Pathologic Basis of Disease, 7th ed. Philadelphia, PA: Elsevier Saunders, 2004.

Maitra A. The endocrine system. In: Mitchell RN, Kumar V, Abbas AK, et al., eds. Pocket Companion to Robbins and Cotran Pathologic Basis of Disease, 7th ed. Philadelphia, PA: Saunders, 2006:567–75.

❖ CASE 50

A 28-year-old woman gives birth to a term female infant. After delivery, the newborn is noted to have a defect in the skin and vertebrae in the lumbosacral region, with protrusion of a segment of flattened spinal cord with an overlying meningeal outpouching. The mother did not receive any prenatal care or routine prenatal screening.

- **What is the most likely diagnosis?**
- **What is the underlying developmental derangement involved?**
- **What are the risk factors and screening methods for this disorder?**

ANSWERS TO CASE 50: NEURAL TUBE DEFECT/SPINA BIFIDA

Summary: The newborn of a woman without prenatal care is noted to have spina bifida.

- **Most likely diagnosis:** Meningomyelocele.
- **Underlying developmental derangement involved:** Failure of the neural tube to close.
- **Risk factors and screening methods:** Multifactorial, including medication exposure, lack of folate, and family history. Screening includes offering a maternal serum α-fetoprotein assay.

CLINICAL CORRELATION

The neural tube closes very early in embryonic life, beginning in the cervical spine region and proceeding both cephalad and caudad. Failure of this normal closure results in a spectrum of congenital abnormalities that range from nearly undetectable abnormalities to those not compatible with life. The etiology of this failure is poorly understood, although it is clearly multifactorial in origin. It is known that deficiency of folic acid in the maternal diet is associated with these disorders and that dietary supplementation with folate will decrease the incidence of neural tube defects significantly. Neural tube defects also are associated with certain medications, specifically the anticonvulsants valproic acid and carbamazepine. A female who has given birth to an infant with a neural tube defect has a greater likelihood of delivering another affected child.

The clinical sequelae of neural tube defects correlate well with the size and location of the defect. In general, larger defects and those more cephalad have a more significant impact on long-term outcomes, whereas smaller lesions and those located more caudally tend to be associated with more normal neurologic function. Typically, open lesions have a poorer prognosis than do lesions that are closed. Impairment of bowel and bladder function and decreased neuromuscular function up to and including paraplegia are typical of patients with neural tube defects.

Prenatal diagnosis for neural tube defects of all sorts is widely available. This primarily takes the form of screening for the α-fetoprotein (AFP) level and frequently is combined with screening for human chorionic gonadotropin (hCG) and estriol levels in the "triple screen" test, which can produce a risk score for neural tube defects; other defects of dermal covering, such as gastroschisis; and chromosomal defects such as trisomy 21 (Down syndrome). The tests are performed routinely as part of normal prenatal care and, when positive, allow for definitive diagnosis by means of ultrasonography and/or amniocentesis.

APPROACH TO CONGENITAL ANOMALIES

Objectives

- Describe the major cause of neural tube defects.
- Know the markers used in prenatal diagnosis and screening of neural tube defects.

Definitions

Anencephaly: Failure of fusion of the rostral portion of the neural tube, resulting in congenital absence of the brain and cranial structures.

Holoprosencephaly: Failure of fusion or abnormal fusion of the most rostral portion of the neural tube. This defect is associated with midfacial defects, absence of the corpus callosum, and significant internal structural abnormalities within the brain.

Hydrocephalus: Increased size of the lateral ventricles of the brain secondary to abnormally poor drainage of the cerebral spinal fluid (CSF); commonly associated with neural tube defects.

Meningocele: A closed neural tube defect that involves two or more vertebral levels in which the meninges protrude into a skin-covered sac.

Meningomyelocele: A closed or open neural tube defect that involves two or more vertebral levels in which a large sac, which may be covered by skin, may be covered by meninges only, or may be open, contains not only the meninges but also the spinal cord itself. This has the worst prognosis for long-term neurologic function.

Spina bifida occulta: A small area of failed fusion of the vertebrae posteriorly. Typically located in the lumbosacral region and frequently covered with a tuft of hair. These lesions are common and are usually of no clinical significance.

DISCUSSION

Epidemiology

Major congenital anomalies occur in approximately 3 percent of **liveborn** infants. Among these anomalies, approximately one-half, representing 1.5 percent of liveborn infants, are identifiable at the time of delivery, whereas the remainder is diagnosed later in life. These anomalies have a variety of etiologies, with approximately 1.2 percent arising from a **single genetic defect.** Examples of these types of disorders are Tay-Sachs disease, cystic fibrosis, sickle cell anemia, and the thalassemias. In almost all these examples the **specific diseases are individually quite rare,** although in the aggregate this category accounts for the largest single group of congenital anomalies. Approximately 1 percent of liveborn infants have an anomaly that is **multifactorial** in origin, which includes

Table 50-1
SELECTED LIST OF CONGENITAL ABNORMALITIES

Single gene mutations	**Chromosomal abnormalities**
Sickle cell anemia	Sex chromosome abnormalities
Cystic fibrosis	(e.g., 45X, 47XYY, 47XXX)
β_1-Thalassemia	Autosomal trisomies
α_1-Thalassemia	Trisomy 13, 14, 15
Tay-Sachs disease	Trisomy 16, 17, 18
Canavan disease	Trisomy 21, 22
Numerous other rare disorders	Translocations
Multifactorial anomalies	Balanced (robertsonian)
Hydrocephalus	Reciprocal (translocations)
Neural tube defects	Unbalanced
Cleft lip with cleft palate	**Teratogenic agents**
Cardiac anomalies	Alcohol
Diaphragmatic hernia	Anticonvulsants
Pyloric stenosis	Phenytoin
Omphalocele	Carbamazepine
Renal agenesis (Potter syndrome)	Valproate
Ureteral anomalies	Phenobarbital
Hypospadias	ACE inhibitors
Defects of müllerian fusion	Vitamin A derivatives
Müllerian aplasia	Chemotherapy agents
Limb reduction defects	Cocaine
Talipes equinovarus (clubfoot)	

the neural tube defects as well as numerous other types of structural abnormalities. Another 0.625 percent of liveborn infants demonstrate **chromosomal abnormalities,** with trisomy 21 being the most common among liveborn neonates. The remainder includes anomalies thought to be associated with the various **teratogenic agents** and anomalies of unknown origin. See Table 50-1 for a partial listing of congenital abnormalities.

Embryology

The neural tube appears at approximately the fifth week of gestational age (third week of embryonic age). It **closes by approximately the sixth week of gestation,** and it is during this period of closure that it is susceptible to the formation of neural tube defects, which primarily take the form of failed fusion of the neural tube (see Figure 50-1). Unfortunately for clinicians, this is typically just when or **before most patients identify their pregnancy;** closure of the neural tube occurs in the first or second week in which menses would be

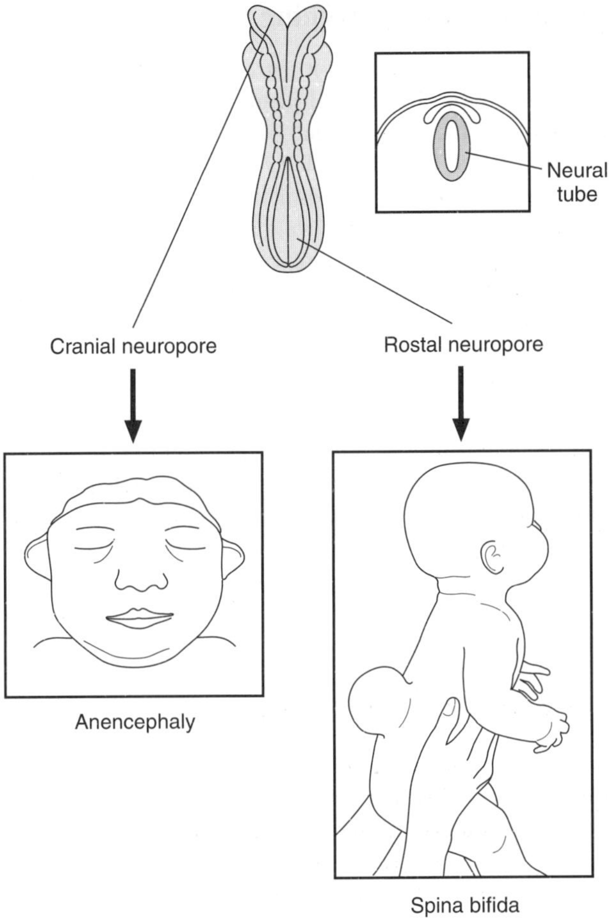

Figure 50-1. Development of the neural tube.

expected. For this reason, therapies during pregnancy have proved ineffective. Fortunately, a **major contributor** to the incidence of neural tube defects is **deficiency of folic acid** in the maternal diet, and **supplementation with folic acid before conception** (which for most females includes the first 5 to 7 weeks of their pregnancies) has proved to **reduce the incidence of neural tube defects at least sevenfold.** The American College of Obstetricians and Gynecologists now recommends that **all females supplement their diets with 0.4 mg of folic acid daily for at least 1 month before pregnancy,** and females with a **prior history of delivering an affected infant** should receive **4 mg of daily folate** supplementation.

Prenatal Diagnosis and Screening

Prenatal diagnosis and **screening** for neural tube defects can be **quite effective** and has become a **routine part of prenatal care.** Prenatal screening typically is accomplished by using multiple biochemical markers found in **maternal serum.** These markers include **α-fetoprotein, human chorionic gonadotropin,** and **estriol,** which form the contents of the **triple screen.** Several other markers are available as well, and their clinical use is being evaluated. These tests typically are performed between the fifteenth and twentieth weeks of gestation. These screening tools unfortunately carry relatively high **false-positive rates,** and when screening is positive, further confirmatory testing is required to establish the diagnosis. Large neural tube defects, including those most likely to lead to long-term neurologic sequelae, and many defects involving the brain are detectable by means of **targeted ultrasonography.** However, failure to diagnose neural tube defects on ultrasound does not rule out the presence of small neural tube defects. Definitive diagnosis at present is made by **amniocentesis** and measurement of amniotic fluid α-fetoprotein levels and acetylcholinesterase levels. Infants with open neural tube defects appear to have better neurologic prognoses when delivered by cesarean section rather than vaginally, although controversy exists about the significance of this difference.

COMPREHENSION QUESTIONS

[50.1] On physical examination, a female newborn is found to have a defect in the lumbosacral region through which a segment of the spinal cord protrudes with an overlying meningeal outpouching. The mother did not receive prenatal care or routine prenatal screening. The abnormality seen in this newborn is associated with a maternal deficiency of which of the following substances?

A. Ascorbic acid
B. Cystathionine
C. Folic acid
D. Vitamin A
E. Vitamin B_{12}

[50.2] A triple screen for neural tube defects entails examining maternal serum for elevated levels of human chorionic gonadotropin, estriol, and which other substance?

A. Acid phosphatase
B. α-Fetoprotein
C. Carcinoembryonic antigen
D. Chromogranin
E. Methylmalonic acid

[50.3] An autopsy performed on a stillborn male fetus reveals the presence of polydactyly, a cleft palate, and a single central eye. Examination of the brain finds fusion of the frontal lobes with a single ventricle. Which of the following is the most likely diagnosis for this abnormality of the central nervous system?

A. Holoprosencephaly
B. Hydranencephaly
C. Hydrocephalus
D. Meningomyelocele
E. Micrencephaly

Answers

[50.1] **C.** The etiology of neural tube developmental defects such as anencephaly and spina bifida is multifactorial in origin, but these defects clearly are related to a maternal deficiency of folic acid. Indeed, dietary supplementation with folate during pregnancy has been shown to decrease the incidence of neural tube defects significantly.

[50.2] **B.** Prenatal screening for neural tube defects has become a routine part of prenatal care. This testing looks for elevated levels of certain substances in maternal serum. These markers include α-fetoprotein, human chorionic gonadotropin, and estriol. The combination of these three substances forms the contents of the triple screen.

[50.3] **A.** Holoprosencephaly is an abnormality that results from failure of the brain to cleave into two hemispheres. The result is the formation of a single frontal lobe and a single ventricle. This abnormality also is associated with midfacial defects such as the formation of a single centrally located eye. Holoprosencephaly is seen with the fetal alcohol syndrome and trisomy 13 (Patau syndrome).

PATHOLOGY PEARLS

- The neural tube closes early in pregnancy, often before pregnancy is diagnosed.
- Folic acid supplementation reduces the incidence of neural tube defects when taken before conception.
- Neural tube defects are quite common and range in clinical significance from minimal to devastating.
- Prenatal screening and diagnosis allow for detection by means of maternal serum screening early in pregnancy. This diagnosis allows informed choices to be made regarding the continuance of the pregnancy and the mode of delivery.

REFERENCES

Anthony DC, Frosch MP. The central nervous system. In: Mitchell RN, Kumar V, Abbas AK, et al., eds. Pocket Companion to Robbins and Cotran Pathologic Basis of Disease, 7th ed. Philadelphia, PA: Saunders, 2006:678.

Gabbe SG, Neibyl JR, Simpson JL. Obstetrics: Normal and Problem Pregnancies, 4th ed. Philadelphia, PA: Churchill Livingstone, 2002.

Langman J. Medical Embryology, 4th ed. Baltimore, MD: Williams & Wilkins, 1981.

SECTION III

Listing of Cases

Listing by Case Number

Listing by Disorder (Alphabetical)

LISTING BY CASE NUMBER

LISTING BY DISORDER (ALPHABETICAL)

INDEX

Note: Page numbers followed by *f* or *t* indicate figures or tables, respectively.

H

M

R